# The Consultation in Phytotherapy

## The Herbal Practitioner's Approach to the Patient

**Peter Conway**  Dip Phyt MNIMH MCPP Cert Ed
President, College of Practitioners of Phytotherapy
The WellSpring Clinic
Tunbridge Wells
Kent
UK

*Foreword by*
**Simon Y Mills**  MA FNIMH MCPP
Secretary, European Scientific Cooperative on Phytotherapy
Former President, College of Practitioners of Phytotherapy
Exeter
Devon
UK

**Dedication**
*This book is dedicated to my beloved Melanie, whose love, support and encouragement made it possible*

First published in 2011 by Elsevier Limited

This reprint published in 2024 by Aeon Books

Copyright © 2011, 2024 by Peter Conway

The right of Peter Conway to be identified as the author of this work has been asserted in accordance with §§ 77 and 78 of the Copyright Design and Patents Act 1988.

All rights reserved. No part of this publication may be reproduced, stored in a retrieval system, or transmitted, in any form or by any means, electronic, mechanical, photocopying, recording, or otherwise, without the prior written permission of the publisher.

British Library Cataloguing in Publication Data

A C.I.P. for this book is available from the British Library
ISBN-13: 9781913274504

# FOREWORD

Herbal medicine has had a terrible 20th century. An evolving relationship between humans and plants ground to a shuddering halt in the industrial world somewhere around the end of the 19th century. This was astonishing: humans had for millennia been articulating and finessing a primal co-evolution with the plant world and all sentient beings. The insights and benefits for health that had emerged were rich and real. However, while suited to living close to the land, these had become increasingly inadequate to meet the needs of urban life, often involving squalor and pandemic diseases, and when the principles of science and engineering became applicable to medicine the old ways were rudely thrown aside.

Where herbal medicine did survive in the industrial West it is usually as a caricature of its former self. Modern simplicities dominated. Could peppermint cure my irritable bowel? Will chamomile or valerian help me sleep? Will ginseng make me good in bed or saw palmetto help me stay in it through the night? Will St John's wort finally make me happy? Herbs became the most banal of nostrums. People resorted to them, uncritically often, as natural recipes to fix things. The fact that time and time again research has shown that such simple hopes are misplaced has sullied the herbal sector: the smart money has stayed away.

Peter Conway has in this book leapt over the bad years and provided a fully 21st century revival of ancient principles. It is a wonderful thing to behold! Peter has made it his business to sit with, often literally, the most remarkable practitioners and thinkers of our time. He has masterfully processed what they share with us into a sweeping and comprehensive insight into the heart of herbal medicine or phytotherapy. On reading this no longer is it possible to say that herbal medicine is primitive and without rationale. Peter has made it truly a strategy for modern times with the added value of also being true to human history and to ancient principles.

There are particular highlights. Peter has absorbed and made relevant the latest insights into the placebo effect, the explosive and largely unprocessed impact on medical thought of Ivan Illich's work 40 years ago, the insights from observing the properties of complex systems, the role of the story or narrative at the heart of medicine, the profound implications on the business of health care of understanding the lived experience of illness, the healing presence in health care, and the interaction between practitioner and patient. His acknowledgement of the work of Bob Duggan in Chapter 3 is personally satisfying, having set up a Master of Science in Herbal Medicine at Bob's Tai Sophia campus precisely because of the extra dimension to practice they provide there. All this leads to a refreshing and muscular riposte to the more absurd manifestations of fundamentalist science that has so undermined core values across all health care.

What emerges is also muscular: a convincing argument for the value of herbal medicine in the modern world. These age-old remedies now have a new role, to help us reclaim our relationship with our own health care. While Peter has focused on the role of the practitioner as channel for these benefits, using her or his skills to tailor remedies to the needs of a patient, the value of his insights are that they can feed us all. Each of us has a relationship with nature to develop. Most of us now have a long way to go in this. The particular properties of the plant world as foods and remedies have often been obliterated by industrial processing and by the remoteness of the natural world from our lives. Plants in their primary metabolism provide us with our most effective foods, and in their secondary metabolism with a range of pharmacological constituents that will always be the envy of the pharmaceutical chemist. Moreover these healing agents are often well known in human history, recurring as healing archetypes through all the main cultures around the world. Peter has reclaimed these ancient principles and brought them to life. This book is immensely important for all those interested in expanding their interests in health care to make them more grounded in our nature.

Simon Mills MA FNIMH MCPP
Secretary, European Scientific Cooperative on Phytotherapy
Former President, College of Practitioners of Phytotherapy

# ACKNOWLEDGEMENTS

I am thankful for my many teachers – especially patients and 'students' – and for those colleagues who have commented on parts of the book, who have discussed issues pertaining to it with me, or have otherwise influenced my thoughts on the consultation – whether they were aware of the fact or not. A far from complete list includes: Simon Mills, Bob Duggan, Kieran Sweeney, Nicky Britten, Jimmy Symmonds, Alex Laird, Olivia Laing, Colin Nicholls, Peter Jackson-Main, Vicki Pitman, Miche Fabre Lewin, Gillian Leddy, Michael McIntyre, Julian Barker and the late Hein Zeylstra. Music was a substantial help in completing this work and some readers may be interested to note that key aids included Terry Riley's *Persian Surgery Dervishes* and Fila Brazilia's *V&A*.

# INTRODUCTION

This book is concerned with the clinical practice of phytotherapy (from the Greek *phytos*, meaning 'plant'); a term, first used by Henri Leclerc (1870–1955), that has been applied to a cluster of approaches to the therapeutic utilization of botanical agents. These range from the use of plant remedies as quasi-drugs in conventional medical practice by some doctors in mainland Europe (see, e.g. Schulz et al. 1988); to the 'terrain' theories of French phytotherapy such as the 'neuroendocrine' or 'endobiogenic' model developed by Duraffourd and Lapraz (2002); to a more recent adoption of the term by some traditional herbal practitioners in the UK who have begun to develop their own particular variation on the theme (see Mills & Bone 2000). It is from the latter group that this author originates.

'Phytotherapy', therefore, includes a number of distinctive takes on the practice of herbal medicine. Although differing, the various phytotherapy schools are linked by a central engagement with the relationship between plant chemistry (phytochemistry) and human physiology. This distinguishes phytotherapy from other herbal medicine practices where detailed pharmaco-physiological considerations are more peripheral, or where they are deemed non-essential or even rejected.

The UK phytotherapists trace one strand of their heritage to the physio-medical approach to herbal medicine that was introduced to Britain from America in the mid- to late-nineteenth century. This combined a vitalist philosophy with an appreciation of the latest discoveries in physiology (including, significantly, that of the autonomic nervous system) and an attempt to integrate psychological methods of healing, as Thurston (1900), one of the key physicomedicalists, asserted: 'suggestive or mental therapeutics or more properly psychotherapeutics, should rapidly find its way into the *legitimate resources* of the general practitioner' [original emphasis]. The UK-based brand of phytotherapy can be viewed as continuing this project on account of: its emphasis on the body as a self-healing organism, representing an ongoing vitalist orientation; interest in the cutting edge of physiology in areas such as psychoneuroimmunology (PNI) and the new perspectives on inflammation; and awareness of the psychotherapeutic potential of the consultation, including a re-casting of the placebo effect as the 'healing-' or 'meaning-response'.

In this variety of herbal practice, pharmacotherapy is entangled with psychotherapy: while the former type of treatment is taken by the patient following the consultation, the latter arises during the consultation itself. Indeed, the phytotherapy consultation (sensitively conducted) may be perceived as constituting a psychotherapeutic act. All healthcare consultations have this potential to some degree. As Balint (1963) points out: 'by far the most commonly used drug in general practice (is) the doctor himself', but the implications of this insight have failed to be substantially registered, developed and integrated into practice – either in conventional or herbal medicine – such that Balint's case still stands in need of response, for example when he states that:

> *In spite of our almost pathetic lack of knowledge about the dynamisms and possible consequences of "reassurance" and "advice", these two are perhaps the most often used forms of medical treatment [original emphasis].*

Yet our appreciation of the dimensions and mechanisms at play in this territory is increasing. Studies within the field of, e.g. PNI, have demonstrated the negative effects of repression (inhibition of strong emotions) and rumination (persistent intrusive thoughts), and the positive effects of disclosure (telling one's story), on the immune system (Kiecolt-Glaser et al. 2002). The consultation helps partly because it is a place where talk occurs: where issues can be identified, matters discussed, emotions released, stories told and disclosures made. PNI-related research shows us that biochemical effects are not limited to the administration of pharmacologically active substances but occur in response to thoughts and feelings too – phenomena that can adapt and thrive in the conducive environment of the sensitive consultation.

A holistic phytotherapy, then, will seek to exploit the healing potential that resides within the consultation in addition to that of herbal medicines themselves – the combination of the two effects constituting a potent therapeutic modality. While many texts have addressed the second aspect of this partnership, few have concerned themselves with the first – an oversight that this volume seeks to contribute towards remedying. Other books have certainly made suggestions regarding aspects of the herbal consultation, such as how the patient might be profiled and diagnosed, that are linked to arriving at a prescription and treatment plan, but the therapeutic potentials of the consultation that run parallel to these outcomes have rarely been scrutinized. While diagnosis (however that notion is framed) is essential in enabling the formulation of a medication, it represents an activity that is frequently largely the agenda of the practitioner, not the patient. As Toombs (1993) expresses it: 'on being presented with a sick person doctors do not attempt to find out what is the matter but, rather, attempt to make a diagnosis. This is not the same thing'. Herbal practitioners may be just as culpable in prioritizing our interpretive and diagnostic models over a raw engagement with the patient's unique situation. How then do we 'find out what is the matter?' That is the key question I will attempt to respond to in the following pages. In doing so, however, issues to do with phytotherapy-specific diagnostic considerations will not be neglected and a number of perspectives on this territory will be offered.

Much of what is contained in these pages is not exclusive to phytotherapy and may appeal not only to other herbal practitioners who categorize themselves differently but also to any health practitioner interested in the therapeutic potentials of the consultation. I will argue however, that the form and capacities of the consultation in any particular modality are profoundly influenced by the nature of the therapeutic tools the practitioner uses. In order to successfully apply them, any practitioner working with whole plant medicines will need to develop a sensibility that accounts for their inherent qualities of complexity, inexactness and multi-system modulation. Operating from such a standpoint is likely to render the practitioner better prepared to work with complicated pictures, particularly those associated with chronic disease, and to cope more comfortably with the uncertainties attending these states, than colleagues trained in the linear dynamics of simpler and more precise interventions. The plant-therapist should therefore be especially well placed to explore and apply ideas about the concept of the 'therapeutic consultation'.

This book contains frequent reference to conventional medicine for three main reasons. First, since it is hard for any marginalized system of medicine to define itself in the absence of comparison with the dominant medical model pertaining in the culture in which it arises; second, out of respect for, and with reference to, the advances in theory and practice made by conventional medical practitioners through concepts such as narrative-based and patient-centred medicine; and lastly, due to the need to critique the limitations and dysfunctions of the dominant consultation model in order to make the case for alternative perspectives. Research into the various domains of the consultation is considered from a number of fields, including orthodox medicine and the psychological therapies but little will be presented from the world of herbal practice itself, since little is available there. There is simply not enough research on the consultation specifically applied to phytotherapy for me to even attempt to maintain an authoritative third person voice. For this reason, I will use the first person to provide myself with the leeway to express my own views and experiences in order to stimulate debate and to encourage others to go into print in this area.

No attempt is made here to provide a substitute for more specific and comprehensive textbooks on diagnosis, examination and investigation; rather a critique of these concepts is offered combined with the provision of supplementary and alternative perspectives for consideration. A wide range of viewpoints will be presented, some of which are of a persuasion that may trigger the kind of reaction in the reader that Gray (2007) had to post-modern thinking: 'Post-modern philosophies that view science as just one belief-system among many are too silly to be worth refuting at length – the utility of scientific knowledge is a brute fact that is shown in the increase of human power'. I am happy to risk being accused of silliness in drawing on concepts and viewpoints that propose a kinder, less brutish approach to medicine. Mary Douglas (1994) has observed that: 'Some friends explain their preference for complementary medicine by saying either that it is "holistic" or that it respects spiritual values, or both … I propose to put this preference in the context of a widespread leaning to what I will call "gentleness".' In responding to Douglas's case a distinction can be made between the perspectives of acute- and chronic-oriented medicine. While the acute model (rapid diagnosis, objectification of the body, aggressive treatment) may be appropriate and gain results in emergency situations it is largely both inappropriate and ineffectual in general practice in working with chronic conditions. Here a different therapeutic perspective and way of being is required, combining a subtle appreciation of the patient's predicament with gentle and sustainable remedial advice and treatment. Although the herbal *materia medica* possesses its own aggressive agents and has a place in the treatment of acute pictures, it is also lavishly endowed with less harsh substances that ideally suit the patterns of chronicity. This book focuses primarily on the latter aspect of herbal practice.

A key perspective that guides the approach taken to the consultation in this book is the notion that illness can be considered as both a journey and a teacher. It represents an opportunity for both patient and practitioner to travel and to learn.

Facilitating the patient in telling, and reflecting on, their story, can lead to more than the fitting of a herbal prescription to the patient's pattern of dysfunction – it can also aid the patient's discovery of meaning and help nurture their self-development. While considering some of the issues and ideas that arise from this kind of approach, it may be helpful to bear in mind Cassell's (2004) counsel for reflecting on deep transpersonal issues in medicine: 'If it has a touchy-feely "new age" sound, do not be put off; good clinicians are strange instruments'.

In this introduction, I have referred to a few core approaches, ideas and concepts that will be discussed in more detail in the following text: PNI; the meaning-response; narrative-based and patient-centred medicine. Other essential reference points that we will explore include those of phenomenology, ethnobotany and complexity theory. In my view, the great strength of phytotherapy lies in its ability to take on board the insights offered by these approaches and to integrate them with traditional herbal practice. This book is written for all herbal practitioners who wish to work in this way, whether they may call themselves phytotherapists or not. It does not provide a definitive portrayal of the phytotherapy consultation, rather it offers one practitioner's perspective based on a long and continuing involvement with herbal practice as well as with the development and provision of herbal education and training in several UK universities. It is hoped and intended that this book will be of practical value and utility to both herbal practitioners and students but also, that it might stimulate reflection and the expression of views on the specifics of the herbal consultation.

Chapter 1 places 'Phytotherapy in context', considering the history, varieties and current status of this modality and describing the type of herbal practice with which this book is concerned. Chapter 2 reflects on the importance of the therapeutic relationship and its central place in phytotherapy. Chapter 3 considers the 'Aims and structure' of the phytotherapy consultation, describing its scope and recommending ways in which its goals may be achieved. Chapter 4 challenges the notion of, and emphasis on 'diagnosis', instead suggesting that phytotherapists are equally concerned with 'appreciating the patient's predicament'. Chapter 5 explores case history-taking as the heart of the consultation and Chapter 6 critiques the role of physical examination and investigation. The final chapter is concerned with how the consultation is drawn together and concluded and how 'case management' can be recast as the 'continuing relationship'. Three appendices are provided, briefly commenting on issues relating to the consultation.

## REFERENCES

Balint M: *The doctor, his patient and the illness*, Edinburgh, 1963, Churchill Livingstone. Millennium Reprint, 2000.

Cassell EJ: *The nature of suffering: and the goals of medicine*, 2004, Oxford University Press.

Douglas M: The construction of the physician: a cultural approach to medical fashions. In Budd S, Sharma U, editors: *The healing bond: the patient-practitioner relationship and therapeutic responsibility*, London, 1994, Routledge.

Duraffourd C, Lapraz JC: *Traité de phytothérapie clinique: endobiogénie et médecine*, 2002, Editions Masson.

Gray J: *Black Mass: apocalyptic religion and the death of utopia*, 2007, Middlesex, Penguin/Allen Lane.

Kiecolt-Glaser JK, McGuire L, Robles TF, et al: Psychoneuroimmunology: psychological influences on immune function and health, *Journal of Consulting and Clinical Psychology* 70(3):537–547, 2002.

Mills S, Bone K: *Principles and practice of phytotherapy: modern herbal medicine*, Edinburgh, 2000, Elsevier/Churchill Livingstone.

Schulz V, Hänsel R, Tyler VE: *Rational phytotherapy: a physician's guide to herbal medicine*, 1998, Springer.

Thurston JM: *The philosophy of physiomedicalism: its theorem, corollary and laws of application for the cure of disease*, 1900, Nicholson Printing & Mfg. Co.

Toombs SK: *The meaning of illness: a phenomenological account of the different perspectives of physician and patient*, 1993, Kluwer Academic.

# Phytotherapy in context

## CHAPTER CONTENTS

**The origins of herbal therapeutics** 1
   The common origins of diet and medicine 1
   Matters of taste 2
   Shape-shifting 5
   Food, medicine and pharmacology 7
   Co-evolution 9
   Wholeness and complexity 11
**The development of herbal medicine as a practice** 14
   The nature of life is change 14
   Ethnobotanical insights 17
   In search of 'the herbalist' 18
**Phytotherapy** 21
   The varieties of phytotherapy 21
   Phytotherapy in the UK 23
   Integration and regulation 24
   Phytotherapy and evidence-based medicine 27
   Moving beyond scientism 30
   Phytotherapy: a personal view 33

## THE ORIGINS OF HERBAL THERAPEUTICS

### THE COMMON ORIGINS OF DIET AND MEDICINE

Using plants to promote healing is an ancient and global practice, referred to in our earliest texts and oral traditions:

> *Spoken stories were the living encyclopedias of our oral ancestors, dynamic and lyrical compendia of practical knowledge. Oral tales told on special occasions carried the secrets of how to orient in the local cosmos. Hidden in the magic adventures of their characters was precise information regarding which plants were good to eat and which were poisonous, and how to prepare certain herbs to heal cramps, or sleeplessness, or a fever.*
> Abram 2004

The search for food by early peoples inevitably led to encounters with plants that were discovered to be either toxic or therapeutic – sometimes both (depending on the amount ingested and the constitution of the individual). The development of herbal medicine thus occurred alongside adventures in determining the diet, so that we might consider herbal medicine to represent a branch, or offshoot, of nutrition. Zysk and Tetlow (2001) have observed that: 'The most traditional source of Ayurvedic medicine is the kitchen. It is likely that, at an early stage of its development, Indian medical and culinary traditions worked hand in hand with each other'. Beyond India, across the planet, we can suggest that the origin of the pharmacy lies in the kitchen.

The human relationship with medicinal plant chemicals is therefore a primary one. *Homo sapiens* emerged into a world long since populated with a great diversity of plant life with which our hominid ancestors already had intimate experience. To put things into perspective – we can compare the origin of our species, currently estimated at around 200 000 years ago, with the origin of the tree – and the now popular herbal remedy – *Ginkgo biloba*, which appeared some 200 million years ago. We tend to overlook, or take for granted, the fundamental essentiality of the plant–person relationship: just as we cannot live without sunlight, our health depends on plants.

The interaction between people and plants is, however, not straightforward. Rather it can be seen as a process of mutual adaptation, a dynamic evolutionary interplay. This deep engagement necessarily involves the full range of plant chemistry, running the gamut from attraction to repulsion, nutriment to poison. The ethnobotanist and professor of nutrition, Timothy Johns (1996), has described how the search for sustenance also laid the foundations for plant medication:

> *The properties of plants that make them unpalatable and toxic are the same properties that make them useful pharmacologically. In exploiting plant foods it is impossible to avoid their defensive chemicals, and I believe that in adapting to them our species has made them an essential part of our internal ecology.*

In this statement Johns touches on three key points:

- The connection between the sense of taste and the perception of pharmacology
- The ability of humans to adapt to and utilize physiologically potent plant compounds
- The profound degree to which the medicinal plant–person interface has evolved.

Human beings are hardwired for herbal medicine.

## MATTERS OF TASTE

Early medical systems were founded on:

- The interpretation of sensory information personally experienced when taking medicinal substances (e.g. did the item make you feel hot or cold, stimulated or sleepy, etc.)
- The observation of the effects of these substances on others
- A close observation of nature and the environment – which provided an explanatory and integrating framework for practice.

The sense of taste is at the core, as the primary sensory engagement with medicinal substances at the point that they enter the body. In the Hippocratic tradition 'eight qualities of taste' are recognized: sweet, fatty, acid, bitter, pungent, salty, bilious and astringent (Ullmann 1978). These are similar to the flavours discerned in traditional Chinese medicine, where herbal agents are classed according to whether they possess such distinctions as sourness, sweetness, bitterness, saltiness, pungency, blandness and astringency. These categories are not abstract or abstruse rationalizations, but rather the representation of clear and direct sensory experience. Each particular taste is associated with certain properties. For example, in Chinese medicine: bitter herbs have 'drying, reducing and downward-moving capabilities. (They) can dry Dampness and dissolve Phlegm … [and] reduce Heat from the internal organs' (Yang 2002). This is a very practical set of correspondences, based on observation and experience. The taste of the herb is associated with its sensed and observed ability to, for instance, warm (pungency, as in ginger) or cool (bitters) the body, or to be drying (astringent) or moistening (saltiness) in character. This range of information provides a pattern of activity, which can then be mapped against, and applied to, patterns of illness. When the patient has a condition that is hot and wet in its manifestation (such as a fever accompanied by sweating), then the requirement for herbal treatment that is cooling and drying is obvious. Such reasoning is at the core of ancient medical systems and constitutes the experiential origin of therapeutics.

That is not to say that classification systems of this type have ever been straightforward or unopposed! Controversy over classifications and the difficulty of making fine distinctions in diagnosis and prescribing has been in evidence since ancient times, as a Hippocratic author (from around the sixth century BCE) demonstrates:

> *I am utterly at a loss to know how those who prefer these hypothetical arguments and reduce the science to a simple matter of 'postulates' ever cure anyone on the basis of their assumptions. I do not think that they have ever discovered anything that is purely 'hot' or 'cold', 'dry' or 'wet', without it sharing some other qualities … It would be useless to bid a sick man to "take something hot". He would immediately ask "What?" Whereupon the doctor must either talk some technical gibberish or take refuge in some known solid substance. But suppose 'something hot' is also astringent, another is hot and soothing as well, while a third produces rumbling in the belly. There are many varied hot substances with many and varied effects which may be contrary to one another.*
>
> Lloyd (1983)

Careful judgement also needs to be exercised in determining when to encourage or oppose the expression of a disease phenomenon. For example, a low grade fever may need to be provoked into an acute manifestation with warming herbs in order to be fully expressed and thereafter fully healed. Suppression of a fever at an early or mild stage may be actively harmful. Therefore, traditional medicine is not exclusively allopathic (contrary in nature) but includes homoeopathic (similar in nature) elements too. The physician's skill lies in knowing how to modulate the pattern of the disorder, drawing on a range of capacities as required.

Returning to taste, we can say that the intensity of sensation derived from a herb or food can provide general indications as to its potency of action, its safety profile and the dosage that might be appropriate for it:

> *A rough indication of the qualities of a food or herb is the strength of taste. This could be seen to represent the relative amount of Qi contained within the food or herb. Generally, mild flavoured foods are consumed as staples (grains and pulses for example), while foods and drinks with stronger taste (tea, coffee, spices and condiments, etc.) are used less frequently because they have more of a medicinal effect.*
>
> Jilin (1995)

Mild flavours typically indicate a broad therapeutic window (i.e. a wide potential dosage range, suggesting the relatively benign nature of the substance) and hence suitability for long-term use in chronic disorders. Mildness occurs in herbal categories such as the 'adaptogens' (e.g. *Astragalus membranaceus* – huang qi) or the nervous 'trophorestoratives' (e.g. *Avena sativa* – oat straw). Strong flavours, conversely, are suggestive of a narrower therapeutic window (where the toxic dose is close to the therapeutic dose) and are more appropriate for short-term use and in acute disorders, e.g. the use of the powerfully bitter herb *Hydrastis canadensis* (golden seal) in sinus or gastrointestinal infections.

'Mild flavoured' foods and herbs may alternatively be classed as 'bland'. The sinologist, Francois Jullien, has used the motif of blandness to provide insight not only into Chinese medical thinking but into the philosophy of Chinese thought in general:

> *First, one accepts the paradox: that to honour the bland – to value the flavourless rather than the flavourful – runs counter to our most spontaneous judgement … But in Chinese culture, the bland is recognised as a positive quality … When the seemingly paradoxical becomes self-evident, when the value of the bland has changed signs, we begin to feel more comfortable with Chinese culture. When we begin to apprehend the stirring – beyond our ideological reflexes and cultural conditioning – of the possibility of a positive notion of the bland, we have entered China: not into its flashiest or most sophisticated realms, but into what is most simple and essential.*
>
> Jullien (2004)

Our direct sensory experience of the world shapes how we interpret it. Jullien's study helps to demonstrate the connection between taste and world-view: between physiological taste and aesthetic taste. In this analysis, blandness is a desirable quality of foods and herbs since it denotes those that are likely to be safe and suitable to take more frequently (or at higher dosage). Bland foods (such as grains, pulses, nuts and seeds – also known as 'earth' foods in Chinese medicine) are considered to be staples since they are gentle, easily digested and generative of a point of stability and potential, around which smaller amounts of more pronounced flavours may be consumed. The correlation is that a bland life, which is to say a moderate life, is the most sustainable way of living and one that can accommodate occasional eruptions of disorder or intensity – either planned or unplanned. Here we detect the 'feast' that is at the root of 'festival'. The traditional yearly cycle of generally ordered yet seasonally varying routine interspersed with occasional festivals/feast days provides an opportunity for short periods of stimulation, indulgence and free expression arising from a ground of moderation. While this pattern of living can be criticized as a means of maintaining feudalism and oppressive social control, it need not be constructed to this end – it also tends to spontaneously arise in successful indigenous cultures.

It is clear that the opposite scenario (i.e. the current mode of living in the 'developed world' where the bacchanal has shifted from sacred event to mundane lifestyle) is unsustainable, i.e. a day-to-day life of general stimulation/indulgence interspersed with short intense periods of moderation (going on a diet; checking-in to the detox clinic), is not robust enough to persist over the long term. Seen from this position, conventional medicines can be understood as a strand of an over-stimulated culture since they share the same intense, strong, unrelenting nature – unsubtle, single-gear agents that are integral to, and which fuel and enable an unsustainable mode of living. Herbal medicines, by comparison, appear relatively bland – notwithstanding the fact that several of conventional medicine's most potent remedies are based on plant compounds (e.g. diamorphine from the opium poppy, *Papaver somniferum*). In reality, plant medicines represent a complex spectrum of healing influences from the totally innocuous to the potentially lethal. Recent mainstream discourse on herbal remedies has tended to oscillate between the poles of this range – either plant medicines are too weak to offer the prospect of genuine healing effects or they are too toxic to be further contemplated as possibly valid medicines. Paradoxically, in societies that have drifted so far from nature and so deeply into an immoderate way of living that the continuing viability of the human (and many other) species is now threatened, herbal medicines (a potential part of the solution to an unsustainable lifestyle) are increasingly seen as wildly unpredictable and potentially dangerous entities. Yet this is *not* a paradox, since cultures that have distanced themselves from nature to the point of becoming nature-phobic will tend to fear and distrust the agents of nature (uncomprehending of their complexity, resistant to their meanings) such as herbal remedies.

## SHAPE-SHIFTING

In order for herbal substances to be accommodated within the dominant nature-phobic medical culture they need to be transformed or disguised. The most radical form of transformation takes place when the multi-compound complexity of a whole herb is reduced to a single 'active constituent', thereby actually becoming a 'real' conventional drug (i.e. a single, simple chemical compound). Whole herbs are not easily included into biomedical practice but the more a herbal remedy is disguised to look and feel like a conventional drug, the greater will be its chance of acceptance. This means that it should ideally be a chemically standardized extract of a solitary herb, presented in a processed coated pill form that is branded, packaged and corporatized. Ernst and Singh (2008) paternalistically advise that herbal medicine users only take single plant remedies, making sure to avoid traditional mixtures of herbs (herbalist's 'concoctions'); in their view only standardized preparations of herbs are to be permitted, and these should be bought in a packaged pill form off a pharmacy shelf. What if we were to suggest that herbs could be picked for free from the wild? Presumably Ernst and Singh would be horrified by the idea, yet their protestations would not travel well outside of the UK where they are based – it would be difficult, for instance, to persuade Danes, Germans and Italians that it is ill-advised to pick wild mushrooms! Following such drug-centric, nature-phobic advice directs one to products in which the herb tends to lose its *taste* and wherein it can no longer be *savoured*: odourless, tasteless, intangible – it ceases to have any connection with food and consequently enters into a changed relationship with the digestive system and, hence, the whole organism.

Despite adjustments in its preparation and presentation, the process of assimilating the herb into the dominant scientific medical culture cannot be completed until a corpus of evidence has been accumulated to mark the change in status from 'herb' to 'drug'. In the course of undergoing research, the plant will have to inhabit the diagnostic and prescriptive territory of conventional drugs so that, for instance, *Hypericum perforatum* (St John's wort) must cease to be a 'nervine tonic' used as an aid in depleted and exhausted nervous states and instead become an SSRI-like antidepressant, only to be used for mild to moderate depression. This type of shift in the meaning and significance of the herbal agent is seen by some as representing the rational validation of plants as therapeutic agents while others consider that it debases, diminishes and perverts the true nature and potential of herbal medicine. The transformation from traditional remedy to ersatz-drug in this type of case means that a profound opportunity is missed. In processing the plant to fit the language and classification systems of medical textbooks and prescription manuals the irony is that, while these texts do not recognize the concept of 'nervine tonics for depleted and exhausted nervous states', doctors and patients readily do! Doctors see people in this predicament daily but have little if anything to offer them from the conventional *materia medica*. Failure to consider the traditional understanding of the properties, indications and cautions for herbs, treating them instead as novel substances without a history, whether due to carelessness, ignorance or arrogance, commonly results in needlessly narrowed and warped interpretations of their capacities.

When researchers approach herbs from the perspective of positivist science, a one-way process generally follows with the herb being assimilated into the conventional model. Little or nothing is learned from the story that the herb brings with it. Typically, when attention is paid to traditional records and practitioners, or even where sophisticated original background ethnobotanical research has been conducted with native healers, pharmaceutical company funded research is only ultimately interested in generating leads that may give rise to a new and marketable drug – at which point the 'back story' is ditched. In his book *Prospecting for Drugs in Ancient and Medieval European Texts*, Holland (1996) talks of: 'The use of folk beliefs and traditional healers as a short-cut to the discovery and isolation of pharmacologically active compounds ...', as opposed to promoting renewed use of the herbs themselves. The assumption is that herbal medicines are of no value in their own right, although they might provide clues that enable the production of 'proper' drugs. Why not just run trials on the herbs themselves and, if the old herbals are proven to be correct, then promote the wider use of herbs in medical practice? In answering that question, fiscal as well as scientific bias needs to be considered.

The absolutist nature of positivist science is typified by Dawkins (2003) who asserts that there are no such entities as 'conventional' and 'complementary and alternative medicine' (CAM) but merely 'medicine that works and medicine that does not work'. He is confident that if so-called CAM practices (such as herbal medicine) are proven to work by means of double-blind randomized placebo controlled trials (RCTs) – if they are able to 'pass that test' – then 'mainstream medicine would simply adopt them'. This is a view of biomedical substance, process and assimilation of cartoon-like quality, that displays either stunning naivety or wilful perversity. In this monotheistic view, biomedicine is portrayed as the only legitimate form of medicine. It has the capacity to incorporate techniques and materials into its scope but only when these comply with its own scientific normative standards – there is no need to question these principles, only to rigorously apply them. In order for CAM practices (or aspects of them) to enter the big tent of biomedicine they merely need to show their passport at the flap – suitably stamped 'RCT'. In fact biomedicine cannot eat CAM practices whole – they first need to be prepared into a suitably digestible form via marination in approved forms of research. Yet even long steeping of this kind may still fail to render them appetizing. Would Dawkins be surprised to find that doctors (in the UK at least) are not prescribing the heavily research-validated St John's Wort for depression? For all its evidence-base, this herb somehow remains foreign, it fails to fit in, and meets with the kind of incomprehension and xenophobia that all too commonly characterize the position of the dominant culture in response to the immigrant. Despite what Dawkins has suggested, it appears that the world of biomedicine is not value free.

Since the dominant medical drug model is inflexible, herbal medicines must change their form and divest themselves of their attached traditional rationales if they are to be incorporated into it. We will return to this territory later as we discuss the varieties of phytotherapy and the ways in which herbal practitioners have engaged with or opposed the biomedical project.

## FOOD, MEDICINE AND PHARMACOLOGY

In Ayurvedic medicine, as in other traditional systems, taste is central to appreciating the qualities of herbs as well as foods. Joshi et al. (2006) equate 'taste' with the Sanskrit word 'Rasa' which 'refers to a complex totality of experience arising from all the perceptory interactions of the material with sensors in the mouth and nasal passages, taste buds, olfactory and chemesthetic receptors'. The notion of 'Rasa' incorporates six primary tastes, similar to those already mentioned in ancient Graeco-Roman and Chinese medicine: sweet, sour, salty, pungent, bitter, and astringent. Each primary taste is said to be composed of specific combinations of the elements and exerts particular influences on the Ayurvedic humoural system (i.e. the three 'doshas' of *kapha*, *pitta* and *vata*). For example, the sweet taste is composed of earth and water, it increases *kapha* and decreases *pitta* and *vata*. Further differentiations of taste are drawn in Ayurveda, including the concepts of 'virya' (which identifies thermal, tactile and other effects with eight descriptions that are formed into four complementary pairs: hot–cold, unctuous–dry, heavy–light, dull–sharp) and 'vipaka' (which describes three types of aftertaste: sweet, sour and pungent).

Beauchamp et al. (2005) found that the drug Ibuprofen and a compound found in extra-virgin olive oil (oleo canthal) both caused a similar stinging sensation in the throat. Although possessing different chemical structures, both agents share similar anti-inflammatory activity as COX-1 and COX-2 inhibitors. Joshi et al. (2006) refer to this research, seeing it as offering modern confirmation of the value traditionally placed on taste, and suggesting that: 'Using "taste" as an additional tool, new phytochemicals of desired therapeutic activity might be more rapidly identified'. Taste is a pharmacological detection tool, since different tastes are triggered by different chemical compounds: bitterness relates to compounds including iridioids, sourness to certain acids, sweetness to polysaccharides, astringency to tannins and so on. In this way, even the most primary, non-technological relationship between people and plants can be rendered to the service of biomedicine. Alongside the plundering of the knowledge of traditional healers and of ancient herbal texts, the very sense of taste itself can be exploited to reductive pharmacological ends. In these realms, the balance between justification and appropriation of herbal medicine is played out: proponents of herbal medicine can use traditional and pharmacological evidence to justify the validity of herbal medicine, while biomedicine can use the same means to appropriate it. This paired agenda is one of the key sites of tension in the interface between herbal and conventional medicine.

A pharmacological perspective reveals a large overlap in the types of chemical compounds found in both foods and herbal medicines. Some substances may be considered to belong in both categories, e.g. garlic and the culinary herbs and spices such as basil and cinnamon have a place in the kitchen and the dispensary. A chemically-based approach to distinguishing between plants as foods and as medicines may begin by acknowledging the considerable overlap between the two groups before making the general distinction that foods tend to be rich in primary metabolites of nutritional value (macronutrients and micronutrients), while medicinal herbs tend to contain less nutritional compounds but a high proportion of secondary metabolites (such as alkaloids, saponins and volatile oils). Foods – when carefully selected and prepared – are generally, and necessarily, extremely low in toxicity and able to provide nutrients to maintain growth, repair and the maintenance of normal physiological functions. Medicinal herbs provide a spectrum of agents from benign to toxic in effect, which can have an adaptive effect on physiology – modulating the response to challenges including those deriving from pathology. This distinction between foods and medicines is essentially the same as that made by the Persian physician al-Majusi (late tenth century), which was in turn based on the writings of Galen (BCE 129–c.216?), which states that:

> *The drug (herbal medicine) changes the physis of the body, while on the other hand the food increases its substance.*
>
> Ullmann (1978)

Ullmann (1978) further describes al-Majusi's distinctions between foods and medicines, which are based on how the body changes, and is changed by, these two types of substances. Al-Majusi's perspective is divided into four categories of relationships:

1. Remedies in the absolute sense are the materials which the body at first changes but which then change the body and transform it into their temperament
2. Deadly poisons are those materials which change the body and gain power over it without the body being able to resist them
3. Remedial food materials are those which at first change the body until the body gains power over them and transforms them into its own nature …
4. Finally, the (pure) foods are those which the body changes and transforms into itself.

This systemization continues to provide a good model for appreciating the differences between, as Ullmann terms them, 'remedies' (i.e. herbal medicines); 'poisons' (certain toxic herbs and conventional medicines); 'remedial food-stuffs' (those possessing gentle therapeutic activity); and 'food-stuffs' (which build the substance of the body). The ability to distinguish between plants that are foods and those that are medicines (as well as those which straddle both categories) in this way has been crucial to human survival. This understanding is also vital in other species, as the science of zoopharmacognosy is revealing (for an introduction to this area, see Engel 2007). The importance of this knowledge is testified to by the number of documents (known as 'herbals') from earliest times, dedicated to listing and explaining the therapeutic properties of naturally occurring substances – principally botanical material. A stunning example is the Ebers Papyrus (discovered by Georg Ebers in the 1870s), which gives some 700 remedies for a wide variety of conditions. This ancient Egyptian text, dating from around BCE 1550, is considered the oldest medical text extant. Numerous other herbals are left to us from around the world from Ancient Greece and Rome, Mediaeval Europe, India, Central America and China.

## CO-EVOLUTION

We might now reflect on the nature of the relationships between plants and animals, including humans, particularly with regard to how these have influenced the production of secondary metabolites, and how tolerance and utilization of these compounds has developed.

According to Wynne-Edwards (2001): 'Evidence of coevolution of plants and herbivores is abundant'. Animals have used plants for food and plants have responded by developing mechanisms to deter them. While some plants may accrue positive gains from being consumed once they have developed seeds (the animal can then spread the seed in useful manure-wrapped deposits), they are at risk of being destroyed without benefit if eaten before this point. Some plant defences are physical (e.g. thorns) but most are chemical. Many chemical defences produced by plants taste unpleasant to us (e.g. intense bitterness) – the unpleasantness *is* the deterrent, while our retention of this sense of unpleasantness helps to protect us from consuming too much. This poses palatability challenges when working with herbal medicines, and relates to such folk wisdom as: 'The worse the medicine tastes the better it is for you'.

Animals have developed a range of strategies in adapting to plant defences, as Wynne-Edwards (2001) describes:

> ... mammalian herbivores often consume a diverse diet composed of sublethal doses of chemical defences or carefully consume only the tissues that are least toxic to them ... (they) can also evolve detoxification mechanisms that allow them to consume specific plants in spite of their chemical defenses ...

Beyond this, animals have evolved to use plant defence chemicals to their advantage, often for the same purposes as the plants themselves. Plants, for example produce antimicrobial compounds for their own needs, which can be used by humans to destroy our bacterial and fungal infections. Plant secondary metabolites may serve multiple purposes within the plant itself, for instance: alkaloids act as a deterrent to herbivores but are also involved in absorption of nitrogen from the soil; flavonoids help to prevent infection in plants but also protect them from UV radiation and play a role in regulating growth. It is important to note that the plant–person relationship works in both directions, animals and plants adapt in response to each other. A major human cause of changes in plant chemistry is that of domestication of food plants. This has led to changes in their chemical composition, including the reduction of more aggressively acting or toxic secondary metabolites. Wild potatoes, for example, are generally too unpalatable and potentially harmful for human consumption but some of their inherent toxicity has been reduced through careful selection and cultivation.

The origins of herbal therapy then, lie very deep – through co-evolution with plants we are hardwired for a dynamic interaction with plant secondary metabolites. This relationship is not limited to the purely physical level. O'Doherty et al. (2001) have shown that both pleasant and unpleasant tastes influence the amygdala (a brain structure associated with emotional and mental activity) and the psychoactive (especially hallucinogenic) properties of some plants can be considered as a particular category of deterrent innovation that have influenced humans profoundly – shaping beliefs about the world.

Much of the literature on herbal medicine (most pertinently the growing body of texts considering herbal safety issues) seems ignorant of this primeval dance. We have learned not only to tolerate a great range of plant chemicals but beyond this we have also been successful in turning many of them to our advantage. We can utilize plant resins in stimulating leucocytosis for instance, or triterpenoid saponins from plants such as ginseng (*Panax ginseng*) to improve our energy, endurance and stamina. Such gains are the remarkable fruits of our long interplay with the botanical realm – we spurn them at our peril.

At a micro-level, we can discuss the relationship between people and plants in chemical and pharmacological terms: referring, for example, to triterpenoid saponins and their ability to induce intracellular generation of adenosine triphosphate (ATP) leading to enhanced energy, endurance and stamina. The macro-tier however, has to do with the relationship between *Homo sapiens* and, in this example, *Panax ginseng*. Many herbs contain triterpenoid saponins but the particular herb in question, in each specific case, is sufficiently chemically and structurally different to be classified as a distinct and separate species. For instance, although they both contain triterpenoid saponins, *Panax ginseng* and Siberian ginseng (*Eleutherococcus senticosus*) do not have exactly identical therapeutic actions since they do not share precisely the same chemical make-up. Successful herbal medicine is practised with an appreciation of both the pronounced and the subtle distinctions between herbs that share key chemical constituents.

Some herbal authorities decry the tendency to focus on herbs at the micro-level at the expense of the macro-aspect. One does not have to choose between the two, however. Both levels of scrutiny possess their own validity and each may be impoverished when it stands alone. Some critics of the phytotherapy approach have associated it with an undue and unbalanced focus on reductive pharmacological scrutiny of the plant. This need not be the case, since it is perfectly possible to view narrow (but potentially helpful) pharmacological insights in the context of a broader appreciation of the whole plant. We will return to the discussion of phytotherapy towards the end of this chapter.

## WHOLENESS AND COMPLEXITY

The comparison of micro-scrutiny via focus on areas such as phytochemistry with macro-perception of the plant in its entirety is pivotal in appreciating the distinctions between the conventional medical utilization of plant products and that of herbal practitioners. It is a tenet of herbal medicine that whole herbs must be prescribed rather than the isolated active constituents derived from them. This is the difference between making a medicine directly from strips of, e.g. willow bark (*Salix* spp.) itself as opposed to extracting acetyl salicylic acid (aspirin) from it. When liberated from the context of the (many) other phytochemicals present in the plant a single active constituent will not behave in quite the same way as the whole plant. Typically, the isolated constituent exhibits one pronounced quality of the whole plant (taken from among many less prominent ones) but does so more aggressively and with greater potential to generate adverse effects. Occasionally, an isolated constituent may show activity that could not be anticipated from knowledge of the whole plant. Commonly then (but by no means exclusively), use of the whole plant compared with isolated active constituents will demonstrate activity which is:

- Slower to accumulate effects
- Safer (generating no or fewer and less severe adverse effects and producing less or no tolerance over time)
- Wider ranging in the scope of effects achieved (often across multiple body systems)
- Productive of more lasting long-term improvements.

(*Note*: Many of the adverse effects generated by conventional drugs signify attempts at detoxification by the body – this includes many rashes, digestive upsets, headaches, nausea and vomiting, etc. Herbal medicines are more 'food-like' in their complexity and are less likely to trigger pronounced elimination responses.)

This combination of attributes makes whole plant herbal medicines particularly suitable for treatment of chronic disorders.

'Whole' is, however, a debatable concept. If we infuse or decoct a herb in water, or prepare it in other ways such as by using alcohol as an extractive medium (in making herbal tinctures), we do not have every constituent in the resulting liquid, since there will be lots of plant material left behind in the pan or press. The only way to get every constituent into the body is to consume the whole herb, e.g. as a powder. Even then, some constituents will deteriorate or transform while the herb is being dried, processed or stored (albeit that some such changes, in particular cases, may serve to enhance the efficacy of the herb). Then again, whatever the number or quality of constituents present in the preparation, it is uncertain how many will actually cross the body's membranes in order to exert physiological effects. Nonetheless, we can still draw a picture of differing chemical complexity between herbal preparations (which will contain hundreds of different chemical compounds) and conventional medicines – whether plant-derived or otherwise (which are generally single compounds). Herbal medicines are chemically complex, whereas conventional drugs are chemically simple.

The search for processes whereby the complexity of herbs could be reduced to release simpler and more potent remedies is an ancient alchemical one, well summarized by Paracelsus (*c*.1493–1542):

> ... *what the eye perceives in herbs or stone or trees is not yet a remedy; the eye sees only the dross. The remedy must be cleansed from the dross, then it is there.*
>
> Griggs (1981)

This vision would come to pass and to fruition in modern pharmacology as alchemy gave rise to chemistry. In zeroing in on ever-finer detail however, the bigger picture is obscured: the most prominent active constituents in medicinal plants are contextualized within a package of many other, more subtly acting, constituents and co-factors that, far from being 'dross', may play a significant role in shaping the overall actions of the plant. Medicinal plants, the herbal practitioner contends, are not mixed ores in need of refining but, rather, the finished article.

Appreciation of the chemical complexity of the 'whole' plant presents pharmacological challenges both technically and conceptually. The complexity can extend to such an extent that a single herb may have a great number of different actions. For example, yarrow (*Achillea millefolium*) is said to be a: diaphoretic, antipyretic, peripheral vasodilator, anti-inflammatory, spasmolytic, bitter tonic, styptic (haemostatic), antimicrobial, anti-haemorrhagic and vulnerary (wound healing) herb (Bone 2003). It is only when one appreciates the great diversity of chemical composition in plants that one can understand or accept the possibility that a single herb might encompass the breadth of actions that would require assembly of a large part of the conventional pharmacy to be matched. It is in the nature of herbs, as 'polypharmacies' in and of themselves, to influence more than one 'target' at a time; their effects are diffuse, complex and wide ranging. Such therapy enables (and, to be optimally successful, *requires*) a broad approach to the patient that allows for the emergence of unique healing pictures since the outcomes of this type of medicine cannot be fully predicted due to the wide variety of body systems that may be modulated. To practice herbal medicine then, it is essential to be comfortable with a degree of uncertainty regarding the form of results (but in which practice of medicine is this not also true?). The key to successful herbal practice is to be highly sensitive and responsive to the patient's changes (no matter how subtle) at each consultation, varying the prescription accordingly. Herein lies a central feature of herbal practice: as the patient's picture changes over time, the herbal prescription they receive will also change to reflect and positively adapt or propel these developments, since a course of professional herbal treatment is a dynamically evolving rather than static process.

A herbal medicine needs to be considered as a different type of pharmacological entity to a conventional drug. The latter are simple chemical *compounds*, whereas herbal medicines are, at least in terms of the whole plant starting material, highly complex *organisms*. In fact, it is beyond the power of current pharmacological knowledge to completely analyse and track the chemistry of whole herbs – or indeed to come anywhere near achieving such a goal. The chemical complexity of herbal medicines increases of course as several herbs are combined in a particular treatment – comprising perhaps 25 herbs in a classical Chinese medicine formula, for example. The chemical make-up, or at least the relative quantities of each compound, in individual species of herbs also varies depending on growing and processing factors, which include:

- Where the herb is grown (habitat, altitude, etc.)
- Naturally varying aspects of the growing conditions (rainfall, humidity, sun exposure, etc.)
- Time of harvesting
- How the herb is processed (drying method, tincture method, etc.).

Attempts have been made to tame the wild complexity of herbs by standardizing preparations with regard to key active constituents (it is impossible to standardize a herb on all constituents – many of which have not yet even been elucidated). Although many herbal practitioners are wary of any attempt to manipulate the chemistry of herbs, standardization in its most useful manifestation merely consists of measuring key constituents and blending different batches to provide a specified minimum level of one or two compounds. The complex nature of plant chemistry is reflected in the practice of herbal medicine with regard to the consultation. The approach to the patient reflects (and is consistent with) the nature of the medicinal materials used:

- Herbal practitioners claim to 'use the whole plant to treat the whole person', with allowance being made for the complexity and variability of the person, just as must occur (to some degree) with the plant.
- Typically, long consultation times in modern herbal practice provide space to explore the patient's history across its full range, giving

credence to information that might in conventional medical consultations be considered 'dross'.

Conventional pharmacology and medical science has forgotten, ignored or overlooked the complex nature of medicinal plant chemistry to such an extent that the following statement can be made without considering herbs:

> In searching for new and effective therapeutics, it might be useful to use a systems-chemistry approach to modify integrated outcomes rather than targeting single molecules with the hope that the desired systemic effect might be generated. In other words, it is likely that creating a 'new homoeostasis' will require the modification of more than one target.
>
> Hotamisligil (2006)

Time to step out of the lab and into the garden.

## THE DEVELOPMENT OF HERBAL MEDICINE AS A PRACTICE

### THE NATURE OF LIFE IS CHANGE

From earliest times, as people have contemplated life and its meaning, they have pointed to change as a central theme. Things grow and perish, the weather varies (sometimes dramatically), empires rise, fall and disappear. From the Native American tradition, we have the insight that: 'Nothing is born, nothing dies, everything changes' (McLuhan 1973).

Around 2500 years ago, Heraclitus (Haxton 2001) wrote:

> By cosmic rule,
> as day yields night,
> so winter summer,
> war peace, plenty famine,
> All things change.

Living in a world that perpetually changes is challenging – it can be hard to know how to steer one's course. Some changes are cyclical in nature however, and by discerning their repetition we gain a sense of perspective, a hold on how to work with change. Observing the turning of the seasons and the movement of the stars enables us to detect patterns of change. Practices such as agriculture are dependent on a highly developed knowledge of such patterns. Ancient and traditional medical systems also developed their rationales based on a close appreciation of the patterns in nature. Ancient Greek, Chinese and Indian (Ayurvedic) medicine, although distinct approaches, are united in devising explanatory models of health and illness that integrate change in the environment with phenomena arising in the individual. Tables 1.1–1.3 give charts of correspondences that illustrate these relationships in these three systems of medicine.

These charts reveal attempts made to connect, classify and systematize a wide variety of factors pertaining to the person and the world in which they reside, including the:

**Table 1.1** *Correspondences in ancient Hippocratic–Galenic medicine*

| Season | Spring | Summer | Autumn | Winter |
|---|---|---|---|---|
| The 4 elements | Air | Fire | Earth | Water |
| The primary qualities | Hot and moist | Hot and dry | Cold and dry | Cold and moist |
| The 4 humours | Blood | Yellow bile | Black bile | Phlegm |
| The 4 temperaments | Sanguine | Choleric | Melancholic | Phlegmatic |
| Development | Childhood | Youth | Middle age | Old age |
| Direction | West | South | East | North |
| Associated emotion | Joy | Anger | Fear/worry/grief | Indifference |

Adapted from Tobyn (1997).

**Table 1.2** *Correspondences in Chinese medicine*

| Category | Wood | Fire | Earth | Metal | Water |
|---|---|---|---|---|---|
| Season | Spring | Summer | Late summer | Autumn | Winter |
| Direction | East | South | Centre | West | North |
| Colour | Green | Red | Yellow | White | Black |
| Taste | Sour | Bitter | Sweet | Pungent | Salty |
| Odour | Rancid | Scorched | Fragrant | Rotten | Putrid |
| Sound | Shouting | Laughing | Singing | Crying | Groaning |
| Zang (Yin organs) | Liver | Heart | Spleen | Lungs | Kidney |
| Fu (Yang organs) | Gallbladder | Small intestine | Stomach | Large intestine | Bladder |
| Sense organ | Eyes | Tongue | Mouth | Nose | Ears |
| Emotion | Anger | Joy | Pensiveness | Sorrow | Fear |
| Development | Birth | Growth | Transformation | Harvest | Storage |
| Climate | Wind | Heat | Damp | Dryness | Cold |

Adapted from Dowie (2009) and Ergil (2001).

- Cycle of the seasons
- Cycle of growth of the human from birth to death
- Physical elements of which the world is made
- Parts of the body
- Character of the person
- Variety of human emotions
- Information provided by the senses.

Amidst this web of interrelations, herbal medicines can be savoured (their pungency and bitterness; their texture and intensity) and their effects experienced – warming or cooling; clearing phlegm; soothing the stomach

Table 1.3  Correspondences in Ayurvedic medicine

| Characteristic | Vata | Pitta | Kapha |
| --- | --- | --- | --- |
| Elements | Air and Space | Fire and Water | Earth and Water |
| Qualities | Dry, cold, light, irregular, mobile, rough, abundant | Hot, light, intense fluid, liquid, putrid, pungent, sour | Heavy, unctuous, cold, stable, dense, soft, smooth |
| Humour | Wind | Bile | Phlegm |
| Taste | Astringent and pungent | Salty and bitter | Sweet and sour |
| Principal seat | Colon | Stomach | Lungs |
| Physiology | Responsible for all bodily movement and nervous functions | Governs enzymes and hormones and is responsible for digestion, etc. | The principle of cohesion and stability. Responsible for sexual power, etc. |

Adapted from Zysk & Tetlow (2001) and Joshi et al. (2006).

or calming our emotions. Herbal medicines stand revealed in this mesh of relationships as part of the fabric of life and wellbeing; as adaptive entities that can help the individual modulate the effects of change on the body, mind and spirit.

At the roots of Chinese philosophy is the *I Ching* (commonly referred to as 'The Book of Changes'), a divinatory system and text originating some 3000 years ago. The book was originally known simply as *I*, the later addition of *Ching* denotes a classic text. The English translation of *I* is usually given as 'change/s', but this is to limit its interpretation, as Ritsema and Karcher (1994) point out:

> ... I *is neither orderly change – the change of the seasons, for example – nor the change of one thing into another, like water changing to ice ... Unpredictable and ... unfathomable, I originates in and is a way of dealing with trouble ... The term I emphasizes imagination, openness and fluidity. It suggests the ability to change direction quickly and the use of a variety of imaginative stances to mirror the variety of being. The most adequate English translation of this is* versatility, *the ability to remain available to and be moved by the unforeseen demands of time, fate and psyche. This term interweaves the* I *of the cosmos, the* I *of the book, and your own* I, *if you use it.*

Let us also talk of the 'I' of the plant. If the nature of life is change (both orderly and chaotic, relatively predictable and wildly unpredictable), then the key to health is to have the flexibility to adapt and to flow with the currents and movements of change. Herbs are key allies in facilitating such adaptation, acting to promote fluidity as they modulate physiology, emotions and mental activity. Their potential to do this essential work (as agents enabling versatility and resilience) has been recognized and prized across world cultures for millennia.

## ETHNOBOTANICAL INSIGHTS

The discipline of ethnobotany (the study of the relationships between peoples and plants) has revealed much about how early and indigenous cultures have utilized plants therapeutically. A comprehensive knowledge of the medicinal uses of a wide range of plants is a characteristic feature of such cultures. This knowledge may be more extensively appreciated and curated by certain trained and experienced individuals but it is not limited to 'experts' – for the most part the medicinal properties of plants are common knowledge, owned by the whole community.

Indigenous peoples have an extensive appreciation of the biodiversity of their locale and how to use and conserve it. In his monumental study of Native American plant use, Daniel Moerman (1998) has discovered that, out of the 31 566 known North American vascular plant (i.e. 'higher plants') species:

> *American Indians used 2874 of these species as medicines, 1886 as foods, 230 as dyes, and 492 as fibres ... All told, they found useful purposes for 3923 kinds of vascular plants.*

Notice here the difference between the number of plants used as medicines and those used as foods – a far greater number of species are used as medicines than for foods. Interestingly, Van Wyk et al. (1997), in their study of indigenous medicinal plant use in South Africa found almost identical figures regarding plant species and the number used medicinally. Out of an estimated 30 000 plant species growing in South Africa, around 3000 species are used medicinally. Hutchings (1996) gives an even higher percentage of plant species used medicinally in a smaller region. Her study of Zulu herbal medicines profiles 1032 species, which represents approximately 25% of the flora of KwaZulu-Natal.

Who used/uses these plants? Arvigo and Balick (1998) have named and described the various types of traditional healers of Belize:

- The Doctor–Priest/Priestess: 'have the ability to contact the spirit world to ask ... spiritual forces for assistance in the diagnosis and treatment of ailments'
- The Village Healer: an experienced father or mother who looks after 'the entire village's health care needs'
- The Grannie Healer: cares for her own family
- The Midwife: cares for women's and children's conditions and utilizes 'a vast number of herbal remedies'
- The Massage Therapist: treats musculoskeletal problems with 'herbal baths, poultices, teas and oils'
- The Bone Setter: uses manipulation and herbal remedies to treat sprains, fractures, broken bones
- The Snake Doctor: treats poisonings from toxins and venoms, stings and bites.

Among these various practitioners, the use of plants as medicines is a common thread, although none are identified as being 'a herbalist' – their function is emphasized on the means they use to achieve their goals.

Outside of these specific types of practitioners, it has long been common for each person in a community to have some knowledge of plants – stemming, at the very least, from being treated themselves. Such appreciation is part of a shared heritage of basic plant knowledge and skills. Gabrielle Hatfield (1999) has studied the vestiges of this kind of individual appreciation of medicinal plant utility in the UK. She describes it as a:

> ... common sense approach to plant medicine, used as part of people's everyday lives ... People did not regard this as specialist information, but took it for granted as common knowledge.

Who would not know that chamomile (*Matricaria recutita*) is good to settle disrupted digestion? Who would not know that peppermint (*Mentha piperita*) will control a fever? Traditional communities who fail to maintain such knowledge are not only intellectually impoverished but physically *at risk*. One of the key challenges for herbal practitioners in the modern, nature-negligent world, is to find ways of helping to re-establish this herbal knowledge base through educational work in self- and community-care. The current impetus towards bolstering the status of herbal medicine as a regulated profession (see discussion towards the end of this chapter) needs to keep in mind the traditional ubiquity of herbal knowledge.

Hatfield's work flags up the degree to which widespread knowledge of the use of plant medicines persisted into the twentieth century in industrialized Britain, and the extent to which this tends to be overlooked. She concentrates on examining 'domestic medicine', which she defines as: 'the history of self-help rather than of official medicine'. This history continues today, where the vast majority of herbal medicines consumed in the UK (and many other Western nations) are self-prescribed rather than taken on the advice of a practitioner – herbalist or otherwise.

## IN SEARCH OF 'THE HERBALIST'

Official healthcare developed out of traditional medical practices (which now tend to be designated, usually pejoratively, as 'folk medicine') but today bears little resemblance to its origins. The use of herbs in official medicine persisted as a large percentage of the conventional doctor's *materia medica* well into the twentieth century – later than many people suspect. Official pharmacopoeias and *materia medica* attest to this fact: Southall's *Organic Materia Medica* (Barclay 1909), for example, profiles over 200 medicinal plants from *Abelmoschus moschatus* (musk seed) to *Zingiber officinale* (ginger); *The British Pharmacopoeia* of 1948 (General Medical Council 1948) still contains a significant number of herbal medicines – some years after the discovery of antibiotics and a few years before the effective deployment of corticosteroids; and even today:

> 25% of modern prescription drugs contain at least one compound now or once *derived* or patterned after compounds derived *from higher plants* [original emphases]

Duke (1993)

If we turn our gaze to try to make out the 'herbal medicine practitioner' as a discrete entity among the diversity of medicinal plant use – the 'herbalist' – then we may have to look long and hard to make sense of what we see. Although modern western herbal practitioners tend to claim a heritage that includes the great male authors in the western medical cannon (Hippocrates, Galen, Dioscorides, Avicenna) it is oversimplifying matters to label these figures as 'herbalists'. Although most of these writers have left us texts demonstrating that the prescribing of plant medicines was a central part of their practice, it is also clear that it was not the only intervention they utilized. These figures were physicians and in performing the functions of this role, they made use of any substance and strategy that fitted with their approach and which appeared to help. In the medicine of antiquity, a wide range of health-modulating factors were addressed under the heading of *Diatetica*. The discipline of dietetics involved more than food and drink however, it incorporated all key areas of human activity including exercise, sex, bathing and sleep (as we shall see in more detail in Chapter 6). Porter (1997) discusses the persistence of this broad and individualized approach extending into the eighteenth century when 'diet' still meant 'a comprehensive ordering of life'.

Similarly, herbal practitioners today will claim that their practice extends beyond the prescribing of plant medicines to include advising on diet and 'lifestyle' – this being the catch-all term perhaps most commonly used today in place of 'diatetica'. So, the distinction between an ancient physician and a modern herbal practitioner may not lie so much in the claimed scope of practice as in the insistence on the centrality and primacy of plant medicines. In antiquity, diet (in the sense of diatetica) was generally the first treatment option; preferred over drugs (which were mostly herbal), with surgery as the least desirable intervention. A restraint in prescribing herbal medicines combined with a primary focus on dietetics, including proper exposure to clean air and sunlight, connects ancient medicine with 'naturopathy' (itself an influence on the development of modern herbal medicine).

In traditional systems of medicine, animal and mineral substances are usually viewed as equals to vegetable remedies and although less numerous, form an essential part of the traditional *materia medica*. We still have the anomaly in Chinese herbal medicine (in translation) that the term 'herbal' can include any natural substance and is not limited to botanical material. Many western herbal practitioners have been vociferous in their condemnation of the persistence of non-vegetable items in traditional pharmacies. This has been partly due to legitimate concerns regarding trade in endangered species and around animal welfare issues but even in cases where these concerns do not apply, criticisms often persist – any presence of a non-vegetable material being interpreted as sullying or degrading the botanical *materia medica*. The objection to including animal parts, especially, as medicines is strongly held by many western herbal practitioners. Such a standpoint might be contended to be logically inconsistent however, if the practitioner is also advising the inclusion of animal products in the diet or prescribing, e.g. fish oil as a 'nutritional supplement'. One practitioner's 'meat' is another's 'potion' …

In a previous volume, I observed that:

> *Western herbal practitioners can be accused of creating a myth of herbal medicine as a pure practice. In reality, globally, herbs have always been used alongside any other substance that might achieve therapeutic benefits.*
>
> Conway (2005)

To what extent then can we consider the practice of herbal medicine, in the modern western sense, as a discrete profession? Certainly there is evidence of professional self-organization going back a reasonable way. In the UK, the National Association of Medical Herbalists (later the National Institute of Medical Herbalists) was founded in 1864 and persists to this day. In a study examining the state of herbal practice in mid-nineteenth century Britain, Brown (1982) discovers: 'Two types of herbalism, the traditional and the Thomsonian' – the latter group were followers (and frequently trained 'agents') of Samuel Thomson, an American who developed and promoted a system of herbal medicine and who was a fierce opponent of the means and methods of conventional medicine.

According to Brown (1982):

> *Traditional herbalism and orthodox medicine could co-exist without too many problems: they had developed from common roots and presumably evolved to meet the needs of different social groups.*

These herbalists mostly lived among and treated the poor, still drew on Culpeper as well as the current pharmacopoeias (which were still largely 'herbals'), commonly had a second job and aspired to equal status with conventional medical practitioners. The Thomsonians by contrast styled themselves 'medical botanists' and proselytized medical reform in books and public lectures, lambasting the errors of conventional medicine to the extent that: 'no easy co-existence was possible with the Thomsonian herbalists'. As conventional medicine increasingly focussed on aggressive treatments based on mineral products and isolated plant constituents, it became possible for proponents of herbal medicine to state their case in opposition, such that the defining features of herbal practice came to include: an insistence on vegetable medicines and a rejection of mineral ones; use of the whole plant as opposed to isolates; advocacy of natural over synthetic remedies, and so forth.

We might suggest then that, actually, the exclusively 'herbal' practitioner, deliberately titled, is a relatively recent construct, given the vast history of human use of medicinal plants – albeit deeply rooted and with many tangled tendrils enmeshing the entire history of medicine across the whole world. Arguably, it is this multiplicity of origins and influences, this complex and non-linear heritage, that adds most interest, robustness and potential to the role of the contemporary herbal practitioner, while at the same time making it unlikely that a single detailed definition of what it means to be such an exponent is ever likely to be universally agreed. The 'phytotherapist' is a complex and contentious notion of one form of modern herbal practitioner.

# PHYTOTHERAPY

## THE VARIETIES OF PHYTOTHERAPY

So why phytotherapy? As if the identity of the herbal practitioner is not already a confused one, why add another term? Does it illuminate or obscure?

The herbal practitioner as an entity (in the sense discussed above) is a relatively local phenomenon. In the UK, Australia and some parts of North America, the herbal practitioner exists as a legal or quasi-legal (but generally tolerated) healthcare provider, operating almost exclusively outside of mainstream healthcare. These practitioners have generally been trained in independent Colleges who have awarded their own, in-house, herbal practice certificates and diplomas. Increasingly, however, they are now emerging with university degrees in herbal medicine – especially in the UK. Should they wish to venture to practice in mainland Europe and beyond though, they will tend to find that their qualifications are unrecognized.

In much of mainland Europe it is common to encounter herbal medicines sold (often with advice thrown in) from market stalls and pharmacies and as a part (either large or small) of the practice of various therapists such as naturopaths and the German *heilpraktikers*. The specific 'herbal practitioner' is a rarity and may be an outlaw. In certain countries, most notably Germany and France, conventional doctors may prescribe herbs in addition to conventional medical treatment and, in doing so, they may describe or advertise themselves as phytotherapists. Some doctor–phytotherapists prescribe herbs in a manner that would be considered limited, reductionist and even ill-informed by many modern western herbal practitioners and traditional medicine practitioners.

This (stereo)type of doctor–phytotherapist tends to use single herb products (as opposed to the multi-herb prescriptions of most traditional and modern herbal practitioners), at relatively low doses, for specific named diseases (as opposed to the individualized approach of herbal practitioners) in standardized preparations (in contrast to traditional herbal preparations), e.g. prescribing *Crataegus* spp. (hawthorn) for hypertension. For these activities, doctor–phytotherapists are scorned by herbal practitioners who argue that the therapeutic potentials of herbs are substantially limited (or even perverted) by being applied within such a framework. One might counter, however, that if such an approach yields benefits (and there is a fair body of research to testify that it does) then surely this style of herb use should be encouraged, especially when the reduced burden of adverse-effects achieved by avoiding the use of conventional pharmaceuticals is factored in? While the contrasting protocols of the herbal practitioner (multi-herb prescriptions, higher doses, traditional preparations, individualized treatment) *may* be even more efficacious, there is less conventionally credible evidence (i.e. randomized controlled trials) available to offer in testimony to this. Incidentally, it should be remembered that many non-herbalist therapists within the CAM bracket use and prescribe herbal products in the same reductive way as just described, yet they are rarely criticized for doing so with the level of intensity directed at doctors!

Other perspectives on phytotherapy are available, however. Kenner and Requena (2001) discuss the use of 'phytotherapy' in France as a banner term that can encompass a number of approaches to herbal practice centred on the concept of 'terrain' which (in France): 'is very much alive and integrated into cultural ideas of health and medicine'. Terrain refers to the biological individuality of people, the unique inner personal conditions (or environment) that determines one's health status and physiological integrity. 'Terrain' is, in effect, a version of the ancient humoural approach (which assessed the state of the body's fluids: blood, phlegm, yellow and black bile), since: 'In the human body, the term has come to refer specifically to the fluid environment of the cells and the way in which the condition of this medium relates to health and disease'. Claude Bernard's (1813–1878) notion of the *milieu interieur* is a terrain model that directly influenced Walter Cannon (1871–1945), the physiologist who coined the term 'homoeostasis'.

Payer (1996), in her study comparing medicine and culture in France, Germany, Britain and the United States has reflected on the meaning of *terrain*:

> There is no really good translation for terrain *in English. The old-fashioned word 'constitution', which has largely gone out of favor in America, probably translates it best ... Many diseases result from a combination of some type of outside insult and the body's reaction to that insult. While English and American doctors tend to focus on the insult, the French and Germans focus on the reaction and are more likely to try to find ways to modify the reaction as well as fight off the insult ... Even Louis Pasteur, who is regarded as the father of modern microbiology, accorded an importance to the* terrain *at least equal to the specific microbe. The late Dr. Rene Dubos, himself a proselytizer for the importance of* terrain, *spoke of Pasteur's views ... 'He even went as far as to suggest that the psychologic state could influence resistance to microbes'.*

This last suggestion is easily accommodated within the more recent systems-view of physiology known as 'psychoneuroimmunology' (for a sound introduction, see Wisneski & Anderson 2005), which is part of the ongoing quest to appreciate the complexities of the interface between the internal and external environment.

Kenner and Requena (2001) maintain that:

> *The most common use of the word terrain is in the different nosologies and whole-system models that have been developed for clinical diagnosis and treatment in phytotherapy.*

These models include some that are little known outside of France, such as:

> *The oligo element diatheses of Menetrier and the neuroendocrine model of Lapraz and Duraffourd. [though] Many French practitioners of phytotherapy feel that the five phase model (of Chinese medicine) is a more digestible introduction to the concept of terrain ...*

Here we have an insight into another dimension of phytotherapy from the 'herbs as quasi-drugs' stereotype outlined earlier. The *terrain* approach to phytotherapy has a number of features that distinguish it as a holistic, person-centred field including that it:

- Places the unique individual at the centre of the therapeutic universe
- Combines traditional and modern insights into the appreciation of patients and the uses of plant remedies
- 'Joins up' knowledge of physiology into whole-systems models
- Represents a continuation of the ancient humoural project.

The varieties of phytotherapy should not surprise us, since all modalities or approaches to medicine take on their own distinctive qualities according to the influences at play in the cultures in which they are situated. This includes conventional medicine, as Payer (1996) has shown. Mainstream biomedical practice is not the same all over the world; indeed in Europe, major distinctions in emphasis and approach can be apparent over the distance of a few miles. A consultation with a GP in Dover is likely to be quite a different experience to that with her counterpart in Calais – with just a short stretch of Channel between them.

Phytotherapy has developed distinctive flavours and characteristics in countries including France, Germany, the UK and Australia. Let us turn now to concentrate on the version that has developed in the UK.

## PHYTOTHERAPY IN THE UK

In English-speaking countries, unlike much of Continental Europe and large parts of Asia, herbal medicine had, by the second half of the twentieth century, been expunged from conventional medical practice. It has now become, instead, a largely over-the-counter phenomenon with people self-prescribing herbal products of varying quality. The basis of this self-care with herbs has changed dramatically, from a tradition of community-acquired knowledge and collection of raw local herbs from the wild or by cultivation to an increasing reliance on books and media sources and accessing of non-locally grown and processed herbs. Herbal practitioners are relatively few in number, typically poorly or loosely organized and drawing on a varied range of influences and traditions.

In the UK, herbal practitioners had done well to survive in the face of a number of potential threats to their survival, including the founding of the National Health Service (from which they were excluded) and the reforming, post-thalidomide, 1968 Medicines Act (from which they were successful in gaining crucial exemptions). By the mid-1960s, however, as Mills (2000) recounts, the number of professional herbal practitioners was critically low, with membership of the National Institute of Medical Herbalists 'down to double figures and declining'. This decline began to reverse in the next decade as herbal medicine was re-discovered as an ecological form of medicine, one that naturally belonged within the growing 'green movement' and which could even be used as a means of transpersonal growth. David Hoffmann (1983), one of the new generation of herbal practitioners, and who once campaigned for election to the UK Parliament as a member of the Green Party, articulated this re-framing as:

> Herbs ... are an interface within the body of Gaia. They are an interface between two realms of nature. Where humanity and plants meet, a synergistic energy can be

*created and exchanged. At such a point inner and outer ecology may resonate and become attuned.*

Hoffmann (1983)

A new language was being applied to the appreciation of plant medicine, including words and terms such as: holism, New Age, consciousness, spirituality, paradigm shift. Few were successful in applying these concepts in a way that illuminated or advanced the practice of herbal medicine amidst what Mills (2000) has elegantly described as: 'a widespread outbreak of philosophical drifting'. The lack of criticality characterizing much of herbal expression, debate and rationale formulation at this time exemplified what Pietroni (1990) characterized as the: '… search for simple and magical solutions'. Some practitioners feared for the mainstream credibility of herbal medicine and worried that it would be tainted by association with the woollier extreme of New Age thinking. In the face of this, the use of the term 'phytotherapy' came to stand for an approach that put the focus back on herbal medicine as a rigorous discipline; one that was open to research and to critical evaluation. Crucially, it did not denote a desire to take on a reductive position in regard to herbal practice, although some construed it so. Instead the group of herbal practitioners who have identified themselves as phytotherapists have maintained an insistence on drawing from an informed appreciation of both traditional and biochemical/biomedical interpretations of herbal activity, practice and potentials, in the spirit of the French phytotherapists. This approach to modern herbal practice has been open to understanding and incorporating modern and ancient, western and non-western, perspectives on herbal practice. The work of Simon Mills and Kerry Bone (see Mills & Bone 2000) has been particularly sophisticated in expressing this approach. Mills' innovative attempt to develop a database that incorporates traditional and modern scientific perceptions of plant medicines (including a rigorous evidence-based ratings system for each) and which contrasts key 'stories' about herbs (including: 'the research story'; 'the human use story'; and 'the expert practitioner's story') provides a Rashomon-type model showing the diversity of perspectives on medicinal plant utility.

## INTEGRATION AND REGULATION

UK phytotherapists have aimed to work collaboratively with colleagues in conventional medicine to the extent that the College of Phytotherapy developed a postgraduate course, training doctors in herbal medicine. An aspiration has been held for plant medicine to return to its former central role in mainstream medicine via increased use by doctors combining allopathic and phytotherapeutic strategies as well as by specialist phytotherapists. Hopes for greater integration between CAM and conventional medicine have been viewed by some as naïve and more likely to lead to subjugation of herbal medicine by the dominant medical model, which has neither the time, taste nor capacity for more complex and subtle interpretations of health, illness and their modulation. Certainly, the journey of any so-called CAM modality from periphery to centre (or from minority to dominant models) is fraught with risks. Malcolm Parker (2003) has delineated some of these dangers in the light of the regulatory process that usually enables/obstructs such navigation. His concerns are worth quoting at length, especially because the herbal profession in the UK is in the throes of negotiating statutory regulation at the time of writing:

> *Ironically, the aspiration of CAM practitioners to be recognised and respected ... chiefly through the achievement of registration status, will be self defeating in terms of maintaining an identity that is distinct from orthodox medicine. The boundaries of those modalities that achieve registration may blur with those of orthodox medicine, as the insistence on evidence forces them to conform and as orthodox medicine appropriates treatments that are demonstrably effective.*
>
> *... modalities that aspire to recognition through registration, and that purport to operate via assessable standards, are taking their first step along the road to scientific assimilation.*
>
> *CAM practitioners will need to choose between the value of preserving their unique identity and offering a true alternative, and the benefits that flow from registration, but they will not be able to have things both ways.*
>
> *CAM practitioners who refuse to violate their professional integrity and identity should be understood as offering no warrant for the efficacy of their claims, apart from the variable dependability of traditions. Conversely, the sign of the effective regulation of CAM practitioners who purport to manage significant health conditions will be the gradual blurring of the boundaries between orthodox and CAM practice.*

Phytotherapy is a controversial form of herbal medicine precisely because it demonstrates this 'blurring' and boundary dissolution by seeking to integrate traditional and biomedical approaches and by valuing traditional and biomedical insights.

While some within both the CAM and conventional medicine categorizations might be hoping for a 'paradigm shift' – a revolution in the way that medicine is essentially understood and practised – on the ground the story so far is, unsurprisingly, less dramatic. Establishment literature (peer-reviewed journals) and the media, in the main, continue to call for CAM to adopt the scientific research methodology of conventional medicine and prove itself on those terms. Only then might aspects of CAM modalities be incorporated into conventional medical practice. We might adapt Parker's assessment to suggest that this process involves:

1. Standard scientific assessment of a CAM approach or specific intervention
2. Appropriation (probably in a limited way) of the 'proven' parts of that approach/intervention into the existing biomedical model
3. Rejection of the 'unproven' parts of the approach/intervention.

In this interpretation, CAM modalities go to the research facility like lambs to the slaughter. Here they are disassembled, scrutinized and then either partially or wholly discarded in a process of appropriation not integration. It is understandable that many CAM practitioners are wary of this possibility, with some completely hostile to exposing themselves to such scientific assimilation. Yet many feel there is no choice but to engage with standard scientific procedures, in spite of the risks, since to do otherwise is to remain, at best, marginalized. Mills (2000) has expressed the view that:

> *Even to survive in the modern world, let alone to be able to take its place again as the most noble form of healing, herbal medicine needs to develop a more muscular pharmacological and therapeutic case for itself. It needs frankly to take on the phenomenon of the placebo-effect, to develop new verifiable models of efficacy that satisfactorily distinguish it from the alternatives. It needs to identify the areas where it can make a valuable contribution and those where it probably has little direct benefit. It can almost certainly withstand the pressure.*

Herbal medicine is a robust entity that has survived from the dawn of therapy to the present day. No sleep need be lost over its capacity to persist; the concerns of herbal practitioners need only be raised with regard to its local form. It will continue in a multiplicity of expressions including reductionist and holistic use by either conventional medics or alternative therapists, traditional use by indigenous peoples and self-care use by individuals. The legal position of practitioners already varies considerably between countries, shaping and limiting the modes of herbal practitioners. In the UK, phytotherapists are campaigning for enhanced legal recognition and professional status from an existing permissive base whereas in America, herbal practitioners have enjoyed less legal licence, instead adapting to imposed restrictions. In some parts of the USA, where practitioners are prohibited from describing their work in orthodox medical language, the notion of the practitioner as a 'wellness adviser' has emerged. In this conceptualization, the therapist is recast as a guide, coach or teacher – a mode that fits well with ideas in decentralized, person-focused medicine. It may be that herbal practitioners elsewhere would gain from considering new ways of doing and describing their work, shifting emphasis from professional self-interest to increasing patient-empowerment and autonomy.

However they style themselves, herbal practitioners have to consider how to engage with the dominant positivist science model. To meekly submit to this model is to allow herbal medicine to be processed into a reduced and perverted form; to aggressively reject it risks ghettoization and limitation of patient access to the benefits of herbal treatment. Rather, a strong critique of the problematic aspects of positivist science is required combined with a sophisticated and coherent justification of alternative perspectives. So far, those within the CAM categorization have had very limited success in effectively articulating a convincing alternative ethos; yet a number of other disciplines and models offer powerful perspectives and arguments that, if drawn together, could constitute a multi-faceted explanatory framework of great capacity and integrity. Examples of these include: the sociology of health and illness; studies in the history and philosophy of medicine and science; the new sciences of complexity and chaos; the new joined-up physiology of psychoneuroimmunology; work on understanding the placebo-effect as the self-healing or meaning-response; and humanistic medical models such as person-centred medicine. These strands need to be woven into the undergraduate, postgraduate and continuing education of herbal practitioners so that facility in cross-linking ideas, concepts and methods can be developed.

A process of boundary dissolution between what may be erroneously portrayed as separate fields of study needs to take place in order to enable more richly informed and diversely capacitated models of herbal practice to emerge.

Herbal practitioners in the UK, aware that their future right to practice was uncertain and fearing that they could lose access to their full materia medica, began to work together from the mid-1990s, forming the European Herbal Practitioners Association (EHPA) and agitating for statutory regulation of their practice. The minds of both herbal practitioners and acupuncturists were further concentrated on this goal when statutory regulation was recommended for these professions by a House of Lords Select Committee Report in 2000 (House of Lords 2000). At this point in time it seemed unlikely that herbal and acupuncture practitioners would be able to ensure their continuing right to practise without such regulation. The consensus in both professions remains that they must participate constructively in attempting to achieve and shape regulation or risk considerable limitations being placed on their legal ability to practise in a climate of increasing healthcare regulation.

Although the UK government initially firmly supported the House of Lords recommendations (DoH 2001) it has subsequently blown hot and cold on pressing for the achievement of regulation – which has not yet been realized as I write, some 9 years after the House of Lords Report appeared. This vacillation has been due to a number of influences, including delays awaiting the outcomes of reports concerning the reform of existing regulated healthcare professions (e.g. DoH 2006, 2007). At the time of writing, a report has recently been published detailing the proposals of a Department of Health Steering Group (DoH 2008) for the regulation of herbal medicine and acupuncture. These include the recommendations that both professions should be regulated by the Health Professions Council (HPC). The report notes that it is a requirement of the HPC that professions aspiring to be regulated by it must 'practise based on evidence of efficacy', returning us to Parker's caution regarding the possible consequences arising from an 'insistence on evidence'.

## PHYTOTHERAPY AND EVIDENCE-BASED MEDICINE

Phytotherapy represents a pragmatic approach for herbal practitioners who both see the need to engage with the call for evidence and take a positive view of the insights and benefits that can accrue from relevant high quality research. Seen from this angle, it is not only untenable to resist calls for rigorous scientific scrutiny of herbal practice but also undesirable, since such research offers one means of enhancing the knowledge base for effective herbal treatment. This leads us to consider the question of how an ancient practice such as herbal medicine responds to the challenge of the emerging research-related practice model in biomedicine – evidence-based medicine (EBM).

Debate continues about the ways in which EBM may have beneficial or harmful consequences for patients, the degree to which it may be relevant to some practice areas, and indeed whether it actually works (e.g. Puliyel et al. 2004; Anthony 2002; Strauss & McAlister 2000). In a highly incisive piece

Klein (1996) described EBM as 'the new scientism' and highlighted the ways in which it could be abused by economists and managers, and how it: 'appears to offer politicians less pain, less responsibility for taking difficult decisions and a legitimate way of curbing what are often seen as the idiosyncratic and extravagant practices of doctors'. Most tellingly (and prophetically), however, he identified what is surely the nub of the matter:

> To the extent that the new scientism, as presently conceived, appears to be a search for certainty, it is an enterprise destined for disappointment. The certainty will most of the time prove elusive, as problems turn out to be more complex than anticipated ...

Nonetheless, EBM has now assumed pre-eminent status as a model for best practice in conventional medicine and inevitably impacts on the perceptions of best practice in CAM modalities too. The definition of evidence-based medicine has developed in response to criticism (see Greenhalgh & Worrall 1997) to be given as 'the integration of best research evidence with clinical expertise and patient values' (Sackett et al. 2000). The authors of this version explained the aspects of EBM as follows:

> By best research evidence *we mean clinically relevant research ... but especially from patient-centred clinical research ...*
>
> By clinical expertise *we mean the ability to use our clinical skills and past experience to rapidly identify each patient's unique health state and diagnosis, their individual risks and benefits of potential interventions and their personal values and expectations.*
>
> By patient values *we mean the unique preferences, concerns and expectations each patient brings to a clinical encounter and which must be integrated into clinical decisions if they are to serve the patient.*
>
> When these three elements are integrated, clinicians and patients form a diagnostic and therapeutic alliance which optimizes clinical outcomes and quality of life.

Understood as such, EBM *should* be easily recognized as an essentially holistic approach that is likely to be compatible with the approach of holistically-minded practitioners from every camp (setting aside the not insignificant matter of what actually constitutes 'best research evidence' for the time being). Unfortunately however, EBM is rarely discussed or enacted in terms of such a synthesis as that outlined above. David Sackett himself (a key figure in developing the concept of EBM, and a medical practitioner) has acknowledged that:

> ... we clinicians who accept the awful responsibility of caring for individual patients with their unique risks, responsiveness, values and expectations have simply failed to communicate key elements of our decision-making to some ethicists and methodologists who don't diagnose and treat individual patients ... their definition of evidence-based healthcare stops with external evidence and ignores the other 2 of its 3 vital elements: clinical expertise and patient values.

Sackett (2000)

EBM can be interpreted in differing ways and used, or abused, to diverse ends – as noted by Klein, above. Pharmaceutical companies have been accused of manipulating evidence to achieve positive profiles for their products and therefore enhanced profits for their shareholders (e.g. Garattini & Liberati 2000; Smith 2003). Governments and their agencies have been accused of selectively drawing on evidence to cut costs, against the best interests of patients (Smith 2000). Clinicians, however, are primarily concerned with the individual before them – for them it is important that EBM has direct clinical relevance and applicability or else it may be seen as an obstacle to good practice. Phytotherapists have common cause with conventional physicians in insisting on applying EBM in its broadest and patient-centred sense.

Critics of phytotherapy, as we have noted, have often taken a rather narrow view of what phytotherapy actually constitutes. Frequently it is assumed to be a practice of herbal medicine that is reductively phytochemically based and predicated on the popular interpretation of EBM as being solely about 'research evidence' – leaving out practitioner- and patient-centred perspectives. Such an interpretation, we said, is associated with certain mainland European doctor–phytotherapists using herbs as ersatz drugs: yet even here the criticisms are somewhat off target. Doctor–phytotherapists are usually general practitioners (family physicians) and GPs seem to share the same types of concerns that CAM therapists may have regarding the potential pitfalls of a one-dimensional (i.e. solely research-based) approach to EBM, e.g. Tracy et al. (2003) found that doctors' concerns about EBM included:

- EBM 'as a devaluation of the "art of medicine" and a threat to their professional/clinical autonomy'
- 'Issues of credibility, bias, and the trustworthiness of evidence (especially) regarding the role of the pharmaceutical industry in the funding and conduct of clinical research'
- The case that 'patients' preferences are often at odds with the evidence'
- The frequent lack of a 'clear consensus within the literature' and the occurrence of 'directly conflicting evidence'
- Lack of fit between research aims and the realities of practice; one interviewee commented: 'I can see lots of conflict between the goals of a study and the goals in real life'.

In the light of the foregoing discussion in this chapter, it may now be possible to see why phytotherapists might stand accused as collaborators in the colonization of herbal medicine by biomedicine. In this scenario, phytotherapists are portrayed as playing a naïve and dangerous game that risks loss of the heart and soul of herbal medicine as its traditions and deeper meaning are gradually compromised out of existence by influences such as EBM. Yet such an analysis fails to account for the complexity and positive potentials of the situation. A holistic phytotherapy has the capacity to use multiple interconnecting explanations of how herbal medicines work and how the practice of herbal medicine achieves results – to integrate various forms of evidence. Strands in this web (echoing earlier arguments) include:

- Indigenous knowledge and experience of the uses of herbs revealed, e.g. by ethnobotanical studies
- Traditional concepts (such as the thermal nature of herbs) and models (such as Chinese medicine theory)

- Reductive phytochemical profiles
- Integrative phytochemical concepts such as 'synergism'
- Modern research from *in vitro* to clinical studies
- New considerations of the 'placebo effect' recast as the 'self-healing response' or the 'meaning response'
- Insights drawn from non-medical disciplines such as the psychotherapies and the sociology of health and illness
- Models of perceiving and facilitating the therapeutic relationship such as narrative-based medicine
- Individual and collective clinical experience
- Consideration of patient perspectives, preferences and wishes.

Many of these issues, as they apply to the consultation, will be explored in the following chapters.

Weaving the varied strands of information and opinion listed above represents a continuing adaptation of herbal practice to the themes, ideas and conditioning of the times. By interpenetrating various approaches and disciplines it is harder to hold to a distinct form and shape of easily recognized 'traditional herbal medicine', yet the potential gains are great – updating, expanding and growing an ancient practice fit for our current era. Wahlberg (2008) has examined the accusation of colonization of herbal medicine by biomedicine and has instead argued that what is occurring is a process of normalization (framing in terms of the dominant cultural model), which:

> … has addressed the ignorance, imprecisions, inconsistencies and incongruences that are seen to surround herbal remedies by attempting to right or square these. And, rather than resulting in some kind of finality or certainty, the process continues to be surrounded and informed by contestation and rectification.

There can be no single definitive model of herbal practice. Phytotherapy, at its best, offers a necessary pluralistic approach to herbal medicine, integrating perspectives and insights from a broad range of sources and critically evaluating qualitative as well as quantitative research and the views arising from the fields of the humanities as well as the sciences, including sociology and philosophy. There is every reason for herbal practitioners to engage dynamically with ideas emerging from within conventional medicine and science since many of these (psychoneuroimmunology, patient-centred medicine, etc.) offer means by which herbal medicine might reassert its relevance and utility.

## MOVING BEYOND SCIENTISM

To engage with 'science', in its various meanings and forms, presents a major challenge for both CAM therapists and conventional doctors, since their training rarely orients or prepares them for such a task. Studies in the 'philosophy of science' offer a critical appreciation of the nature of science and its doctrines and could form a basis to facilitate informed perspectives if incorporated into practitioner education at various levels. The study of 'scientism' that arises in this field is particularly apposite in our review of phytotherapy.

Scientism can be described as a contention that science (meaning positivist science, i.e. an approach that only accepts as valid the observable and measurable, and which rejects metaphysics) is the only credible way of interpreting phenomena – and that other interpretive systems such as sociology, mythology, spirituality, theology and philosophy are inferior or invalid. In its extreme form, this represents a type of secular fundamentalism that fails to account for the meanings and complexities of other sense-making strategies such as mythology, to take one example, which Gray (2007) has described in this way: 'Myths are not true or false in the way scientific theories are true or false, but they can be more or less truthful in reflecting the enduring realities of human life'.

A recent spate of books associating atheism with positivist science and aggressively critiquing religion have been published (e.g. Dawkins 2007; Hitchens 2007), with the same authors also showing a tendency to attack CAM as another example of false-thinking so that two sets of correspondences are laid out to distinguish between the intelligent and the foolish person:

- Foolish people have to do with: pseudoscience, irrational beliefs, religious conviction, use of CAM
- Intelligent people have to do with: 'real' science, logical opinions, atheism, support for conventional medicine and antagonism towards CAM.

A number of journalists and social commentators have subscribed to this line of simplistic and inflammatory dichotomizing, to the point where CAM modalities are now commonly lampooned in the media and an interest in, or use of so-called CAM therapies, is construed as evidence that one is illogical, irrational – a fool likely to believe in any old nonsense. The eminent journalist Francis Wheen (in his book *How Mumbo-Jumbo Conquered the World*) considers that:

> *The swelling popularity of quack potions and treatments in recent years is yet another manifestation of the retreat from reason and scientific method ... The alluring adjectives 'complementary' and 'alternative' are essentially euphemisms for 'dud'...*
>
> Wheen (2004)

Such *faith* in reason and method is as vulnerable to critique as any other tenet of belief, however, as Feyerabend (1993) makes clear:

> *The idea of a method that contains firm, unchanging, and absolutely binding principles for conducting science meets considerable difficulty when confronted with the results of historical research ... one of the most striking features of recent discussions in the history and philosophy of science is the realization that events and developments, such as the invention of atomism in antiquity, the Copernican Revolution, the rise of modern atomism (kinetic theory; dispersion theory; stereochemistry; quantum theory), the gradual emergence of the wave theory of light, occurred only because some thinkers either* decided *not to be bound by certain 'obvious' methodological rules, or because they* unwittingly broke *them [original emphases].*

Positive, nuanced, complex and synthetic messages do not play well in the media. In this zone, the simple, absolute, negative, aggressive and extreme are generally preferred. Dominant media voices are rarely (or rarely allowed to be) insightful, subtle or pluralistic therefore, although the intelligent media consumer can usually be relied upon to discern the lack of these qualities. Absolutist positions on medicine are usually stated by non-practitioners who lack experience in dealing with the complex and varied predicaments of patients and the continuing need for flexibility in helping to meet their expectations and to learn from the lessons they teach.

In challenging scientism, Okasha (2002) attempts to define the limits of scientific understanding and map out the territories where philosophy holds supreme:

> ... the questions that philosophy addresses include the nature of knowledge, of morality, of rationality, of human well-being, and more, none of which seem to be soluble by scientific methods. No branch of science tells us how to live our lives, what knowledge is, or what human happiness involves ...
> [my emphasis]

This is a rather broad sweep of course – science may tell us *some* things about human wellbeing, even *some* things about happiness (e.g. the neurochemistry of happiness; the factors that seem to promote a sense of happiness, etc.), yet these are necessarily partial in nature. Increasing emphasis on specialism has inhibited or disabled many authorities in their ability to take on board perspectives from other disciplines, leading to the failure to take a larger view of any complex phenomenon. So where does the problem in taking a multifaceted view of a particular subject lie? With human wellbeing, for example, why can we not consider the scientific, traditional, indigenous, spiritual, theological, mythological, sociological (and so forth) explanations and insights into the nature of this subject, comparing, synthesizing and interpreting them all? We do not have to choose just one area – instead of 'either/or' we can have 'and'. To move beyond the snares, errors and dead ends of a too-narrow viewpoint requires the open attitude of the pluralist, the polymath, the generalist but during the twentieth century such terms took on negative tones and were often used in a derogatory sense, suggesting 'dabbler'. In the 1930s, the physician Alexander George Gibson, writing a treatise based on a fragment of the philosopher/physician John Locke (1632–1704), bemoaned the move towards narrow specialism:

> *In the age of Locke a man with any pretensions to originality was not accused of being an amateur if he wrote about studies that were not his immediate concern. Inquisitive minds did not hesitate to pursue any branch of knowledge.*
>
> Gibson (1933)

In talking about medicine in the early twentieth century, Lawrence and Weisz (1998) observed that:

> *In Britain around the turn of the century ... many physicians regarded the medical art as built on science but not reducible to it. Such physicians often valued generalism over specialism and a broad cultural background over technical training.*
> [original emphasis]

It is arguable that many doctors, as well as many CAM therapists, still feel the same way.

Sorell (1994) has stated that: 'Scientism is a matter of putting too high a value on science in comparison with other branches of learning or culture'. My argument is that the most useful type of phytotherapy attempts to combine diverse models in science with other sources of perception and explanation – critically engaging with each. The holistic phytotherapist is inevitably a pluralist.

In the light of the foregoing discussion, we can assert that phytotherapy has the potential to represent a contemporary and dynamically adjusting approach to herbal practice that is open, pluralistic, synthesizing and concerned with all aspects of the art and science of plant medicine. Phytotherapists might be accused here of wanting to have it both ways and indeed of indulging in some degree of chicanery – of hijacking the term 'phytotherapy' to assume a veneer of authenticity and scientific respectability (implying a connection with the continental European doctor–phytotherapists) and then subverting it to our own ends – this rather exciting interpretation holds some appeal, although it implies a calculated plan which is hard to trace.

In an entertaining presentation, the phytotherapist Simon Mills characterized two world-views that polarize herbal practice (and which perform a similar role in other fields) as:

1. Romantic: Subjective: Aesthetic: How does this affect me directly?
2. Classical: Objective: Rational: What does this mean?

Through our individual nature, upbringing, education and experiences we all tend, as practitioners, to veer towards one of these poles. The further we are to one extreme, the more likely we are to view the opposite pole as an enemy – diametrically opposed to our entrenched position. The closer we are to the centre, the more we will be able to move between, or combine, the two worlds.

## PHYTOTHERAPY: A PERSONAL VIEW

Given that we have identified phytotherapy as a contested notion within the field of herbal medicine, and one that encompasses a number of possible interpretations, I would like to end this chapter by describing more fully the particular take on phytotherapy that is under discussion in this book, beginning with global philosophical considerations and then moving to the specifics of practice.

My view of phytotherapy is one that is grounded in perceiving herbal medicine as a 'commons' – recognizing that herbs have been used therapeutically by all peoples throughout all times. Helping people to learn how to access (including to grow, harvest and prepare) and use herbs in order to self-treat and treat their families – and in so doing aiding preservation or rediscovery of herbal medicine as an everyday therapeutic event is a core goal. Self-care with herbs is complemented by professional phytotherapeutic care but the latter should not displace or replace the former. Medicinal plants are not 'resources' in the economic sense, they are part of the living environment. This means that in order to work ethically in facilitating the relationship between people and medicinal plants, and to care for the physical environment in which these transactions take place, the phytotherapist will necessarily be a holist, an educationalist and an ecologist. Phytotherapy draws on the broadest possible range of perspectives and information sources in appreciating the interactions between people, plants and their environment, including, but not limited to: science, tradition, indigenous perspectives, ethnobotany, anthropology, sociology, mythology, theology and spirituality. These perspectives can be compared, evaluated and synthesized but most importantly they need to be drawn into discussion with each other. The primary aim of phytotherapy is to engender wellness in the individual and communities. The human organism is essentially self-healing and phytotherapy represents a key means that can be employed to support and promote this capacity. Specifically: phytotherapy may be employed to optimize health, prevent and treat disease and provide palliation. The phytotherapist has an appetite for complexity – in both plant and patient – and seeks to appreciate the patient's predicament in the fullest way possible and, in doing so, aid the patient's search for self-understanding and meaning. Phytotherapy extends beyond plant remedies to include the ancient scope of 'diatetica' – considering diet, balancing activity and rest and so forth. In addition to the plant the phytotherapist is, in and of himself, a therapeutic agent and seeks to apply himself as such by enabling the patient's self-reflection, providing human warmth, care, kindness and bearing witness to the patient's suffering.

In the light of the above conceptualization, the key focus of this book trains on the interpersonal aspects of the phytotherapist's work.

Herbal medicine has always changed with, and adapted to, the times. In the nineteenth and early twentieth centuries, as noted in the 'Introductory' section, a group of American practitioners, known as the 'Physiomedicalists' used herbs as a primary treatment strategy. They combined indigenous Native American plant knowledge with new discoveries in physiology and disease aetiology, being especially influenced by an appreciation of the autonomic nervous system and formulating treatments to regulate autonomic tone in response. Phytotherapy continues to react and adapt to new discoveries and changing conceptions in medical science. Currently, the notion of psychoneuroimmunology (PNI) offers potential to provide one particularly comprehensive explanatory framework for appreciating the actions of herbal medicines on the body. PNI recognizes the key roles that psychology, neurology, endocrinology and immunology play as major regulating systems for the individual person. This developing concept is especially exciting because it provides a link between psychological and biochemical processes showing how influences at the 'psyche' level (mood, emotions, attitude, beliefs) adapt and affect biochemical and physiological activity. The wide-ranging and complex pharmacological effects of plant medicines can modulate these interactions, thereby exerting a profound degree of influence on individual wellbeing. Table 1.4 gives some idea of this net of relationships, providing examples of some herbs that can act on each of the body's major control systems.

Cytokines are now understood to act as important mediators of biochemical responses within the PNI model (integrating neurotransmitter, hormone and immune cell activity) and a particular related area of research at this time

| Table 1.4 *Examples of herbs influencing PNI systems* | | |
|---|---|---|
| **Psychoneurology** | **Endocrinology** | **Immunology** |
| *Valeriana officinalis* | *Vitex agnus-castus* | *Echinacea* spp. |
| *Hypericum officinalis* | *Eleutherococcus senticosus* | *Uncaria tomentosa* |

is that into the influence of proinflammatory cytokines and their connection with the development of inflammatory disorders. A large number of herbs have demonstrated activity in modulating cytokine activity (Spelman et al. 2006), offering potentials to reduce inflammation and enhance immunity. As a resurgence of interest in inflammation takes place and its role begins to be appreciated in such seemingly diverse (though clearly related when seen from the PNI perspective) conditions as stress, obesity, diabetes and other metabolic disorders (Wellen & Hotamisligil 2005) herbal medicine is well placed to add a new pharmaco-physiological rationale for its use.

New broad explanatory models, and new language, to describe and diversify herbal practice continue to emerge in response to research. For example, Rangel (2005) has developed a 'Systemic Theory of Living Systems' utilizing herbal medicines to modulate what he proposes as the three core factors that control physiological health:

> ... *integrity of its structure or organization, O, functional organic energy reserve, E, and level of active biological intelligence, I.*

In this model: *Silybum marianum* (milk thistle) is one of the plant agents that improves O because it is one of the 'organoceuticals that specifically enhance organ function and structure' – here acting on the liver; *Panax ginseng* (Korean ginseng) is an example of a herb that enhances E, due to its ability to increase mitochondrial ATP synthesis; and *Echinacea purpurea* supports I since it is one of a number of 'infoceuticals that enhance bio-intelligence on ... immune levels'.

While it is easy to ridicule the neologisms at play here, the concept is nonetheless worthy of serious study as a new interpretation of the capacities and practical application of herbal medicines.

There are several other examples of contemporary herbal practitioners constructing conceptual frameworks to explain and enable the use of herbal medicines as forms of sophisticated, complex pharmacotherapy. In this book, however, I am concerned primarily with the non-pharmacological aspects of herbal practice – with what else the herbal practitioner, or phytotherapist, does around and apart from her focus on the herbs themselves. This other aspect of herbal practice has been much less explored and it may appear to have much more to do with psychotherapy than pharmacotherapy, e.g. How does the phytotherapist facilitate the evolution of a therapeutic relationship with the patient? And to what extent does this, in itself, have a healing effect?

Before moving on to consider such questions, let us summarize and reiterate that 'phytotherapy' represents a continuing, though disputed, group of adaptations of herbal medicine to the times. It reveals herbal medicine as a living, developing tradition responsive to its cultural setting and able to accommodate to changes in that setting – much like plants themselves as their environment changes. Phytotherapy – its concepts, categories, ideas, viewpoints and capacities – offers a cluster of models of holistic, person-centred, humanistic practice that become ever more popular and necessary as societies, changing under ecological imperatives, become more person-centred, humanistic and nature-oriented. As cultures change in this way, herbal medicine is likely to shift from periphery to centre – a position that, until very recently, it has occupied throughout human engagement with the notion of healing. Advocates of herbal medicine therefore are likely to be found increasingly among the proponents of green politics and ecologically viable alternatives to current ways of living. One such perspective is contained within the 'transition towns' movement which challenges local communities to plan for life after 'the age of cheap oil', envisaging that such a life will need to be based on cooperative activity around sustainable practices. The core 'transition' text (Hopkins 2008) includes 'A vision for 2030': an imagined report on the state-of-the-art in various areas following transition to more sustainable ways of being. Here is part of the report on 'Medicine and health':

> Today (i.e. 2030) our idea of health – how to create it and maintain it – has changed markedly from that of twenty years ago. The Health Service had to rethink itself as the oil price made many of its practices and approaches unaffordable, and it faced the very real threat of collapsing completely ... local healthcare centres are now not just about treating illness but promoting health in many diverse ways. They have forged partnerships with local schools, promoting food growing and familiarising young people with the whole food cycle from seed to salad. The wellbeing of the individual is seen as inseparable from the health of the community. Human biology is now a compulsory school subject, and has expanded to include nutrition and basic herbalism. About half of the medicines prescribed by doctors are now locally sourced, with local farmers growing certain key medicinal plants ...

This scenario envisages herbal *medicines* (i.e. the plants themselves) returning to the mainstream, but if herbal *medicine* (in the form of a discrete *practice* such as phytotherapy) is to occupy a prominent place in future healthcare, it must make a case for itself as an *approach*. The remainder of this book presents part of that case.

## REFERENCES

Abram D: Earth Stories, *Resurgence* 222:20–22, 2004.

Anthony HM: Research aspects of environmental medicine. In Lewith G, Jonas WB, Walach H, editors: *Clinical research in complementary therapies*, Edinburgh, 2002, Churchill Livingstone.

Arvigo R, Balick M: *Rainforest remedies: one hundred healing herbs of Belize*, Poole, 1998, Lotus Press.

Barclay J: *Southall's organic materia medica*, London, 1909, J & A Churchill.

Beauchamp GK, Keast RS, Morel D, et al: Phytochemistry: Ibuprofen-like activity in extra-virgin olive oil, *Nature* 437:45–46, 2005.

Bone K: *A clinical guide to blending liquid herbs*, Edinburgh, 2003, Churchill Livingstone.

Brown PS: Herbalists and medical botanists in mid-nineteenth-century Britain with special reference to Bristol, *Medica History* 26:405–420, 1982.

Conway P: Knowledge and myths of knowledge in the 'science' of herbal medicine. In O'Sullivan C, editor: *Reshaping herbal medicine: knowledge, education and professional development*, Edinburgh, 2005, Churchill Livingstone.

Dawkins R: *The God delusion*, London, 2007, Black Swan.

Dawkins R: *A devil's chaplain: selected writings*, London, 2003, Weidenfeld and Nicolson.

DoH: *Government Response to the House of Lords Select Committee on Science and Technology Report on Complementary and Alternative Medicine, Department of Health*, London, 2001, The Stationery Office.

DoH: *Good doctors, safer patients: proposals to strengthen the system to assure and improve the performance of doctors and to protect the safety of patients, Department of Health*, London, 2006, The Stationery Office.

DoH: *Trust, assurance and safety: the regulation of health professionals in the 21st century, Department of Health*, London, 2007, The Stationery Office.

DoH: *Report to Ministers from the Department of Health Steering Group on the Statutory Regulation of Practitioners of Acupuncture, Herbal Medicine, Traditional Chinese Medicine and Other Traditional Medicine Systems Practised in the UK, Department of Health*, London, 2008, Robert Gordon University.

Dowie S: *Acupuncture: an aid to differential diagnosis*, Edinburgh, 2009, Churchill Livingstone.

Duke JA: Medicinal plants and the pharmaceutical industry. In Janick J, Simon JE, editors: *New crops*, New York, 1993, Wiley.

Engel C: Zoopharmacognosy. In Wynn SG, Fougère BJ, editors: *Veterinary herbal medicine*, London, 2007, Mosby/Elsevier.

Ergil KV: Chinese Medicine. In Micozzi MS, editor: *Fundamentals of alternative and complementary medicine*, Edinburgh, 2001, Churchill Livingstone.

Ernst E, Singh S: *Trick or treatment?: alternative medicine on trial*, London, 2008, Bantam.

Feyerabend P: *Against method*, ed 3, London, 1993, Verso.

Garattini S, Liberati A: The risk of bias from omitted research, *British Medical Journal* 321; 845–846, 2000.

General Medical Council: *The British Pharmacopoeia*, London, 1948, Constable & Co Ltd.

Gibson AG: *The Physician's Art: an attempt to expand John Locke's fragment 'De Arte Medica'*, Wotton-under-Edge, 1933, Clarendon Press.

Gray J: *Black Mass: apocalyptic religion and the death of utopia*, London, 2007, Penguin/Allen Lane.

Greenhalgh T, Worrall JG: From EBM to CSM: the evolution of context-sensitive medicine, *Journal of Evaluation in Clinical Practice* 3(2):105–108, 1997.

Griggs B: *Green pharmacy: a history of herbal medicine*, London, 1981, Robert Hale.

Hatfield G: *Memory, wisdom and healing: the history of domestic plant medicine*, Portland, Oregon, 1999, Sutton.

Haxton B: *Heraclitus: Fragments (trans.)*, London, 2001, Penguin.

Hitchens C: *God is not great: the case against religion*, London, 2007, Atlantic Books.

Hoffmann D: *The holistic herbal*, London, 1983, Thorsons.

Holland BK: *Prospecting for drugs in ancient and medieval European texts: a scientific approach*, London, 1996, Taylor & Francis.

Hopkins R: *The transition handbook: from oil dependency to local resilience*, Dartington, 2008, Green Books.

Hotamisligil G: Inflammation and metabolic disorders, *Nature* 444:860–867, 2006.

House of Lords Select Committee on Science and Technology: *Complementary and alternative medicine, 6th Report*, London, 2000, Stationery Office.

Hutchings A: *Zulu medicinal plants: an inventory*, 1996, University of Natal Press.

Jilin L, editor: *Chinese dietary therapy*, London, 1995, Churchill Livingstone.

Johns T: *The origins of human diet and medicine*, 1996, University of Arizona Press.

Joshi K, Hankey A, Patwardhan B: Traditional phytochemistry: identification of drug by 'taste', *Evidence-Based Complementary and Alternative Medicine* 4(2):145–148, 2006.

Jullien F: *In praise of blandness: Proceedings from Chinese thought and aesthetics*, 2004, Zone Books.

Kenner D, Requena Y: *Botanical medicine: a European professional perspective*, 2001, Paradigm Publications.

Klein R: The NHS and the new scientism: solution or delusion? *Quarterly Journal of Medicine* 89:85–87, 1996.

Lawrence C, Weisz G: Medical holism: the context. In: Lawrence C, Weisz G, editors: *Greater than the parts: holism in biomedicine 1920–1950*, 1998, Oxford University Press.

Lloyd GER: *Hippocratic writings*, London, 1983, Penguin Classics.

McLuhan TC: *Touch the Earth: a self-portrait of Indian existence*, Michigan, 1973, Abacus.

Mills S: Preface. In Mills S, Bone K: *Principles and practice of phytotherapy: modern herbal medicine*, 2000, Elsevier/Churchill Livingstone.

Mills S, Bone K: *Principles and Practice of Phytotherapy: Modern Herbal Medicine*, 2000, Elsevier/Churchill Livingstone.

Moerman D: *Native American ethnobotany*, Portland, 1998, Timber Press.

O'Doherty J, Rolls ET, Francis S, et al: Representation of pleasant and aversive taste in the human brain, *Journal of Neurophysiology* 85(3):1315–1321, 2001.

Okasha S: *Philosophy of science: a very short introduction*, 2002, Oxford University Press.

Parker MH: The regulation of complementary health: sacrificing integrity? *Medical Journal of Australia* 179(6):316–318, 2003.

Payer L: *Medicine and culture*, Amherst, 1996, Owl Books.

Pietroni P: *The greening of medicine*, London, 1990, Gollancz.

Porter R: *The greatest benefit to mankind*, London, 1997, Harper Collins.

Puliyel JM, Baijal N, Narula D: Evidence-based investigation into the relation between sexual intercourse and pregnancy, *Br Med J* Rapid Responses bmj.com 10 November 2004 (Accessed 15 September 2005).

Rangel JA: O: The systemic theory of living systems and relevance to CAM: Part 1: The theory, *Evidence-based Complementary and Alternative Medicine* 2(1):13–18, 2005.

Ritsema R, Karcher S: *I Ching*, Dorset, 1994, Element.

Sackett DL: Equipoise, a term whose time (if it ever came) has surely gone, *Canadian Medical Association Journal* 163(7):835–836, 2000.

Sackett DL, Strauss SE, Richardson WS, et al: *Evidence-based medicine: how to practice and teach EBM*, Edinburgh, 2000, Churchill Livingstone.

Smith R: The failings of NICE: *British Medical Journal* 321:1363–1364, 2000.

Smith R: Medical journals and pharmaceutical companies: uneasy bedfellows, *British Medical Journal* 326:1202–1205, 2003.

Sorell T: *Scientism: philosophy and the infatuation with science*, London, 1994, Routledge.

Spelman K, Burns J, Nichols D, et al: Modulation of cytokine expression by traditional medicines: a review of herbal immunomodulators, *Alternative Medicine Review* 11(2):128–150, 2006.

Strauss SE, McAlister FA: Evidence-based medicine: a commentary on common criticisms, 2000, *Canadian Medical Association Journal* 163(7):837–841, 2000.

Tobyn G: *Culpeper's medicine*, Dorset, 1997, Element.

Tracy CS, Dantas GC, Upshur RE: Evidence-based medicine in primary care: qualitative study of family physicians, *BMC Family Practice* 4(6), 2003.

Ullmann M: *Islamic surveys II: Islamic medicine*, 1978, Edinburgh University Press.

Van Wyk BE, Van Oudtshoorn B, Gericke N: *Medicinal Plants of South Africa*, Pretoria, 1997, Briza Publications.

Wahlberg A: Pathways to plausibility: when herbs become pills, *BioSocieties* 3:37–56, 2008.

Wellen KE, Hotamisligil GS: Inflammation, stress, and diabetes, *Journal of Clinical Investigation* 115(5):1111–1119, 2005.

Wheen F: *How mumbo-jumbo conquered the world*, New York, 2004, Harper Perennial.

Wisneski LA, Anderson L: *The scientific basis of integrative medicine*, London, 2005, CRC Press.

Wynne-Edwards KE: Evolutionary biology of plant defenses against herbivory and their predictive implications for endocrine disruptor susceptibility in vertebrates, *Environmental Health Perspectives* 109(5):443–448, 2001.

Yang Y: *Chinese herbal medicines*, Edinburgh, 2002, Churchill Livingstone.

Zysk KG, Tetlow G: Traditional Ayurveda. In: Micozzi MS, editor: *Fundamentals of complementary and alternative medicine*, Edinburgh, 2001, Churchill Livingstone.

# The therapeutic relationship in phytotherapy

## CHAPTER CONTENTS

The challenge of the therapeutic relationship 39
What is the 'therapeutic relationship'? 41
The variety of relationship models in healthcare 44
Patient expectations: clarification and challenge 52
New perspectives on the placebo effect 53
Setting the context in which a therapeutic relationship can emerge: the importance of practitioner factors 57
Reflective practice: nurturing the 'therapeutic attitude' 64
Evidence-based medicine and the therapeutic relationship 65
Phenomenology: the felt presence of the body in the moment 67
The relevance of the therapeutic relationship in phytotherapy: weaving the loose threads 74

> *And I said that (the cure) was a certain leaf, but that there was a certain incantation in addition to the drug, and that if one chanted it at the same time as he used it, the drug would make him altogether healthy, but without the incantation there would be no benefit from the leaf.*
> Plato, *Charmides* 1986

In the previous chapter, it was stated that: 'the key focus of this book trains on the interpersonal aspects of the phytotherapist's work.' The concept of the 'therapeutic relationship' provides a good place to begin exploring the interpersonal dimensions of the consultation.

The notion of the therapeutic relationship suggests that there is a healing potential residing in the interactions that occur between patient and practitioner that can be considered as both distinct from and complementary to the specified 'treatment' and concrete advice that the practitioner provides. This potential may be realized more effectively when the practitioner is aware that it exists and knows how to work with it. This chapter seeks to explore the concept of the therapeutic relationship, show how it connects with the practice of phytotherapy and consider the ways in which it can be engendered.

## THE CHALLENGE OF THE THERAPEUTIC RELATIONSHIP

Where a patient appears to derive benefit (whether subjectively or objectively defined) from an encounter, or series of encounters, with a healthcare professional we can posit that four major varieties of therapeutic influence are likely to have been involved, overlapping to varying extents across a spectrum of potential:

Influence 1: The individual's innate 'self-healing'
Influence 2: Changes to thoughts, behaviours and activities (attitudinal, behavioural, nutritional, relating to exercise and lifestyle, etc.)
Influence 3: The therapeutic relationship between the person and carer/s
Influence 4: The specific treatment/s applied.

Both conventional and complementary and alternative medicine (CAM) practitioners may assume that, in the cases where it is deployed, the fourth type of influence is usually the most significant, but this is not necessarily (or even usually) the case. Practitioner hubris may ascribe healing to the intervention they have applied, when in truth it has played only a minor part, if any, in the process. Indeed, it may even have obstructed and slowed down achievement of the eventual positive outcome – or prevented it from ever occurring. Although it is self-evident that the animal organism is self-healing (e.g. a small wound will repair without any medical intervention), this fundamental – and most *vital* (I choose this word carefully) – capacity is often ignored or overlooked. Parsons' (1951) observation on the relationship between self-healing and practitioner effects still rings true:

> In general the line between the spontaneous forces tending to recovery – what used to be called the vis medicatrix naturae – and the effects of the physician's 'intervention' is impossible to draw with precision in a very large number of cases.

In herbal medicine, 'Influence 1' is traditionally considered to be central in the philosophy of its practice: it is axiomatic that the human organism is self-healing and the herbal practitioner stands in awe of the body's ability to develop, thrive and repair. This is the 'vitalism' at the core of herbal practice. Plant medicines are applied as triggers, aides or 'nudges' to self-healing. Clearly there are circumstances in which the self-healing capacity of the individual is so severely compromised that decay and death take place. Phytotherapy, and CAM in general, holds little sway at these times and may stand to one side to let nature take its course, though offering palliation as it does so. Conventional medicine, however, is sometimes able to provide strategies that enable life to continue even when innate vital auto-healing capacities are overwhelmed.

'Influence 4' – professionally prescribed or applied treatment – tends to be in the foreground when healthcare professionals concentrate on dealing with a deviation away from normative health parameters (i.e. when 'illness' occurs). The focus of randomized controlled trials (the so-called 'gold standard' in clinical research) is on this zone of influence, usually exclusively so. Qualitative research methods, however, can reveal aspects pertaining to the other spheres of influence, including providing insights into the patient's perception of self-healing and the therapeutic relationship. Combined quantitative–qualitative protocols offer potential to cast a wider net in catching the nuances across the therapeutic spectrum.

We can, however, take the practitioner out of the four proposed spheres of influence. All four can apply without a 'healthcare professional' being involved. The therapeutic relationship in 'Influence 3' may be created with a friend, family member, colleague, cleric, etc. Later in this chapter we will consider the practitioner qualities that help to facilitate the therapeutic relationship as described by the psychotherapist Carl Rogers. He came to realize that these qualities were not specific to healthcare practitioners (and that they can, in fact, occur in anybody in any field or role), and later promoted their application by non-medical practitioners such as teachers (Rogers & Freiberg 1994).

The therapeutic relationship is likely to be the most controversial (and least obvious) of the influences described here and the concept poses certain challenges:

- How can it be defined and studied?
- How can we work with it to maximize its impact?

We will consider these questions below. The greatest challenge, however, may be to ingrained habits and attitudes (cherished or otherwise), which may need to be changed when exposed to the light shed by reflection on this area.

## WHAT IS THE 'THERAPEUTIC RELATIONSHIP'?

All interactions between people feel like more or less positive or negative experiences to those directly involved – as well as for the wider circle of contacts who may be affected in turn by the repercussions and retellings of these encounters. Even rather trivial exchanges may be *felt* quite strongly – a smile from someone passing by in the street may lift our spirits for a whole morning; a rude person at the end of the phone may upset our afternoon. We can suggest a general rule: that the more significant the encounter, the greater is the potential for positive or negative effects to be generated. We are social creatures and the ways in which others treat us strongly affects our sense of self and notions of our place in society. Healthcare encounters are among the most significant types of meetings we may have since the issues at stake are frequently of great import to our sense of identity and our perceptions of personal wellbeing.

Patients may leave healthcare encounters thinking thoughts and feeling emotions in ways that we can broadly categorize as negative or positive:

- Negative: upset, fear, anxiety, uncertainty, confusion, helplessness, hopelessness, irritation, frustration, etc.
- Positive: hope, reassurance, comfort, enlightenment, insight, relief, empowerment, uplifted, focussed, etc.

The ways in which these responses are shaped are not entirely due to the nature of the patient's condition and the availability, or otherwise, of effective treatments. They are also moulded by how the patient has been met, perceived and 'handled'. Practitioners also experience positive or negative reactions following consultations, and reflection (as 'reflective practice') on these thoughts and feelings is one of the key techniques for developing skills as a therapeutic practitioner, as we shall see later.

A number of popular sayings and phrases attest to the potency of positive encounters:

*'A problem shared is a problem halved'*
*'She set my mind at rest'*
*'He took a load off my mind'*
*'I felt the weight lift off my shoulders'.*

These are important statements arising from a common sense that telling our story to a careful listener and hearing their views about it has the potential to reduce the problem we have presented, to calm us and actually to 'lighten' us. We feel freer, liberated, better equipped to progress – to see a way to move forward.

The medical consultation is a process based on storytelling. A ritual is enacted wherein the patient tells a story about their health as the practitioner first listens, then offers an interpretation of the story, perhaps weaving it into a complementary or alternative story of their own creation. The consultation may conclude with the practitioner proposing a master narrative that the patient is invited (or assumed) to subscribe to. This process of reciprocal storytelling and interpretation rarely follows a smooth course. Both parties may cut across each other, fail to hear the other, and seek to impose their own reading of events regardless of the evidence and arguments presented. The initial storyteller ('patient') will tend to have multiple reflections/dialogues regarding their state of health and may withhold information from some listeners/interpreters (including healthcare professionals), presenting the material somewhat differently depending on the audience. The consultation, then, is a complex, partial, particular and potentially treacherous territory in which to roam. Practitioners develop a range of strategies to cope with the dangers that lurk there. The best prepared are those who are able to allow and to coax the patient to tell the most essential story that they can and who have an extensive library of archetypal and individual stories with which to compare the patient's own. The least well prepared are those who know only a few tales and who direct and edit the patient's narrative to fit one of them. Over recent years, the concept of 'narrative-based medicine' (NBM) has been elucidated to describe this type of approach and it offers one model that can help to facilitate the therapeutic relationship. We will return to NBM later in this chapter and at other points throughout the book.

The key proposition regarding the therapeutic relationship at this point, is one that should be fairly non-contentious: regardless of the particular condition and hope of remedy, it is possible to make patients feel (subjectively) better or worse during and following a consultation as a result of the manner in which the practitioner 'handles' the encounter. Most people are likely to agree that if a practitioner deals with the patient in a crass and insensitive manner, they will feel worse, but if they act with respect and kindness, the patient is likely to feel better. Such effects may be thought to be of little lasting consequence if they are believed not to materially affect formal 'patient outcomes' or to have any influence on the healing process. The assertion of the therapeutic relationship, as considered here, is radical however, since it contends that the patient–practitioner encounter, *in and of itself*, has the potential to engender lasting therapeutic benefits. That is to say, that the patient–practitioner relationship should be considered not as an incidental feature of the therapeutic journey, but rather as an integral part of treatment.

We might readily accept this assertion in the context of psychological therapies, where no material remedies are given, yet the patient may nonetheless gain benefit. It could be argued that therapeutic results accrue in the psychotherapies because these approaches use prescribed systems of interviewing, framing and advice-giving that are constructed to constitute a formal 'remedy' and that these are missing from other healthcare approaches. That is to say that the psychological consultation is *designed and intended* to be therapeutic whereas that occurring in the non-psychotherapies is not. The particular format that the psychological consultation follows appears to be of little importance however, since, as Hyland (2005) observes: 'meta-analyses lead to the conclusion that all psychotherapies are equally effective.' Hyland contends that training in particular practitioner skills or techniques is less important than the practitioner's 'therapeutic attitude' or 'therapeutic intent'. The practitioner's belief 'in what they are doing' combined with a warm and caring approach towards the patient are what matters. Hyland cites Rogers (1951) in describing some of the basics involved in the latter of these areas:

> ... complete acceptance ... expression of the attitude of wanting to help the client ... warmth of spirit as expressed by his wholehearted giving of himself to the client in complete cooperation with everything the client does or says ...

We will return to add to the list of practitioner attitudes and behaviours that enhance the therapeutic relationship later in this chapter.

Although much of the literature pertaining to the therapeutic relationship derives from the field of psychotherapy, the concept does not apply in this field alone. The broad principles of the therapeutic relationship can be applied in any healthcare modality – indeed in any helping or caring interaction between people. Hyland (2005) presents one view which states that: 'psychotherapy provides a context that promotes self-healing rather than treats disease, and should coexist with conventional medicine as a parallel but different kind of treatment ...'. Yet is it really necessary to maintain this distinction between psychological and material therapies? McWhinney et al. (1997) have contended that:

> All significant illness is a disturbance at many levels, from the molecular to the personal and social. This implies that some of the skills that are at present considered psychiatric will need to be developed more generally in all clinicians, especially those working in primary care, where so much general, undifferentiated illness is seen.

In the 'Introductory' section, I argued that phytotherapy combined psychotherapy *and* pharmacotherapy and we can now, perhaps, begin to see the crucial nature of this contention.

At this stage, it is worth distinguishing between the concept of the therapeutic relationship and that of 'therapeutic alliance'. Many authorities use the two terms interchangeably but we may consider the latter term as having to do with the specific work of creating a shared sense of positive collaboration between patient and practitioner. This concerns trust-building and other factors that bring the patient 'onside' with the practitioner and enable a course of treatment/therapy to take place. In this sense, the therapeutic alliance may be viewed primarily as a means of improving patient compliance with treatment, which is an especially relevant concern where there may be challenges to compliance such as in treating those who are alcohol dependent (Ernst et al. 2008). The therapeutic relationship can be conceptualized as being much broader than this and as being not just a means to ensuring compliance with the 'active treatment' but of potentially *being an active treatment* in itself. This newer, extended view of the possibilities of the therapeutic relationship is made possible to a great degree by the emerging field of psychoneuroimmunology (PNI), which connects psychology with physiology and offers a way of informing the mind–body question by measuring and correlating the biochemical changes that accompany psychological states. Janice Kiecolt-Glaser, one of the key researchers in this field, contends that: 'The link between personal relationships and immune function is one of the most robust findings in PNI' (Kiecolt-Glaser et al. 2002) and she and her co-workers have studied the 'pathways through which hostile or abrasive relationships affect physiological functioning and health'.

The therapeutic relationship, then, is a positive potential that exists when practitioner and patient interact with each other. Understanding it and knowing how to facilitate it is likely to result in benefits for both parties. A critical appreciation of the concept is necessary, however, e.g. Chew-Graham et al. (2004) have seen a problem in what they consider to be an inappropriate elevation of the practitioner–patient relationship such that practitioners may feel compelled to seek to: 'maintain relationships with patients, even though they felt powerless to achieve useful clinical outcomes and felt forced to collude with illness behaviour that sustained incapacity'. This is the very opposite of a therapeutic relationship and the components and characteristics of the therapeutic approach must be appreciated in detail and in context in order to realize its potential in the consultation.

## THE VARIETY OF RELATIONSHIP MODELS IN HEALTHCARE

In discussing the scope of the therapeutic relationship, Agich (1983) refers to Szasz and Hollender's (1956) classification of the three basic models of doctor–patient relationships:

1. Activity–passivity (the doctor actively does something to the patient, which they passively receive)
2. Guidance–cooperation (the doctor tells the patient what to do and the patient complies)
3. Mutual participation (a collaborative approach).

While the optimally conducive territory for developing the therapeutic relationship would seem to lie with the mutual participation model, Agich (1983) points out that there are times when other models are appropriate, indeed they may be essential, e.g. a coma patient requires application of the activity–passivity model. In fact we can imagine (if we extend the number and types of relationships involved in a particular situation) a scenario where all three models may be employed simultaneously: a practitioner called to a serious accident site may treat an unconscious patient using activity–passivity; direct others at the scene using guidance–cooperation and work with colleagues using mutual participation. The most effective practitioners may be those who are able to move between models as appropriate. We will come back to this notion of adaptability as a key feature distinguishing the practitioner who is better able to form therapeutic relationships later.

Agich (1983) cautions against making the error of seeing the therapeutic relationship as: 'a free-standing relationship between autonomous individuals which abstracts from all social connections'. The autonomy of both practitioner and patient may be limited or constrained to some degree and the patient's situation is impacted by numerous influences besides those that might be considered strictly 'medical' in nature. While many practitioners, especially in the CAM bracket, make broad claims to 'treat the cause, not the disease' and to 'treat the whole person' the difficulties inherent in getting to know a fraction of what constitutes the 'whole person', let alone getting to anything as singular as the 'cause' of a condition (particularly in complex cases), should not be trivialized. In order to gain the fullest possible view of the patient's situation a holistic approach is essential, but in asserting this we may need to pause for a moment of clarification since the term 'holistic' has come to sound trite to many ears due to overuse, misapplication and ill-definition. Gordon's (1982) take on the nature of holism in healthcare still ranks amongst the most concisely useful:

> Holistic medicine is an attitudinal approach to healthcare rather than a particular set of techniques. It addresses the psychological, familial, societal, ethical and spiritual as well as biological dimensions of health and illness. The holistic approach emphasises the uniqueness of each patient, the mutuality of the doctor-patient relationship, each person's responsibility for his or her own healthcare and society's responsibility for the promotion of health.

A practitioner who is thinking and working in a manner that is in tune with this definition will be a person who is oriented to make connections between numerous territories of lived experience and who seeks to synthesize these to a focussed point of understanding, direction or action. Such characteristics tend to lead to greater facility in developing therapeutic relationships, since they enable the practitioner to appreciate the patient's predicament more profoundly.

Looking outside of the narrowly 'medical' consultation zone requires a view of how health and medicine are situated within, and impacted by, sociocultural factors. To enable this expanded way of seeing and knowing the practitioner can look to a wide range of relevant fields of study (many of which tend to be overlooked or underexploited by healthcare practitioners of every stripe) such as that of the sociology of health and illness (see Nettleton 2006, for a solid introduction to this field). Part of the challenge of the therapeutic relationship is that it pushes the practitioner to continually develop and reframe their knowledge and skills as they seek to learn from the patient. To intentionally set up the consultation as a laboratory for personal and professional change and development in this manner constitutes a radical political act that may transgress and subvert both the general model that the practitioner was originally trained in and particular protocols that they may be expected to comply with.

The terms 'healthcare practitioner' and 'political radical' may strike us as antithetical. The dominant conventional medical services deliver the healthcare messages and practices sanctioned by the government and its departments – so that healthcare workers become agents of the state. This places limits on the autonomy of the practitioner. Medicine is an inherently conservative profession – both in its modern and traditional forms. Necessarily so, one might argue, since new approaches and techniques should only be added to the canon once they have been tried and tested. Yet conservatism may both mask and maintain useless or harmful attitudes and practices. It can be very hard for healthcare practitioners (whether conventional or CAM) to see beyond the edges of their own medicalized worldview – within this they live and breathe and have their professional being. Practitioners are restricted by their auto-medicalization, just as society at large is conditioned and constrained by notions of what is medically appropriate and acceptable. In his seminal critique of conventional medicine, Ivan Illich (1976) described the nature of the problem:

> *During the last generations the medical monopoly over healthcare has expanded without checks and has encroached on our liberty with regard to our own bodies. Society has transferred to physicians the exclusive right to determine what constitutes sickness, who is or might become sick, and what shall be done to such people ... The social commitment to provide all citizens with almost unlimited outputs from the medical system threatens to destroy the environmental and cultural conditions needed by people to live a life of constant autonomous healing.*

Since Illich's attack, mainstream medicine has delved more deeply into the body as increasingly penetrating techniques and conceptualizations (e.g. the MRI-revealed body and the genomic body) have been developed. Ever greater reliance on technical means of understanding and reading the body undercuts attempts made elsewhere within medically-related fields (such as public health) to increase patient autonomy since the definitive answers to Illich's questions ('what constitutes sickness, who is or might become sick, and what shall be done'?) still rests with medical experts. We may query, by contrast, the extent to which CAM has been successful in proposing alternative ways of comprehending the body and to what extent it has promoted an ethos valuing greater personal empowerment to evolve. For medical doctor, columnist and noted CAM-critic, Ben Goldacre (2008), CAM is merely part of the problem, another group contributing to the 'medicalisation of everyday life':

> *Alternative therapists, the media, and the drug industry all conspire to sell us reductionist, bio-medical explanations for problems that might more sensibly and constructively be thought of as social, political, or personal.*

General discussions about the role of CAM are flawed where they presuppose that CAM represents a coherent and organized alternative schema to mainstream medicine, i.e. that it is a discrete entity fit for comparison with its supposed antithesis. To proceed in such a way would be to make a category error. 'CAM' is essentially a definition of exclusion – which is to say that all healthcare practices outside of 'conventional/mainstream' medicine (i.e. the dominant model) are bracketed as 'CAM'. Closer inspection reveals the heterogenous nature of the individual therapies constituting the notion of CAM, and differences between the agendas and messages of corporate interests (manufacturers of CAM remedies) and particular groups of practitioners. It may be more accurate to join Kelner and Wellman (2000) in viewing CAM as: 'a complex and constantly changing social phenomenon which defies any arbitrary definition or classification'. How can we gauge the impact of such an amorphous entity on models in the consultation? Most texts that set out lists of the characteristics of CAM assert that a mutual participation model is used by its practitioners, e.g. Fulder (1996) provides eight 'unique features of complementary medicine', one of which is the 'patient as partner'. What is the nature of this partnership though, and how can we know if it has been achieved? In suggesting answers, it may be helpful to return to Illich (1976), noting the distinction he draws between:

> ... two modes in which the person relates and adapts to his environment: autonomous (i.e. self-governing) coping and heteronomous (i.e. administered) maintenance and management.

The former mode Illich associates with positive individual 'powers for healthcare' contrasted with heteronomous adaptation within a 'physician-based health-care system', which is prone to become 'sickening' to the extent that it:

> ... tends to mystify and to expropriate the power of the individual to heal himself and to shape his or her environment.

We can briefly note here that the gradual shift in medicine from paternalistic (heteronomous) to patient-centred (valuing patient autonomy) models that we will explore shortly, reflects what Taylor (2009) has described as a: 'shift that has occurred ... from a culture where beneficence is the dominant ethical principle to one in which autonomy is valued as highly'. (*Note*: Beneficence inclines to paternalism where attempts to benefit an individual are made against their will.)

In any case, CAM practitioners are not immune from the tendency to 'mystify and expropriate' – a potential pitfall for all healthcare professionals. We can suggest, nonetheless, that a key criterion in estimating a practitioner's success in establishing healthy partnerships with patients has to do with the extent to which they are able to empower autonomy and minimize dependency on other-administered 'maintenance and management'. CAM practitioners have an edge here, which may have less to do with the founding philosophies of their particular modality and more to do with the fact and implications of their 'excludedness', especially with regard to what Sharma (1994) has called the 'institutional context'. The differing operating conditions for conventional and CAM practitioners significantly affect their respective capacities for professional autonomy, as Sharma explains:

> ... most orthodox doctors operate within a bureaucratic context and ... this has an inevitable effect on the relationship between healer and patient, being conducive to a hierarchical definition of relationships. Individual physicians may have their own characteristic ways of handling patients and may hold different views on how much information patients ought to be given, but the pressures of the institutional context will do much to determine the range of behaviours which are either permissible or productive both for doctors and patients.

While complementary therapists:

> ... tend to work in settings characterized by a non-hierarchical ethos and minimum of direct control from either superiors or equals. Thus they appear to have the clinical autonomy and freedom from managerial interference which orthodox doctors hold as an ideal ...

Two lacks, then, *may* help engender two positive characteristics in CAM therapists: the lack of statutory authority given to CAM practitioners encourages a less authoritarian style; and the lack of a bureaucratic context enables them to act with greater autonomy. These characteristics (non-authoritarian; highly autonomous) are facilitative of more equal relationships with patients and condition the nature of these relationships. Such an outcome is not inevitable, of course, but the initial conditions of practice set for CAM practitioners make it easier for more autotomizing styles of practice to emerge. Sharma comments that:

> *What transpires in the complementary therapist's consulting room need not be so very different from what transpires in the GP's surgery ... But to the extent that the complementary practitioner usually operates quite independently of the state's interest in the bodies and health of its citizens there is always the potential for a very radical difference.*

The logical conclusion of this line of argument, namely that the non-statutory nature of CAM therapies constitutes a strength (although one that may be offset by a number of weaknesses, such as a lack of accountability); adds a further critical dimension to the discussion of the regulation of CAM professions opened up in the previous chapter. Considerations in this territory relate not only to outcomes for patients but for practitioners themselves, as Moynihan and Smith (2002) make clear as they reflect on the extent of biomedicalization and its impacts on conventional practitioners:

> *Doctors and their organisations understandably argue for increased spending – because they are otherwise left paying a personal price, trying to cope with increasing demand with inadequate resources. Indeed this is one of the sources of worldwide unhappiness among doctors. Although seen by many as the perpetrators of medicalisation, doctors may actually be some of its most prominent victims.*

It is worth noting that 'trying to cope with increasing demand with inadequate resources' constitutes a definition of the cause of professional burnout – a condition characterized by 'exhaustion, cynicism and sense of inefficacy' (Maslach 2003). Approaches that enhance patient autonomy are more sustainable for the practitioner and for national economies such that these two factors are likely to increasingly drive mainstream healthcare in the direction of a patient-centred model of practice and service provision.

At this point, let us add to Szasz and Hollender's (1956) three basic models of doctor–patient relationships by considering later contributions to this subject area in order to better appreciate its scope. In discussing the 'struggle over the patient's role in medical decision making', Emanuel and Emanuel (1992) outlined four models of the physician–patient relationship:

1. *Paternalistic* (alternatively called the 'priestly' or 'parental' model):
    Here the practitioner determines what is best for the patient, with little

explanation given to the patient and minimal patient involvement. The patient is expected to assent to the practitioner's decisions.
2. *Informative* (also known as the scientific, engineering or consumer model): In this model, the practitioner aims to 'provide the patient with all relevant information, for the patient to select the medical interventions he or she wants, and (then) to execute the selected intervention'. In this model, the practitioner is a provider of facts, which the patient interprets according to her values. There is 'no role for the physician's values, the physician's understanding of the patient's values, or his or her judgement of the worth of the patient's values'.
3. *Interpretive*: In contrast to the informative model the practitioner's aim is to 'elucidate the patient's values and what he or she actually wants, and to help the patient select the available ... interventions that realize these values'. Information on the options is provided in conjunction with assistance based on appreciation of the patient's values.
4. *Deliberative*: This model sees the patient's health-related values as open to discussion, such that the practitioner is able to suggest 'why certain health-related values are more worthy and should be aspired to ... the physician aims at no more than moral persuasion; ultimately, coercion is avoided, and the patient must define his or her life and select the ordering of values to be espoused'.

A summary of these four concepts, with correlations including the view taken of the patient's autonomy is provided in Table 2.1.

**Table 2.1** *Comparing the four models of the physician–patient relationship*

| | | | | |
|---|---|---|---|---|
| **Patient values** | Defined, fixed and known to the patient | Inchoate and conflicting, requiring elucidation | Open to development and revision through moral discussion | Objective and shared by physician and patient |
| **Physician's obligation** | Providing relevant factual information and implementing patient's selected intervention | Elucidating and interpreting relevant patient values as well as informing the patient and implementing the patient's selected intervention | Articulating and persuading the patient of the most admirable values as well as performing the patient and implementing the patient's selected intervention | Promoting the patient's wellbeing independent of the patient's current preferences |
| **Conception of patient's autonomy** | Choice of, and control over, medical care | Self-understanding relevant to medical care | Moral self-development relevant to medical care | Assenting to objective values |
| **Conception of physician's role** | Competent technical expert | Counsellor or adviser | Friend or teacher | Guardian |

From: Emanuel & Emanuel (1992).

It is interesting to consider these models in the light of the evidence-based medicine (EBM) discussion, which we began in the previous chapter and will return to again below, particularly around the original definition of EBM as: 'the integration of best research evidence with clinical expertise and patient values' (Sackett et al. 2000). In applying the four models to a hypothetical clinical case, Emanuel and Emanuel (1992) largely interpret 'information' and 'facts' as research so that their discussion focuses on the three territories of EBM, with difficulties in the patient–practitioner relationship occurring particularly when research and/or clinical expertise are emphasized to the detriment of due attention to patient values.

Each of the four models is problematic when viewed as representing a single and permanent way of being as a practitioner. Rather we can assert, as earlier, that the most effective practitioners are likely to be those who are able to move between these models as appropriate – frequently within the course of just one consultation. These are not models of practice, then, but caricatures of practitioner strategies that can be deployed and combined as a given situation requires. As Emanuel and Emanuel (1992) point out, even paternalistic behaviour can be appropriate in situations of medical emergencies.

In selecting which of the four models might generally be preferred as 'the ideal physician–patient relationship', Emanuel and Emanuel (1992) choose the deliberative model, rejecting allegations that it merely represents 'a disguised form of paternalism' – this reading is far from safe, however, since the model suggests that practitioners occupy a position of definitive moral and epistemological authority and little recognition of the role of uncertainty is made. The central issue of uncertainty, that lies within and between the practitioner's and the patient's views of how to proceed in a given situation, tends to be overlooked in discussions of 'shared decision-making' models such as the deliberative.

Shared decision-making (sometimes called 'partnership-centred' medicine) is held as a key tenet of patient-empowering, non-paternalistic relationships but the balance of power and influence is open to question in this concept. The informative model would appear to let decisions rest entirely with the patient but these are in fact limited by the options made available by the practitioner and the manner in which they have been presented; it also tends to leave the patient exposed and unsupported. The interpretive model helps the patient to make their own decisions, providing support but risking excessive deferment to the patient's wishes; while the deliberative model allows the practitioner to be fully engaged in recommending the best course of action but with the danger that the practitioner's worldview and agenda may hold sway over the patient's.

The types of autonomy afforded to the patient within Emanuel and Emanuel's (1992) four models all stand in relation to various ways of negotiating conventional medical care but they are equally relevant in CAM practice. Any discussion of patient autonomy is incomplete of course without referencing ways in which people may care for their wellbeing independently of healthcare practitioners through self-care measures, and the degree to which autonomous healthcare is facilitated or hindered by socioeconomic, political and cultural influences. A full discussion of these factors is beyond the scope of this book but we will return to limited discussion of them at various points in the text.

Kaba and Sooriakumaran (2007) have proposed a time line for the evolution of the doctor–patient relationship beginning with ancient Egypt (c.4000–100 BCE) where the paternalistic priest–supplicant relationship is said to form the basis of the practitioner-relationship; through the Greek enlightenment (c.600–100 BCE) where it is proposed that the roots of the mutual-participation model lie; and on through medieval Europe and the inquisition (paternalism revived) and the French revolution (partial egalitarianism shifting emphasis from activity–passivity to the guidance–cooperation model) to the modern era, where the 'emergence of psychology', including psychoanalytical and psychosocial theories, has led to a refocusing on the patient as a person. The practitioner–patient relationship, they argue, has fluxed from one pole to the other, with a general trend of movement from a practitioner-centred to a patient-centred approach.

Mead and Bower (2000) have discussed the ambiguity concerning the meaning of 'patient-centredness' and have identified five 'conceptual dimensions' that they propose as constituting a model for it that distinguishes it from the biomedical model. These are:

1. *Biopsychosocial perspective*: 'broadening the explanatory perspective on illness to include social and psychological factors'
2. *The patient-as-person*: 'understanding the individual's experience of illness … (and) as an idiosyncratic personality within his or her unique context'
3. *Sharing power and responsibility*: 'concerned to encourage significantly greater patient involvement in care'
4. *The therapeutic-alliance*: '(which) has potential therapeutic benefit in and of itself'
5. *The doctor-as-person*: 'emotions engendered in the doctor by particular patient presentations may be used as an aid to further management'.

This formulation represents a sort of 'coming-out' of conventional medics as sensitive, feeling people who are open to the subjective elements of the consultation – a vulnerable circumstance that Mead and Bower (2000) immediately defend by proposing ways in which patient-centeredness can be *measured*!

McWhinney (1996) contends that: 'The essence of the patient-centred method is that the doctor attends to feelings, emotions and moods, as well as categorizing the patient's illness'. It may seem extraordinary to those outside of medicine that such activity stands in need of emphasis – at least to those who have only had positive experiences of conventional medical care – don't all 'good' practitioners do this? The ability and capacity for practitioners to work in a patient-centred way is influenced by their philosophy of practice and institutional context, as we have previously noted, so that healthier relationships with patients depend in large part on practitioner education and the operating conditions for practice – where either are narrow or constrained it will be difficult for patient-centred practice to emerge. The battle to end paternalism has a long way to go in conventional medicine (Coulter 1999: 'Paternalism is endemic in the NHS') and as CAM therapies gradually enter the mainstream, each modality will need to guard against being subsumed into the still predominantly paternalistic ethos of its culture.

## PATIENT EXPECTATIONS: CLARIFICATION AND CHALLENGE

One way of rationalizing the therapeutic relationship is to suggest that it arises when patient expectations are met. This is a rather lopsided take however, since the core of a positive relationship lies in its mutuality. Furthermore, any given individual patient may have expectations of the clinical encounter that are obstructive to establishing a therapeutic relationship, i.e. if those expectations are too tightly focussed; poorly informed; unrealistic; unduly pessimistic or optimistic. The therapeutic relationship may be most clearly in evidence, and most productive, when patient expectations are transmuted during the course of the practitioner–patient interaction. The door needs to be left open for transformative elements such as surprise and revelation to enter, i.e. for learning to occur on the part of both patient and practitioner.

Expectations vary between patients depending on the nature of their predicament, their experience, character and preferences and the role in which they cast the practitioner. A patient may, for example, visit a conventional doctor with a primary desire to receive a diagnosis but not treatment and then visit a CAM practitioner with the opposite priorities. Practitioners need to cultivate openness and flexibility in approaching each patient as an individual. A key question to ask of patients could be: 'What *especially* would you like me to help you with?'

The fit between the patient's expectations and the practitioner's comprehension of them is frequently a poor one. Britten (2004) has pointed out the dangers that lie in this territory: 'Inappropriate assessments of patients' expectations can result in actions deemed unnecessary by the doctor and unwanted by the patient'. There is no reason to suspect that the situation is necessarily any different in CAM consultations. False perceptions of patient's expectations may lead to a sense of pressure to meet these expectations on the part of the practitioner – even when they consider them unfounded or inappropriate. Britten (2004) cites studies that suggest that: '… pressure from patients may be stronger in the doctor's mind than in the patient's mind. Doctors may be making inappropriate decisions for the sake of maintaining relationships with patients without checking whether their assumptions about patients' preferences are correct'. Therapeutic practitioners need to be on guard against this type of misunderstanding and adopt the strategy of repeatedly asking questions to clarify patients' expectations, desires and wishes. Asking such clarifying questions can move both practitioner and patient out of their comfort zones and occasionally, this type of question may lead to profound moments of insight that can catalyse reflection and change. The potential for such crucial episodes to have negative outcomes is diminished when questions are phrased non-judgementally. An example:

> Practitioner: 'So, would you like me to prescribe something for your migraines or would you prefer for us to tackle it in some other way?'

Patient: 'I'd rather not take a medicine if I can help it, even a herbal one, but what other ways are there?'

Practitioner: 'Well, is there anything you can think of that would help you cope with the migraines better?'

Patient: 'Well if life calmed down and I could get more sleep ... if I could get more time to myself ...'

Practitioner: 'Can we talk about ways in which you might find more time?'

The occasions on which this type of exchange are appropriate are limitless. In an observational study (cited by Britten 2004) looking at perceptions of patient pressure, Little (2004) concluded that: 'To limit unnecessary resource use and iatrogenesis, when management decisions are not thought to be medically needed, doctors need to directly ask patients about their expectations'. Practitioners may not be trained in posing questions of this nature and may refrain from doing so for fear of causing upset or offence. However, it is crucial that such matters are addressed in order to achieve the best therapeutic outcome for the patient. Phytotherapists may not query the need to prescribe a herbal medicine as readily as might a doctor prescribing a conventional drug, since herbal medicines represent a very different scale of risk to the patient's health. Yet, the herbal practitioner still needs to be clear that herbal treatment is justifiable and exploration of patient expectations will help to clarify this.

In discussing patient-centredness, Taylor (2009) contends that:

*We must be weary of always chasing 'satisfaction' – at times the consultation may have to be uncomfortable through the need for confrontation, challenge and refusal. Our aim though should be to work together to navigate a path between collusion and confrontation, between the individual and society, between the absolute and the relative and between narrative and science.*

The consultation is not a comfort zone and the therapeutic relationship is not necessarily an easy one since, by requiring the practitioner and patient to communicate clearly and honestly, it may direct the consultation towards rough or slippery ground. Later in this chapter, we will discuss the skills, attitudes and characteristics that help to enable the therapeutic practitioner to successfully navigate such terrain. Before that we need to consider the therapeutic relationship from a perspective that includes an expanded appreciation of the significance and power of patient expectations: the placebo effect. (*Note*: Patient expectations are also discussed in Chapter 4.)

## NEW PERSPECTIVES ON THE PLACEBO EFFECT

If the interaction between practitioner and patient is capable of producing therapeutic benefits, then is this not 'just a placebo effect'? Such a question calls for clarification regarding the nature and significance of the placebo phenomenon and its role within the consultation.

*Placebo* (Latin for 'I shall please') represents a slippery notion. It is popularly understood as referring to an inert substance (e.g. a sugar pill) that can be presented to patients with a claim that it will exert certain beneficial effects (which it does not possess). If, nonetheless, the patient exhibits a response showing a degree of therapeutic benefit a *placebo effect* is said to have occurred. One reading of this transaction is that the patient has been tricked, deceived or misled so that, despite the fact that benefit may be attained, the practice of consciously using placebo 'treatments' is generally considered unethical – other than as a control in clinical trials (although even here, there are ethical questions regarding its use, see e.g. Miller & Brody 2002). It is important to distinguish between 'placebo' and 'placebo effect', particularly in light of Moerman and Jonas's (2002) assertion that: 'placebos *do not* cause placebo effects. Placebos are inert and don't cause anything' [original emphasis]. We will return to the solution offered by these authors for this conundrum in a moment.

First, let us note that the range of factors that have been considered as contributing to, or explaining, the apparent placebo effect is broad and includes: clinician–patient interaction; natural history of the condition; regression towards the mean; and social desirability (Ernst 2007). In an attempt to order and make sense of these influences, Ernst and Resch (1995) suggested that distinction should be made between 'perceived' and 'true' placebo effects. They contend that factors such as the natural course of the disease and regression to the mean constitute perceived effects, while the degree of the true placebo effect depends on a number of factors, including:

> ... the attitude of the ... therapist (towards the treatment and the patient) ... the attitude of the patient (towards his or her own health, the ... therapist, the type of treatment), on the conditioning of the patient (his or her suggestibility), and on the type of treatment (its mechanism as well as impressiveness, invasiveness, perceived plausibility, experience, cost, etc.).

In this view, the practitioner–patient relationship is considered part of the true placebo effect. The extent of the compound placebo effect is now recognized as accounting for anywhere between 0% and 100% of the therapeutic effect in a given individual case. To illustrate the breakdown of total therapeutic effect, let us suggest a case where the placebo effect accounts for 40% of therapeutic effect, the active treatment contributes 40% and other factors explain the remaining 20%. Influences arising out of practitioner–patient interactions may comprise a larger or smaller part of the total placebo and therapeutic effects depending on the particular case. Placebo effects arising from factors to do with practitioner–patient interaction may be construed as evidence supporting the notion of the therapeutic relationship. This has also been named as the 'iatrotherapeutic effect' and the 'iatroplacebogenic effect', based on *iatros*, Greek for 'doctor'.

The mechanism(s) of placebo effects cannot be fully explained by classical conditioning (i.e. Pavlovian stimulus-response learning), rather they are generally associated with psychological activity on the part of the patient in relation to expectancies, beliefs and desires. Let us return to Moerman and Jonas (2002) at this point. They cite a study where medical students were presented with placebos (inert substances) that they were told were either tranquilizers or stimulants (in reality they were neither). The placebos were provided in packets containing either one or two red or blue tablets. Responding to questions, the students identified the red tablets as stimulants, the blue tablets as depressants, and they considered that two tablets of either were stronger than one. Moerman and Jonas (2002) contend that the mechanism for these results depended on the 'meaning' that the students ascribed to the tablets: 'Red means 'up', 'hot', 'danger', while blue means 'down', 'cool', 'quiet' and … two means more than one'. They proposed using the term 'the meaning response' as being more helpful than 'the placebo effect' to describe this process and defined it as: 'the physiologic or psychological effects of meaning in the origins or treatment of illness'. Extending this idea from pills to practice, it becomes clear that awareness of the meaning content of medical encounters presents a field of opportunity for practitioners to influence patient outcomes. Moerman and Jonas describe a number of elements of practice that can be considered as *meaningful*, including therapist factors to do with their dress, manner, style and language. Such factors should be examined closely, since 'meaning has biological consequences'.

Earlier, Brody (1997a) suggested that meaning in the medical encounter consisted of at least three broad components:

1. Providing an understandable and satisfying explanation of the illness
2. Demonstrating care and concern
3. Holding out an enhanced promise of mastery or control over the symptoms.

These regions are best addressed via a narrative approach given that 'the most fundamental and pervasive way we have of assigning meaning to things is to tell stories about them'. The profound and mutual appetite for meaning shared between practitioner and patient acts as a means of generating therapeutic outcomes. Brody (1997b) underlines the fundamental nature of this key dimension of the practitioner–patient relationship in describing it thus: 'The doctor has this biologically driven need to understand, and the patient has a biologically driven need to be understood'. If practitioners do not possess, or lose, this intense epistemological desire, their power to facilitate healing in the patient is drastically undercut.

The placebo effect, then, when reinterpreted as the meaning response, can be seen to have a great deal to do with how we might appreciate and develop the therapeutic relationship. We can further suggest that the patient's perceptions and insights around meaning leads to mobilization of the self-healing response mediated through psychoneuroimmunology (PNI) pathways. Psychoemotional shifts create stimuli that help the body to self-organize, primarily through the control effects arising from interactions between the neurological, endocrine and immune systems. Benedetti and colleagues (2005) are among those who are exploring the complex physiology of this territory, seeing the placebo effect as a 'psychobiological phenomenon'. The esoteric take is contained in the aphorism that 'energy follows thought'. Mysticism and science can be sent to meet at this place: what we hold in our minds deeply influences what occurs in our bodies. How we understand our world, what we believe, how we make sense of things, how we interpret and ascribe meaning – these are key aspects shaping our total wellbeing and they represent territories that are susceptible to navigation and modulation within the consultation. Especially in the zone of case-history taking, we as practitioners are afforded the awesome opportunity to assist our patients in finding coherence – within and between the body and the world.

Yet there is a darker path that can be trodden and of which we need to be aware. The placebo effect has a disturbing counterpart, known as the 'nocebo effect' (*nocebo* means 'I shall harm'). This is a phenomenon wherein the same types of factors that can produce the positive placebo effect instead produce the negative nocebo effect, causing harm rather than benefit. The change in effect occurs when factors possessing a placebo-generating potential are manipulated in a manner that can facilitate the generation of adverse effects. An example would be the reversing of Brody's (1997a) three meaning components so that they became:

- Providing a confusing and unsatisfying explanation of the illness
- Demonstrating a lack of care and concern
- Leaving patients with a diminished sense of mastery or control over their symptoms.

Here, the practitioner's behaviour puts the patient in a state where negative results may accrue, and the nature of the practitioner–patient relationship shifts from a therapeutic to a pathological one. Awareness of the possibility for inadvertent production of the nocebo effect can serve to spur us on in our efforts to develop therapeutic liaisons with patients, and to bring it home to us that the pursuit of this goal is far from being a trivial one.

Scott and co-workers (2008) have shown that the placebo effect is connected with activation of dopaminergic processes and opioid neurotransmission, while the nocebo effect is associated with the opposite – deactivation of both of these physiological mediators – to the end that, e.g. the placebo response will tend to provide pain relief, whereas the nocebo response heightens the sensation of pain. More broadly, dopamine and opioids modulate PNI activity (immunological and neuroendocrine functions) as well as affective states, thereby potentially influencing a huge range of essential body functions and responses. While biological rationales such as this are now available, Illich's (1976) earlier discussion of these effects in terms of 'magic' remains insightful:

> *To distinguish the doctor's professional exercise of white magic from his function as an engineer (and to spare him the charge of being a quack), the term 'placebo' was created.*

In this interpretation, nocebo is a form of black magic, evidenced most notoriously by the concept of voodoo death. The physiologist, Walter B. Cannon (1957), described this phenomenon, where death was supposed to be caused by 'spells or sorcery' and, suggesting that it 'may be real', volunteered that it could be 'explained as due to shocking emotional stress – to obvious or repressed terror'. One way of interpreting this extreme example is to see it as representing a conspiracy of belief, where the malign magician believes he is able to wield fatal power; the cursed individual believes that the magician possesses such power; and the culture in which the individual resides also shares this faith. In this circuit, shared negative thought-forms driven by fear generate adverse outcomes. The opposite also obtains, with *shared positive thought-forms powered by love leading to positive outcomes* representing one working definition of the therapeutic relationship.

Illich (1976) asserted that: 'Magic works if and when the intent of patient and magician coincides'. We can suggest that at the heart of this mystery lies a mutual need to understand and find meaning.

## SETTING THE CONTEXT IN WHICH A THERAPEUTIC RELATIONSHIP CAN EMERGE: THE IMPORTANCE OF PRACTITIONER FACTORS

In the foregoing discussion we have already mentioned several factors that may help to facilitate the development of a therapeutic relationship. Chief among these are aspects to do with the practitioner's orientation, perspective, beliefs and behaviours. Hyland's concept of 'therapeutic attitude' or 'therapeutic intent' is key here. According to Carl Rogers, the core 'attitudinal conditions that foster therapeutic growth' (Rogers & Sanford 1985), not only in the psychotherapies but in other helping relationships, are: congruence, empathy and unconditional positive regard. These characteristics represent central tenets of Rogers' 'client-centred therapy' (later termed 'person-centred therapy') and, although frequently cited, they remain intriguing, tricky, potent and provocative zones for reflection.

- *Congruence*: also referred to as genuineness or realness; Rogers saw this as the most important of the three characteristics. Practitioners should not attempt to abstract themselves from the consultation but rather they should be aware of their own processes, feelings, thoughts and emotional responses during the encounter. The practitioner should be open and transparent but must exercise judgement in deciding when to express what they are experiencing back to the patient. Crucially, being congruent does not mean that the practitioner should express their thoughts and feelings completely, since this may lead to adverse effects in the client. A filter must be applied because, as Greenberg and Geller (2001) put it: 'therapeutic congruence, as well as involving awareness and transparency, also requires that the therapists' internal experience arises out of attitudes, beliefs and intentions related to doing no harm to clients and to facilitate their development. This is the psychotherapeutic equivalent of a Hippocratic Oath'.
- *Empathy*: Rogers came to consider empathy as 'a process, rather than a state' which represents a 'complex, demanding, strong yet subtle and gentle way of being' (Rogers 1975). The facets of empathy in action (adapted from Rogers 1975) include:
  - Entering the private perceptual world of the other and becoming thoroughly at home in it
  - Being sensitive to the changing felt meanings which flow in this other person
  - Temporarily living in the other's life, moving about in it delicately without making judgements, sensing meanings of which the other is scarcely aware

- Communicating your sensings of the other's world as you look with fresh and unfrightened eyes at elements of which the individual is fearful
- Frequently checking with the other as to the accuracy of your sensings, and being guided by the responses you receive
- Being a confident companion to the other person in their world
- By pointing to the possible meanings in the flow of the other's experiencing you help the person to focus on this useful type of referent, to experience the meanings more fully, and to move forward in the experiencing.

In describing empathy in this way Rogers acknowledged the influence of Gendlin's (1962) work on the relationship between experience and meaning. Gendlin coined the term 'bodily felt sense' and used it in connection with his 'focusing-oriented psychotherapy', which relates to the philosophical concept of phenomenology explored near the end of this chapter.

- *Unconditional positive regard*: Rogers (1967) described this as: 'a warm caring for the client – a caring which is not possessive, which demands no personal gratification. It is an atmosphere which simply demonstrates 'I care'; not 'I care for you if …'. It may also be considered as 'acceptance' of the patient, recognizing their intrinsic humanity.

These three zones have large areas of overlap and entanglement but, taken together, Kahn (1991) considers that Rogers' ideas constitute an unsentimental 'therapy of love'. He uses *love* here in the sense of *agape* from the Greek pairing of agape and eros. While eros 'includes the wish to possess the beloved', agape 'wants only the growth and fulfilment of the loved one' demanding nothing in return – a position of which unconditional positive regard is a reformulation.

The Rogerian view seems to fit well with our foregoing discussion in suggesting, when it comes down to it, that love and the search for meaning are the key issues in the therapeutic relationship. Other perspectives on practitioner factors that facilitate development of therapeutic relationships can be seen in the light of this contention.

Research into 'liking' in the practitioner–patient relationship fits in here, although 'liking' may seem a rather timid version of what Rogers is speaking about. Hall and colleagues (2002) found that:

> The physician's liking for the patient was positively associated with … better patient health, more positive patient affective state after the visit, more favorable patient ratings of the physician's behavior, greater patient satisfaction with the visit, and greater practitioner satisfaction with the visit.

The patient's liking for the practitioner had similarly positive correlations. The authors found a gender difference regarding practitioners, however, in that:

> Female physicians reported liking their patients more than male physicians did … Patients also reported liking female physicians more than male physicians.

Considerations regarding practitioner's attitudes and behaviours in connection with the treatments they offer arise alongside reflection on how they view and act with patients. While the interaction with patients in the consultation *is* the treatment in psychotherapy, other approaches offer an additional form of therapy – herbal medicines in the case of phytotherapists. To engender an optimally positive outcome, the phytotherapist needs to attend to the inter-relationship between themselves, the patient and the plants. At this juncture it may be helpful to return to the issue of patient expectations and aspirations, since patients will normally arrive at a phytotherapy consultation with an agenda that includes expectancies regarding herbal treatment. Coulter (2005) has provided a list of aspirations that patients have regarding what they want to obtain from conventional medical primary care services that we can use as a guide to generic patient hopes and expectations. These include:

- Fast access to reliable health advice
- Effective treatment delivered by trusted professionals
- Participation in decisions and respect for preferences
- Clear, comprehensible information and support for self-care
- Attention to physical and environmental needs
- Emotional support, empathy and respect
- Involvement of, and support for, family and carers
- Continuity of care.

Patients consulting herbal practitioners as an alternative or complementary form of primary care are likely to hold broadly similar aspirations for the clinical encounter, including the hope that any advice given will be reliable and any treatment offered effective. Practitioner behaviour with regard to advice and treatment is crucial to establishing the patient's engagement with it. In discussing the placebo effect, Harrington (1997) talked of particular practitioner characteristics and attitudes that endow them with 'curative manna', including:

- Enthusiasm for treatment
- Warm feelings for the patient
- Confidence
- Authority.

The suggestion is that in order to engender trust on the part of the patient so that advice may be taken on board and treatment complied with, the practitioner needs to be credible as an authority in their specialty; radiate confidence about their ability to prescribe and advise; and promote treatment options enthusiastically. Walach and Jonas (2004) argue that: 'If patients receive clear and positive communications conveyed with trust, credibility, and confidence, healing is more likely'. Moerman (2002) considers that the practitioner's 'demeanor activates medication, inert or otherwise' and that the most significant quality pertaining to this is its 'certainty' explained as 'a quiet assurance, a certainty, that things will turn out well'. Qualities such as enthusiasm and certainty need not be brash, but perhaps more in line with Rogers' 'being a confident companion to the other person' and offering reassurance and encouragement to the patient. Nonetheless, there may still remain a sense of tension around the seemingly conflicting exhortations for practitioners to simultaneously adapt sensitively to the patient's unique set of meanings while also confidently promoting an agenda for remediation or optimization. Phytotherapists are well equipped for this challenge however, given our emphasis on individualized treatment and the flexibility of the *materia medica* to accommodate a vast range of patient scenarios. The herbal prescription can readily be fine-tuned to meet the requirements of the patient and has dramatically greater capacity to do this than in conventional medicine, where many of the patient's subtleties cannot help but remain unaddressed by the crass nature of orthodox drugs. Walach and Jonas (2004) see the individualized approach as being fundamental to working with the meaning response: 'It is in the subtle changes to therapy and how they are delivered by a skilled healer that the meaning response is harnessed to its fullest'. Phytotherapists are also likely to experience little difficulty in being enthusiastic about treatment and letting their passion for herbal medicines shine through.

Before moving on, let us note that awareness of the power of confidence and certainty is not an especially recent insight. Although it can be traced back much further, the following perspective is interesting since it is voiced by a herbal practitioner (a doctor of the American, Eclectic school) under the heading of 'The Psychology of Doubt and Faith' – the date is 1919:

> *Doubt induces pessimism; paralyzes effort and energy; [and] conduces to uncertainty ... While doubt is deplorable, faith is absolutely essential. It makes the prescriber strong, resolute, certain. It establishes confidence on the part of the patient, and materially promotes the results desired from the remedy. Its psychic influence is of the utmost vital importance. Faith brings hope, where doubt only leads to despondency and despair*
>
> Ellingwood (1919)

Patrick Pietroni, medical doctor and proponent of the holistic approach, supplies us with one example of how an individual practitioner has responded to the challenge of working with meaning in the consultation. 'Currently', he wrote (in Pietroni 1987), 'I find myself using six separate modes or languages when faced with the task of ascribing meaning to an illness. The clinical challenge is to be able to speak clearly in each and have the skill to select which one is most appropriate for a patient.' The six modes were:

A. Medical/material/molecular: This is a 'dualistic, mechanistic and reductionist' mode where 'Meaning is pursued only insofar as it can be measured and defined in Newtonian terms', but 'Our patients are no longer satisfied with the meaning we ascribe to their illnesses by continuing to restrict ourselves in this way'.
B. Psychological/psychosomatic/psychoanalytical: Here 'physical illness is seen as the expression of a deeper disorder', where 'psychological conflict (links) with physical embodiment', although, 'As in the previous mode, the meaning of illness is still sought in the past ... in the developmental and historical relationship of early childhood or in learned behaviour and conscious conditioning'.
C. Preventive/promotional/anticipatory: This mode has to do with 'anticipatory care – the union of prevention of disease and the promotion of healthcare', where 'Illness is viewed as a consequence of a failure of

teaching and learning preventive health'. This mode 'seeks meaning through the expression of individual choice, freedom and responsibility'.
D. Cultural/social/political: Considering the patient's situation in the light of this mode reveals how the human experience of health and illness is shaped and medicalized differently between cultures and may expose the practitioner as 'trying to give meaning to a non-existent illness, when really the most important task we can perform is to pronounce that no illness exists – only life'.
E. Archetypal/metaphorical/symbolic: Here, 'the search for the meaning of illness is inexorably intertwined with that of health. Illness and health are seen not only as polarities but also similarities. Meaning is found not in linear, rational, causal explanations, but in intuitive, symbolic synchronistic ones. Health and illness are determined by the laws of nature ... For instance, nature tolerates only a limited amount of one-sidedness'. The concept of Yin and Yang, for example, applies here.
F. Space/time/energy: In this case, 'the meaning of illness is taken a step further and incorporates some of the findings of modern physics', where 'we are seen to live in a participatory world', and 'therapeutic endeavours are focused towards a collective awareness of the relativistic nature of matter and time', returning us to 'some of the oldest forms of healing that man has known'.

Writing in 1987, Pietroni's list omits evidence-based medicine (EBM) as a mode of meaning. Although it might be incorporated in mode A above, it has surely now grown sufficiently to occupy its own category. We will return to EBM later in this chapter. For now let us stay with Pietroni's list as he applies these modes to a single hypothetical case, showing how six different practitioners, each focussed on one of the above modes, might respond. His thoughts here are worth citing at length to provide us with a practical example of the meaning models that practitioners carry with them.

### THE CASE

'A 27-year old Spanish man ... with the classical symptoms and signs of duodenal ulcer .... He had left his native country after a troubled affair with his partner's wife and was unsettled and out of work in London. He was a practising Catholic and was much troubled by his affair. He was eating sporadically and drinking heavily. He had noticed an increasing inability to sit still and ... to concentrate on any one thing for any length of time.'

Practitioner's responses (what they might have done):

Physician:

A: investigated the ulcer ... and prescribed cimetidine

B: discussed the conflict experienced by the young man and explored the issues concerning his extramarital affair

C: focused ... on his diet and alcohol consumption

D: saw the plight of the single, unemployed immigrant and helped to provide stability through housing and employment

E: picked up his guilt and suggested the ulcer was symbolically 'gnawing at his insides' and helped him to repent his sin rather than psychoanalyse his symptoms

F: picked up on his 'time' disorder and assessed his energy levels, prescribing meditation and surely a group activity.

Pietroni questions whether these modes can be reconciled and identifies systems theory as offering a potential integrating framework. A key underlying consideration is that, in order to reject or combine a variety of perspectives on meaning, the practitioner must first be *aware* of them. This challenges the practitioner to make the intellectual effort required to develop multimodal ways of thinking since:

> *If we are to develop a truly holistic approach to the meaning of illness, we need to broaden our minds and increase our perception.*

Taking up this mind-expanding task poses risks, however, since it could threaten (at least initially) the practitioner's sense of certainty about, and confidence in, the best way to proceed in advising patients, thereby undermining the therapeutic relationship. Is it better, in fact, for practitioners to pursue a narrow but certain single meaning mode or to take the plural way, aware that they will constantly encounter multiple route choices as they go along? Well, the choice need not be so stark. Practitioners can work confidently utilizing and combining one or more core interpretive models that represent the basis of their practice orientation (for phytotherapists, these are likely to include vitalist, molecular, psychological and anticipatory modes) while being aware of the limits and potentials of other modes and the occasions when referral to practitioners who are centred in those modes might be desirable.

At this point, our discussion needs a shift of focus from the practitioner to the patient. When the patient's sense of meaning is placed in the foreground, a change in emphasis and activity occurs in the way that the practitioner works. The person-centred holistic practitioner can aim to hold their multiple meaning modes in abeyance as they seek to discover the patient's perspective by asking simple questions such as: 'What do you think is going on?' or 'What do you think has caused this situation?' Some patients may be conflicted or in denial about the nature of their condition but most are able to provide a sophisticated and *meaning-full* account that can form the starting point for the practitioner's search for meaning with regard to *this particular patient*. The practitioner's primary area of confidence in this way of working has to do with a sureness that the most helpful and the most ethical way of proceeding in the consultation is to attempt to appreciate and respond to the patient's predicament rather than forcing the patient to fit a pre-formed inflexible model. The position of certainty in this approach to practice is complex. Practitioners who place the patient's sense of meaning at the centre of things must open themselves up to uncertainty each time they consult, since each patient is different. Yet with experience in repeatedly doing this, an awareness of general patterns (which is shared in human experience and which helps to contextualize that which is unique) in patient situations and perspectives will develop which leads to a growing sense of comfort or ease in dealing with uncertainty that comes to be read as a confident manner. Certainty about treatment, then, arises and is deepened during the course of the consultation and not before it begins. The only certainty that exists, or is required, in advance of the consultation is sure knowledge of caring and of a personal commitment to learning from the patient. Working in the manner just described may seem like a daunting prospect, especially to students and novice practitioners, but simple curiosity will serve well here – and a keen intellectual appetite driven by the 'biological need to understand'.

Further insight into practitioner factors that might engender the therapeutic relationship can be gained through reflection on the variety of possible practitioner roles, as a complement to Pietroni's meaning modes. Ryle (1936) contended that:

> ... the physician is expected to combine in his person the attributes of scientist, healer, priest and prophet. He is suspected of some of the powers of the medicine man.

Space does not permit a full exploration of the practitioner's multiple roles or of the origin of these in the figure of the shaman (such a feat would require a large volume in its own right) but let us at least list some of them as a stimulus to reflection. The practitioner's roles, therefore, may include:

- Teacher ('doctor' from the Latin *docere*, 'to teach')
- Student (a necessary companion to the above; *physician* means 'student of nature')
- Philosopher
- Artist
- Scientist
- Priest
- Healer
- Wounded healer (the counterpart to the healer role)
- Storyteller
- Actor
- Prophet/scryer/seer (prognosis as predicting the future)
- Dream interpreter
- Trickster (playing games to get to the truth – see, e.g. Socrates and the TV detective Columbo)
- Fool (playing dumb to gain information – an aspect of the trickster).

One means of exploring these roles or archetypes that is also helpful in developing appreciation of the variety of modes of meaning and of narrative type and process is for practitioners to engage with the arts, especially literature. Scott (2000) proposes that: 'the arts can contribute to whole person understanding in at least three ways':

- Insight into common patterns of response (shared human experiences)
- Insight into individual difference or uniqueness
- Enrichment of the language and thought of the practitioner.

Reading non-medical texts in fiction, biography and history, for example, may reap the above rewards. A more specific practice that helps the development of the therapeutic practitioner is described next.

## REFLECTIVE PRACTICE: NURTURING THE 'THERAPEUTIC ATTITUDE'

'Reflective practice' is concerned with the act of taking time to be conscious of, and to consider (reflect upon) what we think, feel and do in relation to our work (practice). To many, this appears to hardly need stating: 'But everyone does that, all the time!' Such a position is not easy to defend however, it is clear that, as practitioners, we often fail to identify and to address issues that deserve our attention and which, if effectively worked through, might enhance our practice.

Two types of reflective practice are commonly identified:

1. Reflection *in* practice
2. Reflection *on* practice.

The former occurs during the act of practising and has to do with our second-by-second thoughts and decisions regarding our work. Such reflection may often be of an immediately practical nature where there is little time to entertain more complex, subtle or difficult thoughts and feelings. Reflection *on* practice occurs after the fact of practising and provides an opportunity to engage with specific issues arising out of day-to-day practice, as well as more general and philosophical questions.

Bolton (2005) has written that:

*Reflective practice ... (as a) term has lost some credence, becoming a catch-all name for a wide range of activities from deep life, work and organisation changing critique to rote box-ticking practices seeking to make professionals accountable to and controllable by increasingly bureaucratic and market-led organisations.*

Though at the more profound end of this spectrum, reflective practice can provide:

*... practical and theorised methods for understanding and grasping authority over actions, thoughts, feelings, beliefs, values and professional identity in professional, political and cultural contexts ... The paradox is that reflective practice is required by the masters, by the system. Yet its nature is essentially politically and socially disruptive: it lays open to question anything taken for granted.*

Seen from this perspective, reflective practice offers a substantially useful strategy, not only to enhance our effectiveness as practitioners, but also as a radical means of profound and dynamic personal and even organizational development. As regards the therapeutic relationship, it provides a means of identifying and making sense of issues that arise out of clinical encounters – providing a focus for intellectual activity which may, as Pietroni encouraged, 'broaden our minds and increase our perception'.

The most useful way of implementing reflective practice may be simply to become more conscious of and attuned towards our thoughts and feelings arising during and about practice, coupled with a commitment to set aside the necessary time and space to reflect upon the most interesting, disturbing, strange or wonderful of these. It amounts to us noting mentally (or on paper) experiences and questions such as:

- That didn't feel quite right, I wonder why?
- That went really well, why was that?
- Why am I not gelling with this patient?
- This patient didn't respond well when I made that comment – why?
- Why has this relationship become stagnant?

In attempting to answer these questions, we may frequently identify areas where we need to undertake some research or further reading.

The areas that most require our reflective practice are those lingering uneasy thoughts or feelings that we cannot quite shake off. To venture into these areas may require a degree of courage, as we need to admit to our shortcomings and then to do something about them. In some cases our own isolated reflection may not be enough and we may identify that we need to seek help from a colleague or another advisor. Psychotherapists generally have the benefit of supervision in this regard and this may become more commonplace outside of that field as practitioners, such as phytotherapists, seek to increase their capacity to work in psychotherapeutic territory.

## EVIDENCE-BASED MEDICINE AND THE THERAPEUTIC RELATIONSHIP

We have already introduced EBM in the previous chapter, noting that its definition has evolved to become 'the integration of best research evidence with clinical expertise and patient values' (Sackett et al. 2000). Discussions about EBM tend to highlight longstanding tensions between medical researchers and clinicians. The types of study favoured in generating and assessing evidence in EBM (randomized controlled trials, meta-analyses, systematic critical reviews) deal with people as groups rather than as individuals, whereas clinicians work with individuals not groups. Clinicians tend to generalize from the individual to the group whereas research speculates in the opposite direction, making it hard for the two camps to be fellow travellers.

Mayer and Piterman (1999) conducted a focus group study, discussing attitudes towards EBM with 27 Australian general practitioners (GPs). The authors identified that GPs had two major areas of concern regarding EBM: 'the lack of relevant research evidence in primary care and the failure of evidence-based medicine to take into account the complexity of the consultation'. The study revealed that while most of the GPs had a positive perspective on EBM they were wary as to whether evidence from clinical trials could be readily applied in individual cases and anxious that an undue emphasis on EBM might contribute towards a move away from 'the art of medicine'. One might speculate that these reservations are based on an incomplete definition of EBM, focusing on research alone and lacking the appreciation of, and integration with, 'clinical expertise and patient values'. Several quotations from the GPs in the study call for recognition of these latter aspects of EBM. Two examples are given below:

*In terms of the art of medicine, you can imagine how patients would feel if you said, 'you've got such and such ... now let's review the evidence', and you completely ignore their feelings and everything else.*

*Evidence might be that if you've got breast cancer you do such and such, but some patients, for whatever reasons, it might be that they have some other illness or they're 90 or they've got religious reasons or... it doesn't matter what the evidence says, it's just not the right thing for that person.*

To a clinician such views are obvious and common sense, but to a researcher they present a major challenge – how can EBM provide definitive answers when a multiplicity of individual factors may alter specific management plans? Here questions of what constitutes 'evidence' and how it should be applied come into play. It can be suggested that while a reductive approach to evidence may have appeal when trying to arrive at simple conclusions that aid the promotion of a drug or the design of a policy, such an approach will almost inevitably fall short when it comes to implementation with individual practitioners and patients. At this stage, within the context of the therapeutic relationship, an approach needs to be taken which reflects the richness and complexity of the factors that can play upon the development of a treatment/management plan. Williams and Garner (2002), two practising psychiatrists, have asserted that: 'the proponents of EBM oversimplify the complex nature of clinical care'. What should always be remembered, in their view, is that: '... scientific medical practice must be underpinned by the need to understand and respond empathically to the illness in accord with the patient's experiential perspective'.

The originators of the term have responded to criticisms of EBM. Haynes et al. (2002) clarified the place of patient preferences and clinical expertise in EBM by detailing the steps involved in evidence-based clinical decision-making. Their process begins with 'establishing what's wrong and what treatment options are available', then proceeds to an assessment of the research pertaining to the identified treatment options before presenting them to the patient. This third step is necessary because:

*... given the likely consequences associated with each option, the clinician must consider the patient's preferences and likely actions (in terms of what interventions she or he is ready and able to accept).*

Clinical expertise appears in the fourth and final step since it is needed to 'bring these considerations together'.

The spirit of paternalism is alive and well in this conceptualization of evidence-centred medicine. For medico-legal reasons the practitioner is forced to take the patient's views into account, but only in so far as these relate to 'options' that the practitioner has already identified. The meaning mode operating here is 'research' and leaves little place for the patient's personal sense of meaning, which, if it stands in opposition to 'the research' is likely to be considered irrational and therefore invalid.

Despite this, Greenhalgh (1999) has insisted that: 'Far from obviating the need for subjectivity in the clinical encounter, genuine evidence-based practice actually presupposes an interpretive paradigm in which the patient experiences illness in a unique and contextual way'. This is essential since:

'In reality, medical practice simply does not fit the model in which clinical encounters are reduced to undimensional problems and neatly solved by recourse to research trials and the hierarchy of evidence' (Greenhalgh 1997). She has promoted the use of the narrative-based approach (as narrative-based medicine, NBM) to the consultation in order to provide such an 'interpretive paradigm' (Greenhalgh & Hurwitz 1998) and has suggested that the term 'context-sensitive medicine' (CSM) could be used in place of EBM (Greenhalgh 1997).

Other clinicians have been highly critical of the premises and influence of EBM. Dixon and Sweeney (2000) suggest that a focus on EBM is in fact a cause of the loss of 'the personal touch' in practice and they decry the failure of EBM to learn from reflection on the placebo effect, finding it:

*... odd that modern medicine, which increasingly emphasises evidence, has failed to look at the possibility of exploiting this major effect as a means of not only making patients better but also saving on expensive modern medicines and techniques.*

They argue that:

*... there is no absolute universal notion of science, either in philosophical or historical terms, which should afford a position of unassailable centrality in clinical practice. We accept that the practice and understanding of medicine demands in part a rational appreciation and cognitive evaluation of information. But it goes beyond that to involve inextricably the self, both the practitioner's self and the patient's self. We argue that the clarity (of EBM) so appealing to politicians is illusory and disingenuous, based on an inadequate explanatory model that is predicated on linear thinking, now recognised to be inappropriate for examining the complexities and constantly evolving nature of the human condition.*

The theme of 'complexity' returns again and again as clinicians critique EBM and we will develop our sense of what this stands for in the following chapter when we will consider 'complexity theory.'

Armstrong (2002) sees EBM as representing a means of protecting the autonomy of the medical profession as a whole (by demonstrating 'unequivocally the commitment to high standards of care') at a cost of limiting the clinical freedom of individual practitioners (since they are then compelled to follow tightly drawn EBM protocols). The situation is one of 'defending collective autonomy through restricting individual freedoms' that highlights the profound tension between EBM and patient-centred medicine. Phytotherapists face a tricky task in engaging positively with research while avoiding being overtaken by an EBM agenda that would imperil the prospects for working flexibly and creatively to build therapeutic relationships with patients.

## PHENOMENOLOGY: THE FELT PRESENCE OF THE BODY IN THE MOMENT

EBM tends to have an unsettling effect on practitioners, threatening the sense of their innate gnostic ability, and causing disorientation by abstracting and externalizing the locus of authority in the consultation. Evidence-centred medicine *displaces* patient-centred medicine and *replaces* practitioner-centred medicine as (for all its proponent's protestations to the contrary) a new form of paternalism – but one that alienates both patient *and* practitioner since it originates from a disembodied database. Encouraged to think like a statistician, to place likelihood- and risk-ratios at the core of practice in a world where *'p values'* does *not* mean 'patient values', the practitioner is transformed into a technocrat – unable to deal with the intricacies and subtleties of the complex individual case but rather reduced to an agent of central-planning.

Positivist scientific research has its place, for all this, but the question is 'what place?' If EBM brings a sense of certainty to the consultation then it may, ironically, exert a significant placebo effect (see the discussion above). Perhaps, indeed, the placebogenic nature of EBM (*when* it serves to enhance practitioner confidence) may be its strongest commendation. However, attempts to impose simplistic reductionist solutions on inherently complex and mysterious patient predicaments, especially where these fly in the face of the patient's values, are more likely to create nocebo effects.

Reflection in the light of the therapeutic relationship would suggest that EBM is simply one model among many that the skilled practitioner will draw on as appropriate in particular cases. What then constitutes the *ground* on which therapeutic relationships can be built? A major candidate that might support the weight of patient and practitioner expectations is the philosophical approach known as phenomenology.

Brody (1997a) has said that:

*Biomedical science has reified 'disease' so that we often imagine it to exist as an object; but it does so only at the cost of removing from 'disease' almost all understanding of what the patient experiences phenomenologically.*

The therapeutic relationship depends on keeping sight of the patient as a person while an attempt is made to discern their 'condition.' Appreciation of the patient's experience may be substantially aided by an understanding of the phenomenological approach.

Edmund Husserl (1859–1938) is generally considered to be the founder of phenomenology, which Guerlac (2006) defines as: 'an attempt to found the truth of science in immediate lived experience'. Of the many intriguing questions posed by this project, perhaps the most central, and difficult concerns what we understand 'lived experience' to be. In his work on phenomenology and illness, Svenaeus (2000) draws on Freud and Heidegger with regard to thinking about how people experience being-in-the-world. For these thinkers, Svenaeus concludes: 'to become a human being means to be born to *Unheimlichkeit* – that is, to homelessness'. A sense of the 'unhomelikeness' of the world obtains because of an awareness pervading lived experience that 'this is my world but it is also at the same time not mine, I do not fully know it or control it'. This perception generates the duality of 'mineness' and 'otherness' and is essentially a pathology-inducing perception of the world resulting from an aberrant conceptualization of the human relationship with it – why *should* human beings expect to 'fully know' or be able to 'fully control' the world? Such beliefs reveal a psychotic bent that cannot be found in the indigenous worldview, a key central tenet of which is that people belong to the earth rather than that the earth could or should belong to people. Basso (1996) has explored the way of being-in-the-world of a particular Native American group, finding that:

> *Inhabitants of their landscape, the Western Apache are thus inhabited by it as well, and in the timeless depth of that abiding reciprocity, the people and their landscape are virtually as one.*

There is no fundamental perception of homelessness here; rather an essential awareness and certainty of *belonging* permeates the indigenous existence in the world.

Our relationship with the world determines how we see and experience our bodies. We can contend that the healthy body is one that is enmeshed in what Svenaeus calls the 'meaning patterns' of the world in such a way that the person feels *at home*, whereas 'illness can be understood as unhomelike being-in-the-world'. The 'otherness' of the sick body is experienced as 'uncanny and merciless' (Svenaeus 2000) – as 'still mine' yet 'alien'. In tackling disease, biomedicine seeks to 'fully know it' (but only as regards the anatomico-physiological dimension) and to 'control it'. Baron (1992) has reflected on why the phenomenological approach has not gained ground among conventional clinicians and has identified that this is partly due to the privileged authority given to technological ways of perceiving the body as opposed to human psycho-sensory means, to the extent that: 'the living body of the patient presents an obstruction that hides a deeper truth', one that can only be revealed by the superior capacities of machines such as MRI scanners.

Levin (1994) reminds us of Pascal's phenomenological leaning shown in the quote: 'The heart has its reasons, which reason does not know'. Levin depicts Pascal as 'disturbed by the skepticism that was beginning to take hold in the seventeenth century' and as wanting to 'argue for a logic of the heart, a discourse born of feeling, that could make sense out of connections that reason refuses to recognize'. Levin identifies Eugene Gendlin, whom we mentioned earlier, as a key modern representative of Pascal's vision. Gendlin has applied phenomenology in psychotherapy with regard to the 'bodily felt sense', which he has explained as:

> *By 'feel' we usually mean well-known emotions such as being 'scared' or 'angry'. But one can also have a very distinct feeling that has not yet opened to reveal what it contains. That is a bodily felt sense.*
>
> Gendlin (1998)

We are not talking about immediately identified emotions, but rather about actual physical sensations in the body that contain latent meaning. Gendlin says these somatic sensations are felt: 'in the viscera or the chest or the throat, some specific place usually in the middle of the body …'. The sensations occur in both practitioner and patient – the need is for practitioners to render themselves sensitive and attentive to the felt sense and to encourage the patient to do the same; and to notice when it is occurring in the patient. The effort seems to be directed towards identifying properties at the emergent stage, before they have become properties as such; detecting the flickering of something that is felt but not yet known and, by attending to it, allowing it space to hatch and disperse its meaning.

Gendlin has attempted to describe the process of this most ordinary yet mysterious experience; his effort is worth citing at length since expressions of the actual process of phenomenological activity/experiencing are rarely provided in the literature. Gendlin, though, provides us with eight characteristics of a felt sense and its unfolding for our consideration, as follows (adapted from Gendlin 1998; my emphases):

1. A felt sense forms at the border zone between conscious and unconscious:
   At various moments (in the consultation) the client will turn her attention to something implicit that she directly senses. At those moments she senses the border zone between conscious and unconscious.
2. The felt sense has at first only an unclear quality (although unique and unmistakable):
   What is sensed in this way is at first ... murky, puzzling, not fully recognisable. She can address [it] only by temporarily shelving what she had been saying or thinking. When the therapist first asks her to do this she is unwilling to let go of what she was thinking and still wanted to say ... The process moves between thinking and bodily sensing: both are required. *But to find the bodily sense she does have to turn her attention away from the old information, away from what is clear. Instead, she turns to what is felt unclearly around the clear feelings, and beneath them.*
   ... there is a time during which nothing specific emerges from the unclear felt sense. The client does not instantly discover an answer or move ahead ...
3. The felt sense is experienced bodily:
   You will also see that the sense exists bodily for the client; she is attentive to her inward physical state.
4. The felt sense is experienced as a whole, a single datum that is internally complex:
   What she discovers is a whole, a single entity. And yet, when it opens we can see that there was complexity implicit in it.
5. The felt sense moves through steps; it shifts and opens step by step:
   This shift also includes a feeling of physical relief, a bodily indication that what was said, or recognized, is directly meaningful as it emerges from the murky sense. This does not mean that what was said is ultimately true or right ... Later steps are likely to further change what now seems to be true ...
   Such a step feels good; it releases energy. What one finds may feel good or bad, but its emergence – the step of finding – always brings relief, like fresh air. This kind of effect does not make something painful more painful.
6. A step brings one closer to being that self which is not any content:
   ... although the client discovers a deep part of herself, it is not herself that she discovers. That is, she is interested in it and sympathises with it, but she remains separate from it and greater than the part that is there. In this deeper sense of oneself, the person is not the content.

7. The process step has its own growth direction:
   I believe that neither the client's nor the therapist's values made any difference here. But what emerges is not arbitrary; it has its own direction and its own values.
8. Theoretical explanations of a step can be devised only retrospectively:
   In retrospect, one can make sense of what emerges, and one can form a theory and invent logical steps that could have led to it.
   What happens in a step cannot be predicted from what is said or thought before it occurs. And although it remains logically related to the same topic, problem, or issue that brought it forward, the problem has changed from how it seemed.

Toombs (1993), in a book full of uncommon and powerful insight, has written about phenomenology from her perspective as a multiple sclerosis patient, where she found that:

*In discussing my illness with physicians, it has often seemed to me that we have been somehow talking at cross purposes, discussing different things, never quite reaching one another. This inability to communicate does not, for the most part, result from inattentiveness or insensitivity but from a fundamental disagreement abut the nature of illness. Rather than representing a shared reality between us, illness represents two quite distinct realities ...*

The origin of this 'distortion of meaning in the physician–patient relationship' lies in 'the decisive gap between lived experience and scientific explanation', which the phenomenological approach can expose and illuminate. What is revealed by it is that the practitioner's agenda is primarily concerned with the biological body, whereas the patient's experience and attention lies with disruption of the 'lived body'. For practitioners to meet patients where they are and where they are most focussed, they need to attend to the lived experience of the patient. To appreciate the differing agendas of patient and practitioner, Toombs (1993) suggests drawing a distinction between 'healing' as directed towards the 'illness-as-lived' and 'curing', which has to do with the biological emphasis of the practitioner. The complete practitioner will devote himself to both agendas.

Further insights may be yielded by a phenomenological analysis, including with reference to time-sense. Toombs (1993) refers to Husserl's work on internal time-consciousness which: 'reveals a radical distinction between lived time and objective time'. The patient's experience of time may be very different to that of the practitioner and to that measured by the clock. The very title 'patient' derives from the Latin *patientia* 'endurance' from *pati* 'to suffer'. Temporal difference is one of the features that distinguishes each patient's and each practitioner's unique 'own world' and their sense of what is meant by a 'common world'. In any encounter between a patient and a practitioner, then, at least four world views are thrown into relationship – the patient and practitioner's 'own worlds' and the notion of 'common world' particular to each party. This extends such that we cannot talk of a shared 'reality' between practitioner and patient but should rather consider the intersecting of 'realities'.

The patient's immediate experience of the 'illness-as-lived' is the initial and primal one, whereas the clinician's scientific rationale for it is derived from it by a process of abstraction and formalization. A 'decisive gap' may develop between the patient's experience of illness 'in its qualitative immediacy' and the practitioner's scientific construction of it. Although Toombs (1993) focuses on conventional medicine, we can suggest that a gap opens between patient and practitioner *wherever and whenever* the practitioner's understanding of the patient's predicament is abstracted from the patient's lived-experience – including, potentially, in any form of CAM. Regardless, the 'decisive gap' is prone to be reduced when the practitioner has had experience of significant illness – thereby providing them with insight (providing the experience is remembered and not denied) into what it means, and how it feels, to be ill. Possessing such experience may therefore be one of the most profound contributors to the development of a truly therapeutic practitioner. Spiro and Mandell (1998) consider that: 'The stories of sick doctors force emotion back into medicine, and when sick doctors themselves learn the comfort that comes from attention and devotion, empathy cannot lag far behind'.

Toombs (1993) highlights the clinical narrative as a means of appreciating the patient's lived experience of illness, and of getting at its meanings. She contrasts the conventional case history as a place where the 'voice of medicine' is prioritized with the clinical narrative, which permits the 'voice of the lifeworld' to be heard. This latter expression and registration is of critical importance since 'the act of healing *requires* an understanding of the illness-as-lived' (original emphasis). Drawing on Kleinman, Toombs (1993) asserts that in order to gain a full appreciation of the patient's perspective and of what they want from the consultation the practitioner must obtain the patient's 'explanatory model, as opposed to the biomedical explanatory model'. Key questions should concern the patient's understanding of:

- The reasons for the onset of their symptoms at a particular time
- What gave rise to the symptoms
- The expected course and perceived seriousness of the illness
- The chief way's in which the illness (or its treatment) has affected their lives
- What they fear most about the illness (or treatment).

Toombs (1993) uses the term 'the healing relationship' rather than 'the therapeutic relationship', making clear how potent the relationship is when it succeeds in meeting the patient where they are and of appreciating their lived experience. For Toombs the face-to-face nature of the consultation is important, the intimacy of shared presence in time (however perceived) and space provides the opportunity for us to 'experience one another in our individual uniqueness'. The practitioner's conceptions and intentions as they enter the encounter are crucial – a focus on 'cure' is inadequate; attention to 'healing' is also necessary and should in fact form the primary perspective for practitioners. For Toombs 'cure' implies an approach that sees the disease as an 'enemy and the patient's body as a battlefield'; further, the disease is taken to be 'residing in, but in some way separated from the one who is ill'. Healing, by comparison, is: 'directed at addressing and resolving the existential predicament of the person who is ill – at relieving (to the extent possible) the perceived lived body disruption which the illness engenders'. Crucially, while 'curing' may not always be possible, 'healing' is – even in the dying patient: it is possible to 'die healed'. Ultimately, cure and healing/science and lived experience need not be in conflict, but to bring these dualities into the right-relationship, the practitioner:

> ... must have an adequate understanding of the lived experience in order to bring to bear his or her scientific knowledge in devising effective therapy for the patient.

CAM practitioners may substitute 'healing paradigm' for 'scientific knowledge' but they are not exempted from this general requirement (and cannot be assumed to automatically fulfil it) to place the patient's lived experience at the centre of practice.

Working from a phenomenological disposition is not an easy path to take. By doing so we may, as practitioners, help to facilitate patients in accessing the felt sense of things but the meanings that emerge from this may not come readily and (as Gendlin makes clear) when they do appear they may not be 'ultimately true or right', in fact they are likely to undergo multiple revisions over time. Attention to the patient's narrative may have genuine healing effects yet, as Good (1994) points out, they are also: 'the source of contested judgments' and for 'moralizing judgments'. They may give rise to questions that neither the patient nor the practitioner can answer in any definitive way – the neatness suggested by some descriptions of the power of narrative as a sense-making tool is rarely seen in practice. Rather, as Good again tells us:

> ... efforts to bring meaning (via narrative) requires not only resort to theodicy, in Weber's terms, that is to answering 'why me?' (with an implied 'why me rather than him?'), but to the yet more fundamental soteriological issues. What is the nature of this suffering? What is the moral order that makes sense of it? What are the sources for hope to go forward in this context?

Operating in this territory stimulates us to recall the potential practitioner roles described earlier, especially that of philosopher–priest.

Phytotherapists stand as exposed to the challenges posed by the phenomenological approach as practitioners of any other modality but one particular aspect of our practice bestows something of an advantage. This lies in connection with at least some of the explanatory models we use to make sense of the patient's predicament. While Toombs (1993) has contrasted the patient's personal explanatory model with that of the doctor's biological model, other perspectives are possible. Phytotherapists tend to use the biological model alongside others such as traditional perspectives that appreciate the patient's experience in terms of hot–cold, excessive demands, nervous exhaustion, energy depletion, psychological stress, spiritual crisis, and so forth. These interpretations usually provide a much closer fit with the patient's experience since they constitute authentic phenomenological readings of the dimensions and features of illness which tend to be readily appreciated by, and are acceptable to, the patient.

Since the phytotherapist's and the patient's explanatory rationales frequently overlap the patient may feel more at home in the phytotherapy consultation – and, by extension, perhaps in the wider world.

## THE RELEVANCE OF THE THERAPEUTIC RELATIONSHIP IN PHYTOTHERAPY: WEAVING THE LOOSE THREADS

Let me restate my general case, which is that phytotherapy offers a potent means of combining both medicinal (pharmacological) effects with human (psychotherapeutic) effects. Which of these predominates? Well, that will depend on the individual case, but we can assert that herbal medicines *do* have effects that are independent of the placebo effect and of the healing generated by the therapeutic relationship. Anybody who seriously doubts this need only devote a moment's reflection to whether they would, if offered one, be prepared to drink a cup of hemlock or belladonna tea.

Let us return to Hyland (2005), who compared CAM therapies and psychotherapies and concluded that:

> *The evidence leads to the conclusion that the personality of the therapist has a therapeutic effect on the patient. This human effect seems to be the most important aspect of both psychotherapy and CAM, and is certainly greater than the specific effects that therapists believe they are delivering. It is not the skill of technical delivery, but the person that matters.*

Although this particular analysis was limited to CAM and psychotherapies Hyland adds that:

> *… it is evident that the argument applies to all therapists, including physicians. The fact that physicians achieve genuine specific effects in their therapy may obscure the very real therapeutic effects that are mediated via the therapist.*

There are difficulties of generalization in this analysis arising from the implication that conventional medicine has specific (i.e. non-placebo generated) effects on patient health but CAM does not. Earlier in his paper, however, Hyland acknowledges that specific treatment effects have been shown for herbal medicines. There is no justification therefore for suggesting that it is a feature of *all* so-called CAM therapies that they possess no specific effects. The insistence on this point is important in light of the previous discussion of practitioner certainty and confidence – the practitioner *must believe* that their tools work. It is at this point of realization that practitioners may be wary of exploring the placebo effect and the therapeutic relationship in any greater depth lest the journey ends in a crisis of confidence in the potency of their chosen modality. Happily, phytotherapists can rest easy, absolutely certain in the knowledge that herbs *really* do work …

In addition to phytochemicals, however, herbs are also packed full of 'meaning'; a circumstance that provides an extra dimension of therapeutic effect, as Moerman and Jonas (2002) explain:

> *… as we have clarified, routinized, and rationalized our medicine, thereby relying on the salicylates and forgetting about the more meaningful birches, willows, and wintergreen from which they came – in essence, stripping away Plato's 'charms' – we have impoverished the meaning of our medicine to a degree that it simply doesn't work as well as it might anymore.*

As patient expectations change regarding the qualities that they desire of medicines – especially under the influence of growing ecological imperatives – the origins, mechanisms and significances that attach to herbal medicines become ever more evident and ever more *therapeutic*. As the meanings that herbs possess become cherished, so they become more potent. Although I will maintain (and of course, as a herbal practitioner, I *must*) that herbal medicines have always possessed specific effects, we can nonetheless allow that such effects may become more apparent to the degree that they become more highly valued.

We have made the case in this chapter for a fundamental connection between the therapeutic relationship and the pursuit of meaning. Earlier, Brody (1997a) suggested that meaning in the medical encounter could be generated by three broad strategies:

- Providing an understandable and satisfying explanation of the illness
- Demonstrating care and concern
- Holding out an enhanced promise of mastery or control over the symptoms.

Phytotherapists are well positioned to meet all of these requirements. The first is met by sensitivity to the patient's explanatory model and flexibility in the use of multiple explanatory rationales on the part of the practitioner, emphasizing ones that readily fit the patient's lived experience of illness. The second arises from the herbal practitioner's patient-centred focus and is expanded to the extent that the practitioner operates from a position of holding unconditional positive regard for the patient. The third is realized not only by the vast and complex scope of the herbal *materia medica* but also by recourse to a range of accompanying strategies that the practitioner may deploy to promote healing – we shall consider some of these in the next chapter.

## REFERENCES

Agich GJ: Scope of the therapeutic relationship. In Shelp EE, editor: *The clinical encounter: the moral fabric of the patient-physician relationship*, London, 1983, Kluwer.

Armstrong D: Clinical autonomy, individual and collective: the problem of changing doctors' behaviour, *Social Science and Medicine* 55:1771–1777, 2002.

Baron RJ: Why aren't more doctors phenomenologists? In Leder D, editor: *The body in medical thought and practice*, London, 1992, Kluwer Academic.

Basso KH: *Wisdom sits in places*, 1996, University of New Mexico Press.

Benedetti F, Mayberg HS, Wagner TD, et al: Neurobiological mechanisms of the placebo effect, *Journal of Neuroscience* 25(45):10390–10402, 2005.

Bolton G: *Reflective practice: writing and professional development*, London, 2005, Sage.

Brody H: The doctor as therapeutic agent: a placebo effect research agenda. In Harrington A, editor: *The placebo effect: an interdisciplinary approach*, 1997a, Harvard University Press.

Brody H: Placebo: conversations at the disciplinary borders. In Harrington A, editor: *The placebo effect: an interdisciplinary approach*, 1997b, Harvard University Press.

Britten N: Patients' expectations of consultations: patient pressure may be stronger in the doctor's mind than in the patient's, *British Medical Journal* 328: 416–417, 2004.

Cannon WB: 'Voodoo' death, *Psychosomatic Medicine* 19(3):182–190, 1957.

Chew-Graham CA, May CR, Roland MO: The harmful consequences of elevating the doctor-patient relationship to be a primary goal of the general practice consultation, *Family Practice* 21:229–231, 2004.

Coulter A: Paternalism or partnership? *British Medical Journal* 319:719–720, 1999.

Coulter A: What do patients and the public want from primary care? *British Medical Journal* 331:1199–1201, 2005.

Dixon M, Sweeney K: *The human effect in medicine: theory, research and practice*, Oxford, 2000, Radcliffe Medical Press.

Ellingwood F: *American Materia Medica: therapeutics and pharmacognosy*, Portland, 1919, Eclectic Medical Publications.

Emanuel EJ, Emanuel LL: Four models of the physician-patient relationship, *Journal of the American Medical Association* 267:2221–2226, 1992.

Ernst E, Resch KL: Concept of true and perceived placebo effects, *British Medical Journal* 311:551–553, 1995.

Ernst E: Placebo: new insights into an old enigma, *Drug Discovery Today* 12(9/10): 413–418, 2007.

Ernst DB, Pettinati HM, Weiss RD, et al: An intervention for treating alcohol dependence: relating elements of Medical Management to patient outcomes with implications for primary care, *Annals of Family Medicine* 6(5):435–440, 2008.

Fulder S: *The handbook of alternative and complementary medicine*, ed 3, 1996, Oxford University Press.

Gendlin ET: *Experiencing and the creation of meaning*, New York, 1962, The Free Press.

Gendlin ET: *Focusing-oriented psychotherapy: a manual of the experiential method*, New York, 1998, The Guilford Press.

Goldacre B: *Bad Science*, London, 2008, Fourth Estate Ltd.

Good BJ: *Medicine, rationality and experience: an anthropological perspective*, 1994, Cambridge University Press.

Gordon JS: Holistic medicine: advances and shortcomings, *Western Journal of Medicine* 136:546–551, 1982.

Greenberg LS, Geller SM: Congruence and therapeutic presence. In Wyatt G, editor: *Congruence: Rogers' therapeutic conditions; evolution, theory and practice*, Ross-on-Wye, 2001, PCCS Books.

Greenhalgh T, Worrall JG: From EBM to CSM: the evolution of context-sensitive medicine, *Journal of Evaluation in Clinical Practice* 3(2):105–108, 1997.

Greenhalgh T, Hurwitz B, editors: *Narrative based medicine: dialogue and discourse in clinical practice*, London, 1998, BMJ Books.

Greenhalgh T: Narrative based medicine: narrative based medicine in an evidence based world, *British Medical Journal* 318:323–325, 1999.

Guerlac S: *Thinking in time: an introduction to Henri Bergson*, 2006, Cornell University Press.

Hall JA, Horgan TG, Stein TS, et al: Liking in the physician–patient relationship, *Patient Education and Counseling* 48:69–77, 2002.

Harrington A: Introduction. In Harrington A, editor: *The placebo effect: an interdisciplinary approach*, 1997, Harvard University Press.

Haynes RB, Devereaux PJ, Guyatt GH: Physicians' and patients' choices in evidence based practice: evidence does not make decisions, people do, *British Medical Journal* 324:1350, 2002.

Hyland MA: Tale of two therapies: psychotherapy and complementary and alternative medicine (CAM) and the human effect, *Clinical Medicine* 5(4): 361–367, 2005.

Illich I: *Limits to medicine – medical nemesis: the expropriation of health*, London, 1976, Marion Boyars.

Kaba R, Sooriakumaran P: The evolution of the doctor-patient relationship, *International Journal of Surgery* 5:57–65, 2007.

Kahn M: *Between therapist and client: the new relationship*, New York, 1991, WH Freeman and Co.

Kelner M, Wellman B: Introduction. In Kelner M, Wellman B, Pescosolido B, Saks M, editors: *Complementary and alternative medicine: challenge and change*, Newark, 2000, Harwood Academic.

Kiecolt-Glaser JK, McGuire L, Robles TF, et al: Psychoneuroimmunology: psychological influences on immune function and health, *Journal of Consulting and Clinical Psychology* 70(3):537–547, 2002.

Levin DM: Making sense: the work of Eugene Gendlin, *Human Studies* 27: 343–353, 1994.

Little P, Dorward M, Warner G, et al: Importance of patient pressure and perceived pressure and perceived medical need for investigations, referral, and prescribing in primary care: nested observational study, *British Medical Journal* 328:444, 2004.

McWhinney IR: The importance of being different, *British Journal of General Practice* 46:433–436, 1996.

McWhinney IR, Epstein RM, Freeman TR: Lingua medica: rethinking somatization, *Annals of Internal Medicine* 126(9):747–750, 1997.

Maslach C: Job burnout: new directions in research intervention, *Current Directions in Psychological Science* 12(5):189–192, 2003.

Mayer J, Piterman L: The attitudes of Australian GPs to evidence-based medicine: a focus group study, *Family Practice* 16(6):627–632, 1999.

Mead N, Bower P: Patient-centredness: a conceptual framework and review of the empirical literature, *Social Science and Medicine* 51:1087–1110, 2000.

Miller FG, Brody H: What makes placebo-controlled trials unethical? *American Journal of Bioethics* 2(2):3–9, 2002.

Moerman D: *Meaning, medicine and the 'placebo effect'*, 2002, Cambridge University Press.

Moerman DE, Jonas WB: Deconstructing the placebo effect and finding the meaning response, *Annals of Internal Medicine* 136:471–476, 2002.

Moynihan R, Smith R: Too much medicine? *British Medical Journal* 324:859–860, 2002.

Nettleton S: *The sociology of health and illness*, Cambridge, 2006, Polity.

Parsons T: *The social system*, London, 1951, Routledge & Kegan Paul Ltd.

Pietroni P: The meaning of illness – holism dissected: discussion paper, *Journal of the Royal Society of Medicine* 80:357–360, 1987.

Plato: *Charmides* (West TG, West GS, trans.), Cambridge, MA, 1986, Hackett Publishing Company.

Rogers C: *Client-centred therapy: its current practice, implications and theory*, Edinburgh, 1951, Constable.

Rogers CR: *On becoming a person: a therapist's view of psychotherapy*, Edinburgh, 1967, Constable.

Rogers C: Empathic: an unappreciated way of being, *The Counseling Psychologist* 5:2–10, 1975.

Rogers CR, Sanford RA: Client-centered psychotherapy. In Kaplan HI, Sadock BJ, Friedman AM, editors: *Comprehensive textbook of psychiatry*, ed 4, London, 1985, William and Wilkins.

Rogers C, Freiberg HJ: *Freedom to learn*, Princeton, 1994, Merrill.

Ryle JA: *The natural history of disease*, 1936, Oxford University Press.

Sackett DL, Strauss SE, Richardson WS, et al: *Evidence-based medicine: how to practice and teach EBM*, Edinburgh, 2000, Churchill Livingstone.

Scott PA: The relationship between the arts and medicine, *Journal of Medical Ethics: Medical Humanities* 26:3–8, 2000.

Scott DJ, Stohler CS, Egnatuk CM, et al: Placebo and nocebo effects are defined by opposite opioid and dopaminergic responses, *Archives of General Psychiatry* 65(2):220–231, 2008.

Sharma U: The equation of responsibility: complementary practitioners and their patients. In Budd S, Sharma U, editors: *The healing bond: the patient-practitioner relationship and therapeutic responsibility*, London, 1994, Routledge.

Spiro H, Mandell H: When doctors get sick, *Annals of Internal Medicine* 128(2):152–154, 1998.

Svenaeus F: The body uncanny: further steps towards a phenomenology of illness, *Medicine, Health Care and Philosophy* 3:125–137, 2000.

Szasz TS, Hollender MH: A contribution to the philosophy of medicine: the basic models of the doctor-patient relationship, *AMA Archives of Internal Medicine* 97(5):585–592, 1956.

Taylor K: Paternalism, participation and partnership: the evolution of patient centeredness in the consultation, *Patient Education and Counselling* 74:150–155, 2009.

Toombs SK: *The meaning of illness: a phenomenological account of the different perspectives of physician and patient*, London, 1993, Kluwer Academic.

Walach H, Jonas WB: Placebo research: the evidence base for harnessing self-healing capacities, *Journal of Alternative and Complementary Medicine* 10(1):103–112, 2004.

Williams DDR, Garner J: The case against 'the evidence': a different perspective on evidence-based medicine, *British Journal of Psychiatry* 180:8–12, 2002.

# Aims and structure of the consultation

**3**

**CHAPTER CONTENTS**

**Concerning aims** 80
**Interim thoughts** 90
**Notions of health and illness** 91
**Engendering wellbeing** 98
    *Accept the gift of one's own symptoms* 100
    *If you feel 'dis-ease' ask yourself 'why?'* 101
    *Your illness is your teacher* 101
    *Observe your own behaviour – what does it signify?* 101
    *Be able to decline a request* 101
    *Be able to receive as well as give* 102
    *Speak your fears to another* 102
    *Avoid creating expectations that generate pain* 102
    *Shift your perspective* 102
    *Make space for silence and reflection* 103
    *Doing things is easy: getting round to doing them is the issue* 103
    *Distinguish between excuses and reasons* 103
    *Listen to the stories you tell about yourself* 103
    *Cultivate happiness (tend your personal relationships like you would a garden)* 104
    *Cultivate a relationship with nature* 105
    *Choose BIG MIND over small mind* 106
    *Challenges are inevitable but upset is optional* 106
    *Listen to your heart* 106
    *Cultivate an attitude of openness to change (since too much order is dangerous)* 107
    *Choose love over fear* 107
    *Seek novel experiences* 109
    *Be a lifelong learner* 109
    *Exercise your senses* 110
    *Look to your death* 111
    *Be able to surrender* 111
    *Be open-minded, open-hearted and open-handed* 112
    *Walk through life as if it were a labyrinth not a maze* 112
    *Balance activity and rest across the four aspects of being: physical, emotional, mental, spiritual* 112

*Remember that your body believes every word you say* 112
*Energy follows thought* 112
**The practitioner as teacher** 113
**The setting for the consultation** 113
**The structure of the consultation** 116
  Outline format for an initial consultation 116
  Outline format for follow-up consultations 116
**The consultation as labyrinth** 119
**Complexity and the consultation** 124
  Acknowledgements 129

## CONCERNING AIMS

If we state that the overarching aim of the phytotherapy consultation is to arrive at an enhanced understanding of the patient's predicament in order to be better positioned to offer ease in coping with it – that tells us little that is distinctive about phytotherapy, since all healthcare modalities could commit to such a goal. We might go further and claim that the guiding driver of the consultation is a notion of health in its three-fold nature: prevention of deviation from health, remedy of current flaws in health and optimization of wellbeing. That is to say that the phytotherapist has her mind on these three potentials during the consultation:

1. Which avenues can be glimpsed from the main street of the consultation that suggest the need for preventive action?
2. Which are the pressing issues that may be susceptible to, or which urgently require, treatment?
3. How might this person's health and wellbeing be improved overall?

Yet again, however, one is unlikely to find a healthcare approach that would not recognize the need to focus on these three personas of health, although one could debate the degree to which each actually addressed these in practice and achieved success in attaining them.

There may in fact be little that is distinctive in terms of the overall aims of the phytotherapy consultation, broadly stated, in comparison with other healthcare modalities. This should not surprise us since all such modalities will be able to subscribe to global statements about the aims, not just of the consultation, but regarding the intentions of their overall approach. Differences in emphasis and outcome emerge only when more detailed scrutiny is made of the individual therapy – its ethos, practice, scope, nature and culture. Analysis of these individual tints and twists generate the prospect not only of revealing difference but also of showing deviance from the dominant medical model. While both conventional and CAM therapies may be able to sign up to a campaign slogan summarizing the aims of 'good healthcare', the detail of a joint manifesto on how to deliver this might be fiercely debated.

The directional tendencies of the consultation in any healing modality will be largely shaped by the capacities and capabilities of the particular *therapy* being practised. This generalized orientation is then further specified by the personal beliefs and qualities of the *therapist* and in light of the particular expectations, wishes and predicament of the *patient*. In focusing on the former of these three territories we can assert that the distinguishing features of phytotherapy that influence the aims and process of the consultation have to do, in great part, with the nature and properties of herbs themselves. These include:

- The complex chemistry of herbs which enables them to act on multiple levels and aspects of the patient's being
- The non-linear nature of plant medicines which means they act more like networks exerting broad systems effects rather than 'magic bullets' hitting precise and predictable targets
- The vast scope and capacity to formulate helpful strategies drawn from the *materia medica* due to the hundreds of herbs used and the large number of potential herb combinations that can be generated
- The tendency of herbs to work subtly, gently and cumulatively
- The tendency of the prescription to adapt, change or evolve from consultation to consultation rather than remaining a fixed entity
- The tremendous plasticity and adaptability of herbs to meet patient requirements in terms of the type of external and internal applications that can be prescribed (teas, tinctures, creams, lotions, liniments, syrups, baths, inhalations, rubs, gargles, paints, tablets, capsules, pills, compresses, poultices, plasters, etc.)
- The ability of herbs to:
  - Exert thermal and other core effects such as cooling or warming, moistening or drying
  - Tonify or restore organs and tissues
  - Stimulate or relax physiological functions
  - Enhance vital functions such as immunity.

Such treatment potentialities need to be reflected and embodied in the structure and practice of the consultation so that there is a harmony and integrity between the two, and in order that the consultation process may lead to the most appropriate and effective treatment outcomes. The aims and processes of the consultation in any modality are fundamentally shaped by the therapeutic tools and strategies that the particular modality makes available. The consultation is usually directed to the possible outcomes that such tools and strategies will allow. If the therapeutic options are narrow, then this will tend to be reflected in the consideration of the patient in terms of the consultation.

Some of the echoes and resonances from the above list that reverberate in the phytotherapy consultation, and which represent consultation practices formed by plant potentials, include:

- Recognizing, and working with, the patient's inherent complexity and the complex nature of the processes of the consultation
- Embodying the principle of non-linearity in a flexible approach and ability to follow the patient's lead in a flowing consultation style

- Excitement and experimentation in the creative engagement with the huge range of patient predicaments that herbal medicine can potentially aid
- Openness to embracing and working with change in the patient's condition over time
- Attention to subtle detail, markers and outcomes
- Attention to non-conventional factors such as whether a condition is hot or cold and whether a function needs to be tonified, protected or strengthened.

A key theme here is that of complexity. There have been a number of publications by conventional medical practitioners in recent years exploring the implications of complexity and chaos theories for medical care (e.g. Plsek 2002; Holt 2004; Sweeney 2006). Although many of these publications are excellent and offer groundbreaking insights, few of the authors have noted and explored the issue of the inherently linear, non-complex nature of conventional drugs themselves. Non-linear drugs (such as antibiotics) have awesome capacities to provide rapid healing effects in specific conditions at specific points in time, yet they possess profound limitations. Conventional medicine has limited success and may be counterproductive or cause harm in many complex conditions. It is also the simple chemical nature of orthodox drugs that is their Achilles heel, e.g. in antibiotics where the absence of molecular complexity enables the development of microbial resistance. Conventional medical practitioners seeking to embrace the implications of complexity and chaos theories and to use pharmacologic agents that are complex and chaotic in nature would be well advised to train in phytotherapy since their ability to work in this way is limited by the nature and capacities of the conventional *materia medica*.

Herbal medicines offer genuine and exciting potentials as agents of preventive medicine and as modulators of physiological response, leading to optimizing of critical functions, as well as being effective remedies to treat many established conditions. Some key herbs can work across these three aspects, e.g. *Echinacea* spp. (cone flower) can modulate and enhance immune function (leading to both preventive and optimizing results) as well as being a treatment for upper respiratory tract viral infections. Other plant agents can initiate or exert broad dynamic responses in the body that lead to generalized complex and chaotic effects – the results of which are not specifically predictable but rather cause general healing trends that may produce unpredictable, yet positive, effects. An example of this would be circulatory stimulating herbs such as *Zingiber officinale* (ginger) which can enhance blood flow (and hence improve the rate and efficiency of gaseous exchange; delivery of nutrients, hormones, clotting factors, immune cells; removal of waste products of metabolism, etc.) to a range of tissues and organs leading to modulation of systems performance and global changes in physiology and health/illness. A second example would be within the class of herbs known as adaptogens which enhance physical and mental performance, endurance and stamina and protect from the effects of stress – whether physical, psychological or environmental. One of the most famous herbs in this category is *Panax ginseng* (Chinese or Korean ginseng), which is able to trigger such broad and complex consequences in part due to its propensity to increase the generation of ATP within cells, therefore modulating cellular performance. By influencing ATP generation in multiple cells complex and chaotic changes arise leading to the emergence of new properties or qualities within the body's integrated physiological processing.

We will return to more fully consider the ideas and assertions developing here around complexity and chaos, towards the end of this chapter. For now let us propose that phytotherapists have good cause to enter into the consultation process optimistically, with a realistic expectation that they may, on its conclusion, be able to proceed in the majority of cases to offering a herbal intervention that is capable of helping the patient to achieve greater ease at least, and frequently much more than this. Such positivity can energize the consultation and is likely to exert a healing influence in its own right (see the discussion on placebo in Ch. 2).

Let us shift focus at this stage, however, to consider a negative perspective on the question of the aims of the consultation. This would seek to identify the potentialities that are undesirable and therefore which we should consciously avoid generating within the consultation. Chief among these would be to avoid misunderstanding the patient in order to subsequently escape giving inappropriate advice and treatment that might fail to provide benefit where benefit is otherwise possible or, at worst, actually harm the patient. Awareness of the capacity for iatrogenesis (harm caused to the patient by the practitioner or by treatment) is an essential part of the make up of the advanced practitioner. The weight of this vital appreciation should not oppress the practitioner; rather a nuanced realization of its dimensions and implications can act as an anchor to provide grounding amidst the powerful currents of the flow of the consultation. While most practitioners have an understanding of the notion of clinical iatrogenesis, Illich (1976) has identified two other, less recognized, facets of the problem – social iatrogenesis and cultural iatrogenesis. By 'social iatrogenesis', Illich means: '… a term designating all impairments to health that are due precisely to those socioeconomic transformations which have been made attractive, possible or necessary by the institutional shape health care has taken'. For example, social iatrogenesis:

> … *obtains when medical bureaucracy creates ill-health by increasing stress, by multiplying disabling dependence, by generating new painful needs, by lowering the levels of tolerance for discomfort or pain, by reducing the leeway that people are wont to concede to an individual when he suffers, and by abolishing even the right to self-care …. when all suffering is 'hospitalised' and homes become inhospitable to birth, sickness, and death; when the language in which people could experience their bodies is turned into bureaucratic gobbledegook; or when suffering, mourning, and healing outside the patient role are labelled a form of deviance.*

It would be an error to see this type of iatrogenesis as being limited to institutionalized mainstream medicine. CAM practitioners are not exempt from accepting particular dominant ideas, practices and values as normative and therefore the 'correct' or 'right' ways of thinking or acting. For example, women who breastfeed long-term (for years rather than months) may be considered deviant by practitioners from any field who are unaware that in ancient indigenous cultures it is usual to breastfeed for 3–5 years and that, not only does this seem to have been the norm for our species until very recent times, but additionally a number of benefits have been shown for both mother and child accruing from such a duration of feeding. It is plausible to suggest that, since CAM courses are now increasingly provided by conventional academic institutions, CAM students and graduating practitioners are likely to take on the normative values and concepts fostered by institutions of the state to a greater degree than before. We are therefore likely to see an increased blurring between so-called conventional and alternative medical thought than in recent decades. There are few signs yet that the direction of this thought is moving substantially to a more holistic take. The cries of many a disgruntled academic and social commentator that CAM courses do not properly belong in the state's learning centres and that if they are to persist there they must be subject to the correcting influence of 'science' do not help to foster an environment where open philosophical discussion can occur.

Illich considers that cultural iatrogenesis:

> … sets in when the medical enterprise saps the will of people to suffer their reality. It is a symptom of such iatrogenesis that 'suffering' has become almost useless for designating a realistic human response because it evokes superstition, sadomasochism, or the rich man's condescension to the lot of the poor. Professionally organised medicine has come to function as a domineering moral enterprise that advertises industrial expansion as a war against all suffering. It has thereby undermined the ability of individuals to face their reality, to express their own values, and to accept inevitable and often irremediable pain and impairment, decline and death.

This deeper insight calls into question the global positive aims of the consultation that we began with. To what extent, and in which ways, is it possible and even desirable to give ease? Are we correctly oriented if our focus is on 'health', its optimization, and the prevention or remedying of any deviance from its true path? Such questions lead us into a critique of the notions of health and suffering which we will attempt to sketch later in this chapter. At this point it is worth pausing to consider the breadth of Illich's conception of iatrogenesis and let sink-in the implications for practitioners if we wish to minimize the risk of causing harm to, or hindering the free-expression and development of, patients. While clinical iatrogenesis (the risk of causing harm due to medical procedures and treatments) seems a relatively clear and straightforward concept (though arguably deceptively so) for practitioners to address and work with, the social and cultural forms of iatrogenesis are much more subtle, complex and challenging to connect with. In attempting to learn about, and from, these latter two forms of iatrogenesis the practitioner is required to engage at an advanced level of scrutiny of self, environment, society and culture. A philosophical and political engagement with these territories is necessary. The exercise of reflective practice is perhaps the most powerful tool we have to work in this way but the suggestion of the need for advanced practitioners to be fully-faceted resurfaces here. The pluralist philosopher–physician may be equipped to take up the gauntlet thrown down by Illich. Any lesser intellectual engagement with the fascinating challenges of attempting to tread Illich's iatrogenesis labyrinth limits the practitioner's ability to make progress on the patient's behalf and arrests development at the level of technician. This is not to denigrate the value of the technical aspects of healthcare but to flag the limits and dangers inherent when technical aspects are not informed by the broader, deeper contextualization that may be achieved by a critical engagement with influences and issues on the grandest scale. The cultivation of such a wide-ranging view may not be a goal for everyone, yet the practice of medicine is a traditional home suited to those who require a non-abstract laboratory in which to explore the meaning of life. Joseph Needham (1948) commented on the restrictions placed by conventional science on diverse intellectual exploration and got to the nub of the radical nature of those who refuse such limitations in an essay first published in 1941:

> *Even today there are many professional scientists who look askance at the action of a colleague who dares to speak out from time to time on general topics ... The overt rationalization of this feeling is that a scientific worker can hardly be thought to have sufficient intellectual energy for his scientific work unless he is careful to use none outside it ... But the real meaning of this feeling is that to enquire too curiously into the structure of the world and society and the history of society is potentially a menace to the stability of society. The innocent scientist who harbours no 'dangerous thoughts' is a far more wholesome member of the community (from the point of view of its de facto rulers) than the scientist who prefers to prowl ... I am glad to confess that ... I have always been a prowler, an explorer, among ideas.*

Such prowling can only be driven by passion and desire, a hunger for knowledge and connection. In this sense the health practitioner, while striving to help the patient find meaning in their individual predicament, is simultaneously searching for meaning in her own appreciation of the world. The practice of medicine (by which I mean any type of healing modality) in this conception, is intimately part of and indeed is a central strategy in the practitioner's own development as a person, seeking to make sense of the world and to make a helpful contribution towards suffering humanity.

We have already emphasized the extraordinary potential of herbal medicine to play a fundamental role in enabling positive patient outcomes. Yet there are limits as to the degree to which any form of medicine can help relieve and transform suffering. Each practitioner must gain an informed perspective on this if they are to cope with feeling for the suffering of their fellows and in order to be maximally useful to them in their situation. The conventional view of suffering in the modern west is an entirely negative one – suffering has no purpose or redeeming features and is always to be eliminated. This perspective stands in the shadow of the spectre of the modern western secular view of death. Death is the end, oblivion – nothing survives it. Death is the ultimate enemy of life therefore and must be resisted and fought at all costs – as must any form of suffering, which is the intimater of mortality. Of course a healthcare system or medical approach that is founded on conquering death is setting a hard target to achieve! Standing in opposition to death is a flawed ground for working with patient's health challenges. The practitioner must therefore gain a perspective on death too.

Let us return to Ivan Illich at this point and recall that he was a Roman Catholic priest. A key feature of religions and other spiritual belief systems is that they offer a perspective on death. Illich (1976) points out that:

> *The major religions reinforce resignation to misfortune and offer a rationale, a style, and a community setting in which suffering can become a dignified performance. The opportunities offered by the acceptance of suffering can be differently explained in each of the great traditions: as karma accumulated through past incarnations; as an invitation to Islam, the surrender to God; or as an opportunity for close association with the Saviour on the Cross.*

A large body of (contentious) research is now available on the healing influence of faith and prayer. The benefits arising from faith and related practices seem in large part to relate to the elements we can pick out from Illich's statement above:

- Rationale (arriving at meaning)
- Style (methods of coping)
- Community setting (support and sense of belonging)
- Dignity (self-worth/self-value).

The particular article of faith may be less important than the act of faith itself since any belief system may potentially furnish these elements of healing which help one to make sense of and gain some control over suffering as well as decreasing the loneliness and isolation that tend to accompany suffering.

For Rosenberg (1998), Illich's thinking represents: 'a different realm of holism, the explicitly religious and mystical'. He argues that, while this type of holistic approach is shared by some of those involved in biomedical work and has shaped some branches of conventional medicine, it is not integral to it:

> *Spiritual commitment is not explicitly a part of medical thought – even though it has been a fundamental component in the shaping of modern health care institutions and a significant factor in the determining of individual medical careers and worldviews.*

Impulses and insights of a 'religious, mystical, spiritual' nature are accorded value as influences on medical thought and practice but they are far from being seen as central. One calls to mind the little hospital chapel, lost somewhere within the brutal maze of medical architecture.

Illich has been criticized for the alleged extremism of his position in placing individual autonomy and self-care at the centre of 'medicine' and for according little space to modern technological biomedicine. Greaves (1996) asserts that:

> *Imbuing the individual with a vital autonomy sufficient to ensure his own health is not only implausible, but confers grave disadvantages … Most notably the endurance of suffering and pain becomes viewed by Illich as ennobling in itself, even forming part of the definition of a healthy life: and death is seen as better than a life lived through reliance on medicine. While Illich may hold such personal values, there would seem no good reason for claiming that others should share them.*

This is a (uncharacteristically for Greaves) crude analysis, since there lies implicit within it the suggestion that biomedicine has the capacity to relieve all types of suffering and pain and that the notion of living through reliance on medicine is generally non-contentious. The first of these implicit suggestions is obviously unsustainable and the second palls when we consider, e.g. the debate about euthanasia in the aspect of the withdrawal of life-perpetuating medical treatment. For most people, the matter for reflection is not a stark choice between absolute rejection or total acceptance of biomedicine but rather a nuanced consideration of the available options and how they might be combined, including self-care, community care, conventional medical services and CAM approaches.

Certainly, some working in conventional medicine are questioning the limits of biomedicine and identifying its insufficiencies. In a *Lancet* Editorial (2009), the successes of the National Health Service in the UK are acknowledged before reflecting that:

*Infectious diseases, seemingly conquered by antibiotics and vaccination, have resurged. The pain and decrepitude of chronic illness are widespread. Industrial injuries have largely been replaced by the illnesses of unemployment and despair – chronic pain, depression and substance abuse.*

Considering how to move forward from this position, the Editorial continues:

*… perhaps we need to ask what health is, and how to achieve it. Do mechanical and material models adequately capture health, or care? Which suffering can clinicians alleviate, and how? And how can patients avoid suffering alone, and unconsoled?*

These are key questions that demonstrate recognition of the failures (as well as the successes) of biomedical positivism and the need for a renewed meditation on first principles – examining what 'health' is and how it might be best achieved. Perhaps now is the time for 'spiritual commitment' to be shown, and to be prized, in discovering and creating solutions.

A further take on the context for such questions would be the suggestion that, precisely because conventional biomedicine has succeeded in keeping people alive for longer with conditions from which they would formerly have perished but at the cost of a permanent health deficit, the potential for prolonged suffering in the modern age has been dramatically increased. As people have been preserved and partially restored by 'mechanical and material' methods, they continue their lives in a society shaped by the same philosophical principles that gave rise to these methods – a materialist culture wherein community has been diminished and the search for higher meaning devalued. This is not a culture that supports or nurtures health – it is one where those who have health impairments are disadvantaged by the shift from interdependence to independence that occurred over the course of the twentieth century and now continues in the twenty-first. Illness, bereavement, profound personal challenges and losses – such experiences forcefully remind us of Donne's insight that 'No man is an island, entire of itself'. Yet what passes for community support today is often a sham, manufactured, institutionalized form that serves to further a personal sense of separateness from the 'normal world' that continues to take place elsewhere.

The general practitioner Kieran Sweeney (2006) tells of a single transforming consultation he experienced with an 85-year-old widow where, after he had explained how he could prescribe medicines to help with her diabetes, high blood pressure and raised cholesterol, she paused and said to him: 'Well, Jack's dead and the boys have gone'. For Sweeney this statement moved the consultation:

> ... from being doctor-centred to being patient-centred. It moved ... from the biomedical domain to the biographical domain, or from clinical, evidence-based medicine to a consultation predicated on narrative-based evidence. But the shift was profound. When the consultation moved from its biomedical phase, it shed its parameters of p-values, absolute risk and numbers needed to treat. These were replaced by the parameters of the biographical phase of the consultation ... despair, hopelessness, regret, guilt perhaps, and defeat were the parameters. Physical parameters had been replaced by metaphysical ones – two intellectual worlds seemed to have collided.

There is no reason, of course, why these two worlds should not co-exist – there is no requirement to reject one in place of the other. Such a shift to a broader embracing and integrating of explanatory and experiential models does, however, require the practitioner to be able to incorporate and synthesize different perspectives. Cassell (2004) has observed that:

> Since antiquity there has been a prejudice in favour of reason and against experiential knowledge. The long-standing dichotomy of medicine into its science and art is a medical expression of this bias. Knowledge, however, whether of medical science or the art of medicine, does not take care of sick persons or relieve their suffering; clinicians do in whom these kinds of knowledge are integrated.

This false dichotomy of reason/experience substantially underlies the antagonism between conventional biomedicine and CAM. Ironically (and inevitably) at the present time, just as in conventional medicine the wave of recognition of the limits and pitfalls of scientific rationalism is growing and gathering momentum, CAM professions are being exhorted to deny their experiential basis and prove themselves with reductionist science. This is partly embodied in the movement of CAM courses from independent learning centres to state academic institutions as mentioned above. If conventional medicine gets more art and CAM gets more science it may become increasingly difficult to tell the two apart, and perhaps they will meet each other halfway along their gradually developing trajectories. In the meantime it is open to individual practitioners to integrate art and science in their work right now, whatever their discipline, and in so doing to participate in an age-old project.

One approach to helping a patient such as the one just described by Sweeney would be to try to facilitate improved socialization, and thereby the development of a supportive community of care for the patient, by such means as joining a club or activity group, participating in classes or taking up volunteer work. Such solutions may not always be acceptable, practical or achievable however. Yet, there is always the capacity for the practitioner to remember and employ that most basic and powerful act – to bear witness to another's suffering and to communicate one's care, love and support; to be kind and to convey human warmth and integrity.

Egnew (2005) in his exploration of the meaning and definition of 'healing' has observed that as biomedicine became more technically successful in treating a number of diseases:

> ... cure, not care, became the primary purpose of medicine, and the physician's role became 'curer of disease' rather than 'healer of the sick'. Healing in a holistic sense has faded from medical attention ...

The practitioner operating from the cure perspective may feel a sense of failure when full recovery is not achieved and may not feel competent in providing care since that has not been the focus of her training and ongoing development. Care takes place elsewhere – in nursing and in non-medical specialties and in CAM modalities where sceptics might assert that Egnew's critique could be reversed: some might allow that the business of CAM practitioners is to offer care (perhaps), but that they are incapable of offering cure. Again there is a need to transcend such simplistic dichotomies. It is possible for many therapeutic approaches to offer both cure *and* care – to varying degrees and in differing combinations, depending on the individual case. Certainly phytotherapists, given the extended and rounded nature of the consultation; the commitment to provide continuity of care (see Ch. 7); and the flexibility of medicinal plants as complex pharmacological therapeutic tools, should feel confident in their ability to work in both territories.

Egnew (2005) concluded that healing is: '... associated with themes of wholeness, narrative and spirituality'. He cites Frankl (1963) who observed that: 'Suffering ceases to be suffering in some way at the moment it finds a meaning'. Egnew asserts that:

> *The role of the physician–healer is to establish connexional relationships with his or her patients and guide them in reworking of their life narratives to create meaning in and transcend their suffering.*

But he acknowledges that doctors may be ill-prepared to take on this task since:

> *Physicians are not trained to hear patients' stories, often fail to solicit the patient's agenda or pick up on the patient's clues, and often limit storytelling to maintain diagnostic clarity, support efficiency, and avoid confusion and unpleasant feelings.*

While it may be tempting to suggest that CAM practitioners are more open to hearing patients' stories and are less limited or restricted in exploring them, such an assertion is hard to sustain in light of the diversity of so-called CAM approaches, some of which may be more open and some of which may not. To many, Egnew's description of the role of the physician–healer will seem to fit that already ascribed to the various psychological therapies. Surely the 'reworking of ... life narratives to create meaning' belongs with those who have training in this realm – counsellors, clinical psychologists and so forth? Certainly such practitioners operate in this territory but to assign all psychological work to such specialists is to miss the opportunity for psycho-emotional-spiritual insight and development that may arise in all caring relationships, including those that develop in phytotherapy and conventional medicine. One does not have to be a qualified clinical psychologist to aid patients in exploring their narratives. On the other hand, it is important to be aware of the implications of entering into psychological dimensions with patients that may be more fully explored by the specific psychological professions. This brings us back to education and training concerns, which, though legitimate, need not overwhelm us. Simple human warmth and bearing witness are natural caring instincts that require no instruction.

The ability to join with the patient in the moment and to 'feel' alongside them is key. Clinical abstraction detracts from this ability to experience what Gendlin has called 'the felt presence of the moment' – to participate phenomenologically with the patient. Yet clinicians who aim to contextualize and diagnose must attain a perspective from which those twin aims can be realized, hence the ability to step back at the same time as stepping in needs to be cultivated. Again, we need to beware the suggestion from scientific positivism and classical dualism that it is only possible to operate in one state at any given time. The therapeutic practitioner is able to be with the patient in the felt presence of the moment but also, simultaneously, to contextualize, calculate, diagnose and attempt to make sense of what the patient is communicating. To operate deeply, smoothly and effectively across these overlapping zones of emotional and intellectual activity requires practice, and facility in doing so increases over time and with experience. Students and novice practitioners commonly struggle with this synthesis and need to be reassured that time and persistence will bring rewards as well as being taught and trained in ways that facilitate working in this multidimensional way – which should be one of the key goals of practitioner education and ongoing development.

## INTERIM THOUGHTS

It might be timely to pause at this point and consider some of the aims of the consultation in phytotherapy that are emerging from the foregoing discussion. I will now attempt to state the case concisely.

The phytotherapy consultation is a locus or method that has the potential to realize a number of aims, depending on the predicament and preferences of the patient and the dynamics of the interactions between patient and phytotherapist that occur on any given occasion on which they meet and engage together. The aims and outcomes of particular consultations will shift in response to the varying needs of the patient and the changing dynamics of the relationship between patient and phytotherapist. A general list of potential aims would include to:

- Map the dimensions of the patient's predicament as fully as possible
- Detect early signs of illness/disease
- Discern capacities for illness/disease, so as to advise modulation to foster prevention
- Identify aspects that require immediate remedial treatment
- Discern structures/functions that would benefit from support and which might need to be strengthened/nurtured/optimized

- Enable the patient to present their narrative
- Seek to explore, understand and interpret the patient's story
- Assist the patient in finding meaning in their narrative and their predicament
- Bear witness to the patient's suffering and provide human warmth and care
- Aid the patient to determine ways in which they may move towards enhanced connectedness and wholeness.

## NOTIONS OF HEALTH AND ILLNESS

As the scope of the consultation in phytotherapy is now clarifying and opening up, it might be helpful to return to the question of what is meant by 'health'.

'Health' and 'illness' may be contrasted as poles reflecting the degree to which the individual is able to flexibly adapt to the changes and challenges of life and to weave their experiences into a fabric or text that can be made sense of and which has meaning. This ability to dance with the flux of life, retaining a perspective of meaning may be considered to apply across physical, emotional, mental and spiritual aspects of the individual. Illness in one of these personal dimensions may be contrasted with wellness in another. A person may be said to be physically well yet emotionally in turmoil, whereas another may be said to be physically ill yet to possess a serenity of spirit. Properties of health and illness then are not mutually exclusive and they need not be seen as opposing forces. They have been envisaged by some as points along a continuum from an extreme of ease (comfort and dynamic wellbeing) to an extreme of 'dis-ease' (pain and helpless suffering). An alternative perspective would be to see health, illness and disease as overlapping and intersecting fields which commonly co-exist, e.g. patients with some types of cancer may consider themselves to be 'well despite the disease'.

'Disease' can be conceived as a concrete manifestation of illness showing clear breeches in the physical integrity or organization of the body (e.g. something abnormal can be seen in a blood test or MRI scan). Disease then can be equated with organic medical conditions where a lesion or disturbance in physiology of some type can be demonstrated. In contrast illness may be considered a collection of symptoms that exist in the absence of physical correlates such as changes in biochemical values or abnormalities revealed by imaging techniques. Disease therefore acquires legitimacy within the positivist worldview, whereas illness may not. Those who are ill but have no demonstrable lesion may sometimes be dismissed as 'the worried well'. For Kleinman (1988), disease is essentially a medical biological phenomenon that is the concern of medical practitioners whereas illness relates to the experience of, and response to, disease on the part of the ill person, their family and wider community of associates. Conventional medical practice is predicated on treating disease but it is not as comfortable with, or competent in remedying, the state of illness.

Fowler and Christakis (2008) contend that 'people are embedded in social networks and … the health and wellbeing of one person affects the health and wellbeing of others. This fundamental fact of existence provides a conceptual justification for the specialty of public health. Human happiness is not merely the province of isolated individuals'. Indeed the authors found that: 'Happiness is a network phenomenon, clustering in groups of people that extend up to three degrees of separation (for example, to one's friends' friends' friends)'.

The fields of health, illness and disease are ones of essential human concern and experience that are at the core of our self-image and self-understanding. They are also commercial territories to be exploited by the provision of products and services.

Foucault (2007) suggests that:

*The natural locus of disease is the natural locus of life – the family: gentle, spontaneous care, expressive of love and a common desire for a cure, assists nature in its struggle against the illness, and allows the illness itself to attain its own truth.*

Two themes are especially interesting here – first, that illness and disease are an intimate, and natural, part of family life and second, the assertion that illness may be able to 'attain its own truth'. This intriguing latter point may be interpreted in at least two ways. First, that by making sense of and discovering meaning in the illness, the 'truth' of the illness is constructed by the ill person and their family and wider group of friends and associates. Second, though related to the first point, a teleological interpretation may be made – that the illness has a life of its own and a purpose for being; the condition arises for a reason and towards a goal. People's perception of where illness comes from and to what end are commonly expressed in the consultation, especially where such reflection is requested and welcomed by the practitioner. Questions around this area are in fact essential in a holistic consultation and may be posed along the lines of: 'Tell me why do you think you have this condition?' 'Do you think there is a point to your condition? Is it there for a particular purpose do you think?' Replies to these types of questions are frequently highly revealing and insightful. Common responses include such expressions as:

*I haven't been taking care of myself properly, I've been doing too much ... this thing is telling me to slow down.*

*Ever since my marriage ended I haven't been right, I think my body is telling me it's time to move on.*

Here notions of causality and purpose are linked and it is clear that while conventional science tends to be reluctant to conflate aetiology and teleology, patients have no such hesitations.

Herzlich (2004) has suggested that notions of the cause of illness fall between two extremes:

*On the one hand, illness is endogenous in man, and the individual carries it in embryo; the ideas of resistance to disease, heredity and predisposition are here the key concepts. On the other hand, illness is thought of as exogenous; man is naturally healthy and illness is due to the action of an evil will, a demon or sorcerer, noxious elements, emanations from the earth or microbes ...*

Interestingly, these two extremes can be viewed from a Christian perspective as being consistent with worldviews pertaining after and before the fall.

Endogenous causes relate to the concept of original sin, with exogenous causes prevailing in the garden of Eden – before the fruit of the tree of the knowledge of good and evil (an archetypal dual noxious/healing element presided over by a demon/teacher) was consumed. These two extremes can be posited as 'naturephobic' and 'naturephilic' standpoints. To be naturephobic is to distrust nature; to see it as something that must necessarily be controlled and contained lest it cause harm. Here the universe is a dangerous, purposeless place. This is consistent with the dominant scientific–positivist paradigm and is a perspective that allows the justification of the manipulation of nature in aggressive and invasive ways such as the development of conventional drugs, genetic modification and nuclear energy. The naturephilic position is that nature is inherently good and wise and can be trusted, the universe is a safe and purposeful place, we should aim to learn from and live in harmony with nature and not harm it. Such positions can be contrasted with modern and aboriginal relationships with the planet – in the modern view land can be owned, bought and sold; in the aboriginal view, the people belong to the land, are owned by the land if you will, therefore it is impossible for land to be bought and sold. Kingsley (2009) has explored the enduring importance of the relationship that indigenous people have with the land in Victoria, Australia, concluding that it is a 'key determinant of the health and wellbeing of Indigenous people'. These are the words of the Native American leader Smohalla (c.1815–1895) presenting a traditional view of the sacred nature of the land:

> *You ask me to plow the ground. Shall I take a knife and tear my mother's breast? Then when I die she will not take me to her bosom to rest.*
>
> *You ask me to dig for stone. Shall I dig under her skin for her bones? Then when I die I cannot enter her body to be born again.*
>
> *You ask me to cut grass and make hay and sell it and be rich like white men. But how dare I cut off my mother's hair?*
>
> McLuhan (1982)

Such a worldview is compatible with the notion among some CAM practitioners and patients that the human body is similarly sacred and inviolable and which interprets such interventions as surgery, radiotherapy, conventional drug therapy and vaccination as aggressive and unnatural assaults to be resisted.

Such deep trends and convictions underlie the differences between conventional medicine (essentially naturephobic) and CAM (essentially naturephilic). These currents also underlie the antagonism that occurs when a naturephobic practitioner meets a naturephilic patient, and vice-versa, as we shall see below.

Health, illness and disease can be perceived as emergent properties of living, their relative expression depending on a host of factors, including:

- Socioeconomic factors
- Parenting
- Education
- Environmental influences

- Nutrition
- Socialization
- Political influences
- Personal attitudes, behaviours and beliefs.

Concepts relating to health, illness and disease have been created throughout time and across cultures. Both religious and secular explanations have been proffered to explain their presence – particularly the suffering that arises with illness and disease. Utopian visions of a world without suffering also have a long history. The project of biomedicine can be seen as utopian, especially because it is essentially set up in opposition to disease and death. There are no more extreme utopian visions than those seeking immortality, however, with the powerful effects of conventional drugs such as antibiotics and corticosteroids in the mid- to late-twentieth century, along with advances in surgical techniques and social measures such as improved water hygiene, such a vision may have seemed to be finally materializing. In companion with delivery from our physical ills, perhaps Freudian psychoanalysis and newer approaches to the mind would reveal ourselves to ourselves and open the door to permanent joy. Expectations of attaining a higher degree of health in any case had been raised to a new level – which was not sustained for very long. Even as statistics showed improved health-related outcomes for first-world populations, individuals continued to suffer. In an article entitled 'The paradox of health', Barsky (1988) set out four factors (summarized below) that he saw as influencing the perception of a gap between individual health and the health of the group:

- Advances in medical care have lowered the mortality rate of acute infectious diseases, resulting in a comparatively increased prevalence of chronic and degenerative disorders
- Society's heightened consciousness of health has led to greater self-scrutiny and an amplified awareness of bodily symptoms and feelings of illness
- The widespread commercialization of health and the increasing focus on health issues in the media have created a climate of apprehension, insecurity, and alarm about disease
- The progressive medicalization of daily life has brought unrealistic expectations of cure that make untreatable infirmities and unavoidable limitations seem even worse.

Although sound and important, Barsky's list is open to an alternative reading as an apologia for biomedicine as it hits the barrier and fails to deliver year-on-year growth in health achievements. Nonetheless, Barsky helps to clarify the limits to medical expansion and the generation of new territories for suffering that accompany medical 'progress'. Other authors have explored the notion of 'healthism' – an excessive and misguided preoccupation with health that is unrealistic, unhelpful and perhaps irrational. Herman (1996) discussed institutional healthism and considered that it has: '… almost become a new morality' that is coercive in nature such that: 'submitting to preventive measures, diagnosis and therapy is part of what the upstanding citizen owes himself, his family, the State and even his God'.

Herman questions the validity of equating longevity with health and calls for discussion of the motives that underlie biomedicine's 'war on death'. He proposes that: 'Perhaps we should be using what have been slightingly referred to as our "pastoral skills" to make peace with the inevitable'. By contrast, Greenhalgh and Wessely (2004) see healthism embodied in certain perspectives and behaviours of the individual. They maintain that: 'Healthism in the consultation ... is a common source of irritation and stress to health professionals'. What then might the characteristics of the healthist be? They are (adapted from Greenhalgh & Wessely 2004):

- Typically young or middle-aged, from university educated, information-rich, semi-professional backgrounds
- Vocal and articulate (aware of, and keen to exercise, citizen and patients' rights)
- Health-aware and enthusiastic in seeking information about health and illness *via* books, magazines, the internet
- Generally makes positive lifestyle choices, e.g. takes regular exercise, diet aligns approximately with official recommendations, tends to avoid alcohol
- Consumes food supplements, alternative medicines, and tonics, all of which are attributed 'natural' and 'holistic' qualities
- Concerned about 'unnatural' substances (chemicals, vaccines, drugs, additives), especially when there is a civil liberties dimension (e.g. fluoridation of water, mass vaccination, pollution, GM foods)
- Particular fear of small, unseen, insidious threats capable of penetrating the body's boundaries
- Associates science/medicine with danger rather than safety
- Exercises a high degree of consumer choice (hence, seeks multiple opinions), often in the private sector.

Can this really be what the stress-inducing healthist looks like? Certainly this list has a lot in common with many identikit pictures of CAM users. Perhaps we just have a CAM patient entering the wrong surgery door? Let us return to our earlier contrasting of the naturephobic and naturephilic worldviews. Greenhalgh and Wessely's upset would seem to arise from a clash of ideologies. If doctors are irritated and upset by such patients, then this surely arises from a failure to intellectually appreciate and practically accommodate the patient's ethos and predisposition. A strange twist has taken place here. In rejecting Herman's coercive institutional healthism the patient has been labelled a healthist for taking the trouble to pursue an alternative agenda. But could Greenhalgh and Wessely's profile of the deviant healthist not just as readily be taken as a portrait of a well-meaning citizen trying to take some responsibility for their own health and willing to question authority? How do we understand the absence of this perspective in their article then? Clearly there continue to be differences of opinion as to which health practices and health perspectives are deemed to be legitimate and which are not. General principles may be agreed but specifics are open to controversy; yes it is good to question received wisdom, *but not that particular bit of it*! Indeed it is great to take responsibility for your own health, *but just not in that way*! Medical paternalism continues in fact but under the guise of medical rationalism – they shall be taken seriously who approach health rationally.

A similar gap in understanding may occur when a more conventionally medically-orientated patient visits a CAM practitioner. The CAM practitioner may well experience stress if the patient rejects their advice and questions the premises of their worldview: 'That patient wasn't prepared to take any advice or change their lives in any way, they just wanted a quick fix – I can't work in that way!' The suggestion is that the advanced practitioner, working in any healthcare field, should be able to work with a wide range of patients without self-inducing irritation and stress by:

- Listening carefully to the patient's story
- Discerning the patient's health orientation, ethos and values (drawing on a deep personal appreciation of the breadth of possible perspectives)
- Respecting this orientation even if it differs from the practitioner's own world view
- Conveying the practitioner's opinion of the best course of action for the patient's predicament and discussing these as fully and as strongly as is appropriate to the case
- Accepting the patient's personal choices, even if these mean rejection of the practitioner's advice (accepting without upset through respecting the patient's autonomy)
- Advising the patient on the options available to seek advice/help elsewhere.

Let us return once again to 'health'. The widely known World Health Organization definition of health (WHO 1948) remains an interesting catalyst for discussion: 'Health is a state of complete physical, mental and social well-being and not merely the absence of disease or infirmity'. This may easily be dismissed as post-war utopianism but let us linger a moment and see if we can conceive of what such a state might look like. In doing so we might be accused of archaic romanticism if we suggest that some indigenous peoples may once have enjoyed this state. Perhaps some members of some Native American tribes, for instance, achieved this harmony within their own relatively small social groups for some extended periods of time. Perhaps we all have and shall again, *a la* Warhol, achieved this for 15 min or so – here and there, from time to time. Yet it is hard to imagine as a steady continuing state, and perhaps now – more than ever – we are the furthest away from this potential due to what is implicit in the word 'social'. If we are now aware of ourselves as a global society, then how can any one person be well in one place while having knowledge of the inequalities and suffering of people in other parts of our society? Indeed how can human beings living on an ecologically disrupted planet with massive disparities in health measures between nations and facing huge challenges such as climate change and population growth achieve such a level of personal health perfection? And why should we? We need to return to where we started this discussion – the WHO definition ultimately fails to be a reliable definition of health because it is oppositional, it requires the eradication of disease and infirmity from life, which is not in the nature of things.

The great source of practical and philosophical insight that ancient peoples draw on is nature itself. As we observe nature, we see (as noted in Ch. 1) that it is in the nature of things to change – either rapidly (e.g. sudden changes in weather) or slowly (geological and cosmological change). Yet around these changes sometimes patterns may be observed – such as seasonal and lunar cycles – which help us to orient ourselves in our world. So life is to do with change and cycles and to be in tune with nature we need to be able to adapt to change and to work with cycles. In Zen philosophy and practice, the aim is for the person and their environment to 'move together' and one translation of Zen is just that. This is a similar insight to that provided by the sociologist Aaron Antonovsky where he associates wellbeing with the individual's ability to establish and maintain coherency between the internal and external environment, particularly in the face of stressful situations. Antonovsky's ideas became known as salutogenesis – the origin of health – which focuses on how health is generated rather than on the processes of pathology. For Antonovsky (1987) the key to resilience and good health lies in possessing a sense of coherence which can be defined as:

> *A global orientation that expresses the extent to which one has a pervasive, enduring though dynamic feeling of confidence that (1) the stimuli from one's internal and external environments in the course of living are structured, predictable, and explicable; (2) the resources are available to one to meet the demands posed by these stimuli; and (3) these demands are challenges, worthy of investment and engagement.*

Item (1) corresponds to 'comprehensibility' (that the stimuli can be understood); item (2) concerns 'manageability' (that one has the resources to cope) and item (3) relates to 'meaningfulness' (that the challenge makes sense and is worth meeting) (Lindstrom & Eriksson 2005).

It may be difficult to maintain comprehension in the light of life's biggest disruptive events and critics (e.g. Endler et al. 2008) have questioned elements of Antonovsky's model such as the insistence on the importance of predictability. Arguably, resilience in the face of challenge would be crucially facilitated by the ability to find a way of making sense of unpredictable events.

Illich (1976) has it that: '"Health" after all, is simply an everyday word that is used to designate the intensity with which individuals cope with their internal states and their environmental conditions …'.

This intensity is diminished when energy is depleted (physical, emotional, psychological, spiritual) and a key to conserving and generating energy seems to lie in Antonovsky's view of meaningfulness – essentially, if we cease to see 'the point' of the situation we are facing then we are unable to produce and invest the energy required to deal optimally with the challenges it poses.

Traditional medical systems such as Chinese Medicine assess that if the nature of life is change then the nature of health will be the ability to adapt to change and disease will develop where this ability is lacking. So health is associated with words such as: flow, movement, flexibility; and illness and disease with words such as: blockage, obstruction, stagnation. The Tao Te Ching of Lao Tsu (sixth century BCE) provides examples of this connection between observation of natural phenomena and reflections on how to live:

*A man is born gentle and weak.*

*At his death he is hard and stiff.*

*Green plants are tender and filled with sap.*

*At their death they are withered and dry.*

*Therefore the stiff and unbending is the disciple of death.*

*The gentle and yielding is the disciple of life.*

Trans. Feng and English (1973)

Illich (1976) contends that: '... the cultivation of health ... to a large extent depends on innate and inbred mettle'. Mettle may be considered here as the ability to cope well with challenges and difficulties. The word is associated in dictionary definitions with qualities and characteristics such as: courage, spirit, character and resilience. Mettle is often considered an inherent property and Illich terms it 'innate and inbred', but might it not be possible to acquire skills, knowledge and practices which propagate mettle, enabling the individual to more ably deal with life problems? Such enabling work can constitute a major aim of the consultation, which in turn shapes the thought and questioning of the practitioner during the consultation and generates forms of advice, teaching, ideas and reflection arising spontaneously and creatively during the consultation and gathered together for emphasis at the end of the consult. We will now consider and propose ways in which 'mettle' might indeed be developed.

## ENGENDERING WELLBEING

The consultation provides an opportunity to identify areas where changes in attitude and behaviour (and not just consumption of medication – herbal or otherwise) might lead to enhanced self-care and wellbeing, as well as movement towards a greater degree of meaning-perception, coping ability and resilience. Strategies for change and movement can be proposed by the practitioner and then negotiated with the patient. In order to work in this way the practitioner must possess three qualities or capacities:

1. An orientation towards facilitating achievement of enhanced self-care and wellbeing in patients as a primary goal of the clinical encounter
2. A frame of reference that makes possible the recognition of the characteristics of a patient's thinking and acting that might benefit from adaptation
3. A fund of concepts and practices that can be taught by the practitioner and applied by the patient to achieve such adaptation.

The practitioner's orientation is profoundly influenced by the particular school of thought and practice in which they are trained and inducted but is not limited to this. It is additionally coloured by a complex array of factors, including:

- Upbringing and early life experiences
- Sociocultural influences

- Ongoing education, study, training and personal development work
- Exposure to influential teachers and ideas
- Work context, environment and ethos
- Personal convictions, beliefs and faith
- Political persuasion
- Clinical and life experience
- Critical personal episodes such as bereavement.

In its natural healthy and dynamic state the practitioner's perspective is not a fixed point but one that is continuously expanded, deepened and modulated in the light of experience, study and reflection. An orientation towards propagating self-care, wellbeing, meaning-perception and resilience does not lie especially on either side of the biomedicine/CAM divide, it is a way of seeing that is independent of any particular healthcare modality and therefore may arise in any or all practitioners, although its application may be inhibited by factors such as the limitations of institutional requirements or operational restrictions.

The dimensions of the practitioner's frame of reference with regard to facilitating self-care, wellbeing, meaning-perception and resilience are set in proportion to the degree of the practitioner's orientation, emphasis and commitment to these goals. The detailed features and contours of the map used to describe the territory of these regions of patient ability are drawn over the course of the practitioner's career. Maps vary according to their users then, and the terrain revealed in each map changes over time, yet in order to assist the patient in arriving at enhanced self-care and wellbeing there *must be a map* of some sort. In other words, the practitioners will only be able to fully engage with the type of advice and teaching described below if they possess a personal broad explanatory model, which aids in understanding and making sense of the world. Some ancient traditional medical systems, such as Chinese medicine, come ready supplied with such an explanatory model. Foundational concepts in Chinese medicine, such as those of Qi and Yin/Yang, power insights not just into the practice of medicine but into the nature of the universe and all that it contains. Many other medical systems however (including phytotherapy), are not so richly endowed with such perceptual aids. Yet, even if we are provided with a broad philosophical head-start built-in to our medical training, it always falls to each practitioner in their personhood to discern and create their own unique conceptual habitat and sense of meaning. The practitioner who is following such a path is likely to be better equipped to help patients discover their own provisional truths.

What follows is a number of concepts, strategies and practices that *may* represent relevant discussion and teaching opportunities in response to the detection of patient attitudes and behaviours that are considered by the practitioner to be in need of modulation in order to further the patient's potential to care for themselves, find personal meaning, develop coping abilities and resilience and engender enhanced wellbeing. Some readers may rebel against or reject some of the standpoints that are explicit or implicit in the reasoning underlying some of the ideas/practices given below. The plan here is not to give a universally applicable set of concepts/strategies (this would be tricky given that there is no globally agreed position on all, or indeed any questions in philosophy) but rather to provide some examples that can be accepted, adapted or replaced by the reader as desired.

It is difficult to frame, or at least I have found it challenging to frame, some of the ideas below without them appearing rather pat or *glib* on the page. The use of 'glib' here is perhaps most appropriate when one thinks of its probable origin in the Middle Low German *glibberich*, meaning *slippery*. Many of the items below reference complex and slippery notions and it is not the intention to suggest that their nature is easily discernible or their implications easily soluble. Nonetheless, these ideas at least represent discussion points – both within and without the consultation space – and I have found them to be easy to work with in practice. The examples given below might be criticized and diminished by categorizing them pejoratively as techniques for stress management, self-help or self-improvement or they may be dismissed as hackneyed homilies, new-age clichés or psychobabble. If so we might need to question our prejudices – why would one sneer at the concept of 'self-help' for example? We need to get over allowing these terms to prevent us taking a broader, and more helpful view.

### Accept the gift of one's own symptoms

Bob Duggan (2003) refers to symptoms as a 'marvellous resource' since they are messengers conveying vital information about our bodies, which, if we can listen to them properly can guide us to enhanced wellbeing. Patients can learn to pay attention to small changes and ask themselves 'What is my body telling me?' This is not to transform people into hypochondriacs but merely to help them take account of commonplace useful information that can enable helpful adjustments in attitude and behaviour. Practitioners tend to get worried about this, since it appears to advocate breaking the taboo on self-diagnosis. What if a patient tells themselves a story about a serious symptom that delays them seeking 'proper' medical help leading to treatment being applied too late? Well, the majority of people are likely to seek expert advice if their symptoms are unusual, severe or persistent and it seems probable that they are more likely to do this if they are in the habit of paying attention to what their body is telling them and asking – what does this mean? Even if this is so, it may still be the case that patients interpret symptoms 'incorrectly' from a medical perspective, e.g. a person may ask, 'What is the meaning of this headache?' and self-reply, 'Well, I haven't slept much for the last week, perhaps I need to lie my head down and rest'. This is not a 'correct' textbook medical diagnosis but it is common sense and is the kind of advice a practitioner is likely to give in any case. People will need to consult practitioners to help them interpret and understand their symptoms on occasion but many of the everyday niggles and tugs of our bodies can be consciously registered and understood by people if they are encouraged to do so, rather than ignoring, repressing or medicalizing them. Such everyday reflection can powerfully increase the personal sense of meaning and control over our health and wellbeing.

### If you feel 'dis-ease' ask yourself 'why?'

Although we may not describe them as symptoms, feelings of discomfort, awkwardness and 'dis-ease' are also messengers that have useful insights to impart to us. Rather than ignoring or pushing through such feelings we can ask ourselves: 'Why am I feeling uncomfortable?' and then: 'What can I do to change this?' before taking appropriate action. Although such practice may seem absurdly simple and we might assume that we think in such a way all the time, it is clear that this is not the case for everyone.

In practising the art of asking: 'What is this symptom and what does it mean?' (as above) and 'Why am I feeling uncomfortable and what can I do to ease this discomfort?', the underlying principle is that the body has a language of feelings and sensations as well as thoughts that we have often learned to tune out but which repay attention with increased self-knowledge and wellbeing.

### Your illness is your teacher

We are relating here to the concept of illness as teacher – what is your condition telling you about your life and how you live it?

### Observe your own behaviour – what does it signify?

*I go to bakeries all day long, there's a lack of sweetness in my life.*
Jonathan Richman (1976)

Becoming aware of our own behaviour patterns and reactions enables us to reflect on them and consider why we do what we do and whether there are areas where we need to make changes. It is useful to focus this scrutiny on areas of life where problems occur or where there is repeated dissatisfaction with performance or outcomes. How do we react in certain situations or in response to certain issues? How might we amend our attitude and behaviour? What is preventing us from making progress?

### Be able to decline a request

Many people are living under excessive pressure because they are unable to place boundaries around their commitments to time, energy and emotional outputs. Being able to decline a request, when appropriate, to conserve these outputs can enhance wellbeing. This is not to say that one should refuse every request that one would rather avoid, since there may be occasions when this is inappropriate. Rather, it is about declining requests that one considers unreasonable or exploitative but which we might do in order to 'keep the general peace' at the risk of disturbing our personal peace. If we are unable to decline requests we develop the reputation of a person who can be 'put upon' and who consequently may become overburdened by unnecessary and unfair demands. Such a tendency runs deep and may take time and skilled help to change, yet the concept of declining a request is easy to grasp and merely discussing this with patients may empower them to attempt to apply it as a practice.

### Be able to receive as well as give

A lot of people find it hard to receive thanks, praise, gifts and other acknowledgements of their contribution and value. The roots of this may be complex and profound but it is frequently a cultural practice of misplaced modesty. Being able to gratefully and warmly receive genuine thanks and compliments creates a harmonious circuit with the bestower that enables a dynamic flow of human consilience and vitality. To spurn or play down this positive attention is to diminish the power of one of life's most enjoyable and necessary exchanges.

### Speak your fears to another

It is a commonplace truism that it is better to speak about what worries you than to keep things pent-up inside. Even during the consultation however, it is frequently the case that the patient leaves significant fears unvoiced. The practitioner can address this in the consultation by asking, at a relevant point, a question along the lines of: 'Aside from what we have already discussed, do you have any worries about anything at all? Is anything causing you anxiety or even fear?' The practitioner can also encourage the patient to tell their fears to an appropriate confidante within their family or friends, or to write them down. Again, the act of identifying and reflecting upon issues can increase understanding and help empower expanded life control.

### Avoid creating expectations that generate pain

This is not to advocate resignation or abandonment of one's hopes or desires but rather to adapt our expectations so that they are realistic, or to section a large goal into achievable intermediate stages. It is also important to accept that in all our endeavours we are likely to receive a measure of criticism as well as praise. If we expect that we are going to receive universal adulation for everything we do, we are likely to feel pain when this does not materialize. This pain is compounded if we focus on negative comments to the exclusion of more positive ones.

### Shift your perspective

Although we are unavoidably entangled in the dominant cultural worldview pertaining in the society in which we live, this does not prevent us from shifting our perspective to a more positive position, if such is required. This is not to suggest that we should deny the realities taking place around us – but rather to recommend that we keep in mind the fact that, as The World Social Forum slogan has it, 'another world is possible'. Perspectives can shift on personal and global issues. We can select and filter the ideas and messages we are exposed to. Passive consumption of newspapers and TV news, for example, tends to give the impression that the world is a dangerous and disordered place and can induce a sense of futility, depression and powerlessness in the individual. Choosing to read books (fiction and non-fiction, ancient and modern) that provide a broader picture and insights into human nature and potential and selectively using online media that presents alternative views may help us to arrive at a place where the individual can make greater sense of their place in the world. From this position, life may be lived in a more positive and rewarding way.

Considering your illness as your teacher, as mentioned above, is a profound technique for shifting perspectives on health and disease.

### Make space for silence and reflection

It is difficult to make sense of one's life and world in the absence of reflective space in which to review and consider thoughts, experiences and occurrences. Prioritizing exposure to thoughtful silence is one way of allowing our exposures to settle, cohere and come into focus.

### Doing things is easy: getting round to doing them is the issue

Most of the tasks we set ourselves, or goals we wish to achieve, are within our capacity to realise. The stumbling block is rarely our ability to perform the task so much as our ability to actually knuckle down and work at it. It is generally good practice to spend less energy on worrying about our competence to perform a task or realize a goal and more on the practicalities of putting a timetable in place and freeing up the space to do the work itself.

### Distinguish between excuses and reasons

If we are failing to make the progress we would like with a particular project or area of life or self-development, we can write down the factors we believe account for our position. These factors can then be divided into excuses (pretexts that need to be recognized for what they are and discarded) and reasons (genuine explanatory factors that need to be tackled).

### Listen to the stories you tell about yourself

It is useful to listen to, and to critique, the stories we tell about ourselves in order to distinguish between those that promote our development and those that inhibit it. We can tune in to the parts of the stories that do not 'ring true' and therefore strike a 'false note'. When we hear the jarring notes we can halt and edit our stories, e.g. 'Actually, that's not right – it's more like this …'. We can listen out for erroneous and discordant themes and details such as those to do with blame or transference of responsibility. With repeated practice we can tell stories that are more 'true', which enable us to be more congruent as individuals and to make stronger connections with others, meeting them at their own place of personal 'truth'. The connections are stronger because the nature of the threads of the stories that enable the connections to be made have greater integrity and toughness to withstand impacts.

## Cultivate happiness (tend your personal relationships like you would a garden)

Some factors contributing towards a sense of personal happiness may be cultivated. Research on happiness (summarized by Layard 2006) suggests that its attainment is facilitated by:

- Personal freedom and a set of personal guiding values
- Physical health
- A supportive network of friends and community relationships
- Meaningful and personally rewarding work (not necessarily a 'job' or paid work)
- Adequate financial situation
- Positive and satisfying family relationships.

Within this framework, we can posit that personal freedom; guiding values, physical health and adequacy of finances provide the foundation on which happiness can flourish in proportion to the degree that the individual is occupied with meaningful work or activity and enjoys a range of satisfying relationships. In light of this we might surmise that, in promotion of the patient's personal happiness, the practitioner should place emphasis on supporting the patient's efforts to:

- Liberate themselves from oppressive situations such as negative personal relationships (where these cannot be transformed into more positive ones) and unsatisfying work
- Pursue a personal understanding of the world and develop personal guidelines for living
- Attain physical fitness
- Participate in social and community activities and prioritize friendships
- Develop knowledge and skills leading to meaningful and satisfying work that provides an adequate financial return
- Prioritize and nurture family relationships.

Fowler and Christakis (2008) consider that: 'Like laughter and smiling, the emotion of happiness might serve the evolutionary adaptive purpose of enhancing social bonds'. The process appears to be two-way in that happiness enhances social bonds while at the same time positive social bonds create happiness. Simply spending time with people who are happy induces one's own happiness by means of what Hatfield et al. (1994) have called 'emotional contagion'. This appears to be mediated not only by exposure to positive emotions but also, in part, by mimicry of the happy person's posture, facial expressions and vocal presentation. Human beings are social creatures and thrive within a network of satisfying interpersonal relationships. The potential to create such relationships depends in large part on the individual's tendency towards conviviality or proximity to persons who possess this quality. The patient may be encouraged to join a group organized around a topic of interest to her where she may expect to meet people who are happy and enjoying themselves – such as a dancing class or walking club. The variable dynamics of groups means, however, that several may need to be tried before finding one that is truly convivial and 'happiness-generating'.

In a culture in which happiness has become commodified, the cultivation of human relationships in opposition to the consumption of products constitutes a radical act. The practitioner must also engage radically with a critique of her own practice behaviours. There may be little difference between prescribing St John's wort or Cipramil to treat depression where the cause of unhappiness is left unaddressed and, moreover, where the strategies for renewal are not also taught and then coached.

## Cultivate a relationship with nature

Abstraction from nature is, in the words of Terrence McKenna (p.o.d.) 'the knife poised at our hearts'. The result of this abstraction is that many people no longer feel at home in nature, which increases personal feelings of isolation and alienation as well as allowing the abuse and destruction of nature. By spending time in nature we can help re-establish a sense of belonging in this world and, through observation and participation, begin to discern nature's patterns and messages. Our abstraction from nature is of such a degree that we might consider an indigenous perspective such as the one below to be tantamount to the ravings of a lunatic:

> *Did you know that trees talk? Well they do. They talk to each other, and they'll talk to you if you'll listen. Trouble is, white people don't listen. They never learned to listen to the Indians so I don't suppose they'll listen to other voices in nature. But I have learned a lot from trees: sometimes about the weather, sometimes about animals, sometimes about the Great Spirit.*
>
> McLuhan (1982)

How do we make sense of a statement like this? Is this romanticism, anthropomorphism or schizophrenia? Or does it speak of a sophisticated sensory relationship with the world that we have some potential to develop?

The ways in which we can interact with nature, and that we can recommend to patients, are numerous and include:

- Sitting in the garden
- Visiting gardens
- Gardening
- Walking in the countryside
- Walking along the beach
- Watching the sea or a river flow
- Hiking or climbing in the hills and mountains
- Camping out in the wilderness
- Sailing or boating
- Watching the night sky
- Observing clouds, sunrise and sunsets
- Celebrating the changes of season
- Being aware of the phases of the lunar cycle and the shifting constellations.

Milligan (2004) has explored the significance of communal gardening in allotments for older people in northern England and observed that: 'gardens and gardening activity may offer a key site of comfort and a vital opportunity for an individual's emotional, physical and spiritual renewal'. She also refers to the notion of the 'therapeutic landscape' developed by Gesler (1992), although Gesler's initial use of this theme was predominantly concerned with the built rather than the natural healing environment. Still, we may talk of the stillness, relaxation and insight that can be found in wild or cultivated outdoors environments.

Nature is the original and ultimate source of human inspiration and creativity and, as Emerson (2000; first published 1844) puts it: 'Art and luxury have early learned that they must work as enhancement and sequel to this original beauty'. Appropriate ways of being with nature have the capacity to open us up to the healing power of beauty, the perspective-generating potential of awe and wonder, the loneliness-dispersing effect of connecting with the natural world, and the meaning-enhancing result of this connection.

### Choose BIG MIND over small mind

In every difficult, challenging, frustrating or irritating situation (whether major or minor) we have a choice between reacting in a 'small-minded' or a 'big-minded' way. Small mind gets stuck in the detail while BIG MIND steps back and sees the larger picture. Whenever there is a choice between small mind and big mind, one should ALWAYS CHOOSE BIG MIND! With practice, the voice of small mind becomes quieter and BIG MIND becomes the default reaction. In the course of any given day, there are usually numerous opportunities to practise this technique.

### Challenges are inevitable but upset is optional

Problems, difficulties and challenges will inevitably arise in our lives. A number of small irritations can occur every day with larger challenges happening less commonly, although still, for most people, sufficiently often to cause frequent upset. We cannot prevent problems arising but we can modulate our reaction to them – the challenges will come but the upset does not have to accompany it. If we become used to dealing with minor everyday irritations without succumbing to upset, then we will cope better with the bigger issues when they happen.

Among the key conclusions about what matters in living one's life reached by Hans Selye, the famous researcher of stress, is that 'it's not what happens to you, it's how you deal with it' (Selye 1978).

### Listen to your heart

*We have to re-learn, in order, perhaps too late, to attain even more: to re-feel.*
Nietzsche (1982)

It is commonplace for people to refer to a conflict between 'what my head says and what my heart tells me'. This reflects a cultural inability to synthesize emotional and intellectual information and reactions, with intellect being awarded primacy over emotions. Emotional reactions to events and phenomena tend to be seen as irrational and dangerous – needing to be controlled and over-ruled by the mind. Denigrating emotional information as inferior can prevent us hearing important signals from our bodies and diminishes our experience of life. Patients can be encouraged to recognize their emotions as legitimate agents of communication – paying attention to what they have to say. *Feeling emotions* and *thinking thoughts* are equally valid activities and inform each other.

## Cultivate an attitude of openness to change (since too much order is dangerous)

We discussed, in Chapter 2, the proposition that the nature of life is change, suggesting that developing versatility in order to flow with change was a central strategy for successful living. Being open to change, to experiencing the new in a mode that is fully engaged and possessed of a desire to learn, enables one to gain benefit from both pleasurable and painful events. When the response to change is closed, disconnected and directed away from learning, a picture of stagnation of, or deviation from, the vital coursing of energy in the body (the learning-developing trajectory) is present. With deeply painful change (such as bereavement) it may be necessary to rest in the closed zone for a little while as we recover the capacity to move with change again, but permanent habitation of this realm as a life-attitude or mode of living prevents the growth of the self.

Resisting change and striving to maintain a fixed point of equilibrium, beyond a certain degree of effort and appropriateness, becomes draining of energy in addition to being futile. Excessive control and ordering of life is contrary to the nature of life and the malign influence of this stance reverberates through the holder's physiology. Conceptualizations of the nature of physiology have developed from simple 'homoeostasis' (the body needs to be kept within narrow physiological parameters in order to maintain stability); to 'homeodynamism' which states that 'biological systems are ... [able] to dynamically self-organize at bifurcation points of their behaviour where they lose stability' (Lloyd et al. 2001); and to McEwen's notion of 'allostasis' which he defines as: 'achieving stability through change' (McEwen & Wingfield 2003). We will return to this area towards the end of this chapter when discussing complexity but for now let us assert that wellbeing has more to do with the ability to adapt in the face of change than to maintain a fixed position in spite of it. Goldberger et al. (2002) has dramatically illustrated the difference between fixed patterns of physiological reactivity and dynamically fluctuating ones with a study of a 30-minute heart rate time series taken from four different people (shown in Figure 3.1). Person B is the only one without a heart pathology but detection of this heart rate record as the healthy one is, as Goldberger puts it, 'perhaps nonintuitive', since we are so disposed to view the records that appear more regular and ordered as normal.

## Choose love over fear

With regard to change we can associate openness to it with the pattern of worldview and life-engagement that is representative of a state or way of being that has to do with love and a closed attitude to change as the corresponding pattern that is shaped by fear. Operating from a love state or from

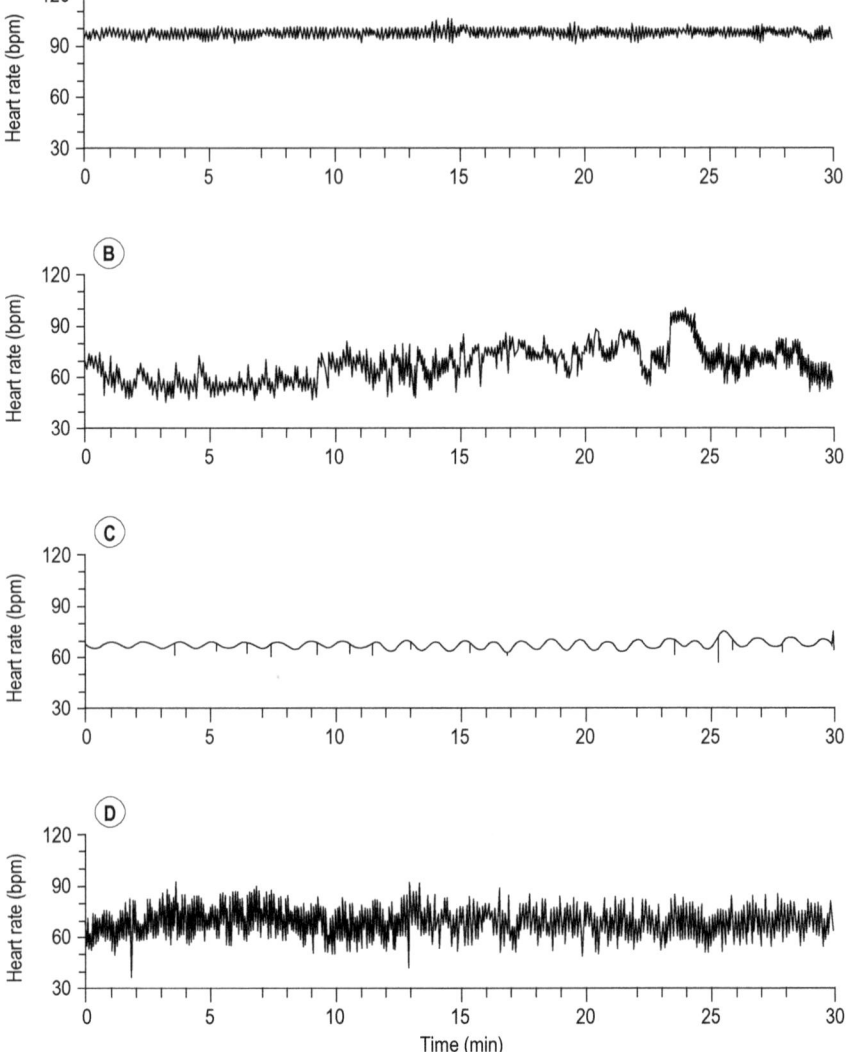

**Figure 3.1** ECG analysis. Representative heart rate recordings in health and disease in four people, presented as four unknowns. One record is normal; the other three represent severe pathologies. Can you identify which is normal?
Answers: (A) and (C) are from patients in sinus rhythm with severe congestive heart failure, (D) is from a subject with a cardiac arrhythmia, atrial fibrillation, which produces an erratic heart rate. The healthy record, (B), far from a homeostatic constant state, is notable for its visually apparent non-stationarity and 'patchiness'. These features are related to fractal and non-linear properties. Their breakdown in the disease may be associated with the emergence of excessive regularity (A) and (C), or uncorrelated randomness (D). Of note in (C) is the presence of strongly periodic oscillations ($\approx$1/min), which are associated with Cheyne–Stokes breathing, a pathologic type of cyclic respiratory pattern. Quantifying and modelling the complexity of healthy variability, and detecting more subtle alterations with disease and ageing, present major challenges in contemporary biomedicine. *(Adapted from Goldberger et al. 2002, with permission.)*

a fear state has broad implications since we can associate love with an open, responsive and expansive engagement with life that is reflected in a fluid dynamic physiology (homoeodynamism), while fear is connected with a closed, unresponsive and contracted picture of functioning that centres on core survival mechanisms (homoeostasis). Both expansion and contraction are necessary for a heart to beat but whereas love has the capacity to accommodate fear; pure fear is anathema to love. Love is the life promoting and enhancing force associated since ancient times with Eros whereas fear is connected with the death orientation of Thanatos; love inclines to life and growth whereas fear leans towards deterioration and death. To *be* from the place of love is to be open to life, a condition we may fear because we perceive this as rendering us *vulnerable*, the origin of which means 'to wound' (hence, incidentally, the categorization of wound healing herbs as 'vulneraries' of course). A conviction that sustains the state of fear is that, by operating from it, we are more able to protect ourselves. While an undiscriminating approach to the world based on a naïve loving trust might have dangers associated with it and the appropriate registering of fear may indeed have a protective capacity, the key issue is to do with enjoying a healthy and proportionate relationship between these two ways of being and reacting. Many patients live in an unwarranted and unnecessary state of fear that negatively impacts their wellbeing and contributes to the development of illness and disease. In such cases, the encouragement to choose love over fear when reacting to events (similar to choosing big-mind over small-mind) may help to promote a more positive and pleasurable engagement with the world.

The reasons why a patient is fundamentally and/or currently predisposed to live from a position of love or fear may lie deep but the practitioner can, nonetheless, raise awareness of these two poles and encourage the patient to reflect on their background and choices with regard to these two dimensions of being. The following set of correspondences may provide a trigger for such reflection (see Table 3.1).

### Seek novel experiences

A way of going out to meet change, rather than waiting for it to arrive, is to actively seek and engage in new experiences. Placing oneself in new situations that have the potential to lead to positive outcomes is a means of propagating learning.

### Be a lifelong learner

Many of us have grown up with the idea that education is a matter for children and adolescents and, in terms of higher education, young adults. Once we have come fully into maturity then formal education and learning is at an end. In recent years this conception has been changing, partly as a result of political interest in encouraging people to take a positive view of further education and re-training as a means of mitigating the backlash against poor job security and the need for re-employment. The term 'lifelong learner' has come into use to describe the role people are now increasingly expected to take on by the state in order to be flexible in finding new work to replace the

**Table 3.1** *Set of correspondences for 'Love' and 'Fear'*

| Love | Fear |
|---|---|
| Expand | Contract |
| Relax | Tense |
| Open | Closed |
| Expose | Conceal |
| Let go | Hold on |
| Receive | Reject |
| Accept | Oppose |
| Trust | Doubt |
| Eros | Thanatos |

job that has been lost. Yet there is a positive aspect to this concept (particularly when its application arises out of choice rather than necessity) for it does describe a key helpful approach to life – we are always learning and always have the potential to achieve something fresh and new. Cultivating an attitude of openness to self-directed learning will greater enable us to achieve autonomy and personal development.

### Exercise your senses

Human beings are social and sensual creatures. Recognizing and exercising our innate sensuality increases our pleasure in life and heightens our overall sense of wellbeing. Practitioners can help patients find their own ways of awakening or, when necessary, calming, their sense of: smell, touch, taste, hearing, seeing.

In contemporary western and westernized cultures audiovisual input is generally aggressively overemphasized, while taste may be demeaned by poor diet, smell assaulted by noxious synthetic odours and touch generally neglected.

It may be helpful to reduce or soften visual and auditory sensory activity by:

- Reducing exposure to television/computer screen imagery
- Paying closer attention to sights and sounds in nature
- Listening to more subtle musical forms
- Spending time sitting or lying with eyes closed.

The sense of taste is most joyfully developed by improving the diet and exposing the palate to freshly cooked ingredients and to a range of spices, herbs and other natural flavours. Variety, quality and intensity are the keys to enabling taste. It is also useful to avoid aggressive toothpastes, mouthwashes and so forth.

Smell is a fleeting sense that quickly tires of registering conscious signals. It is insulted by cigarette smoke and crude artificial odours such as are found in most washing powders and other cleaning products, room 'fresheners' and so forth. It delights in the subtle smells of nature: sea breezes, the night air, the warm exhalations of flowers, the pheromones of others. It is generally beneficial to reduce synthetic odours around the home by using ecological unperfumed cleaning products.

Many people are starved of touch from other human beings. Touch is given and received in many ways: touching hands, hugs and cuddles, the baby naked on the mother's chest, caressing, sexual activity, massage, stroking a cat or dog, simply holding someone. A number of studies have suggested that oxytocin and endorphin levels are raised by touch and lead to outcomes including decreased blood pressure and better stress control, as well as playing an important role in social bonding (Dunbar 2010). The practitioner can help the patient find appropriate ways of enhancing touch, including:

- Becoming more of a tactile person – expressing oneself more through the medium of touch, e.g. becoming more able to hold another's hand, give and receive hugs, etc.
- Giving and receiving massage with family and friends
- Engaging with nature in a more tactile way – touching the earth, walking barefoot, swimming, etc.

### Look to your death

Gaining a perspective on death and living in the face of the inevitability of death is a difficult challenge for many of us. Perspective is aided by a personal explanatory model or spiritual or religious conception that helps to make sense of dying – but this will not always prevent anxiety and fear arising in connection with the subject area. The practitioner can help by at least being open and able to discuss death and dying with patients, thereby lessening the taboo on broaching this topic. Beyond this, accepting that we will die can have a fecund influence on our life, helping us to relish the time in which we tread the earth.

### Be able to surrender

*Grasp, it cannot be held – it is intangible.*

Lao Tsu. In Feng and English (1973)

There are occasions when we need to let go, to surrender to an issue or situation when we are unable to make progress. Not to surrender in despair but rather to relieve ourselves of the burden of unproductive effort. Painful and difficult as it may be to open our hands and let go for fear of losing and falling, even so, surrender may enable us to move on and to release the blockage and stagnation that has built up around the issue of concern. It can help to surrender to 'something' – to God, the Universe, the Great Spirit, the earth, to mystery or love or healing. It is easier to surrender when we trust and have faith that good will follow, since this is the natural way of things – releasing one's grip allows movement, flow and change so that the natural processes of the universe can be re-established.

### Be open-minded, open-hearted and open-handed

The mind is opened by curiosity and humility; the heart is opened by love; the hand is opened by trust and generosity.

### Walk through life as if it were a labyrinth not a maze

A labyrinth appears convoluted but leads to the centre if one just keeps following the path. A maze has dead ends and trick turnings. Life is a labyrinth, it only appears to be a maze when we cease to move and change.

### Balance activity and rest across the four aspects of being: physical, emotional, mental, spiritual

We each have four aspects to our being which require activity and rest. Many methods of activity and rest affect more than one aspect of being. It is helpful to explore with patients which aspects are in need of stimulation or relaxation and find ways to provide the appropriate remedial influence. We will explore this idea in the next chapter.

### Remember that your body believes every word you say

We need to be careful what we tell ourselves about ourselves, what we choose to incorporate or exclude from the stories we create and repeat. Beliefs shape physiology through the pathways of psychoneuroendocrinoimmunology (what we think and feel impacts the body primarily via the nervous, hormonal and immune systems).

### Energy follows thought

The last point relates to the occult statement that 'energy follows thought'. What we think and believe about ourselves and the world will influence what we encounter and experience. If we accept this as a working hypothesis then it becomes imperative to questions one's thoughts and direct them to positive goals.

The advice above may be seen as largely psychospiritual and therefore properly belonging to (and only to be administered by) counsellors, clerics, philosophers and spiritual advisers. What territory is left to the phytotherapist then? Should we be content with prescribing complex pharmacological agents for physical ills? Clearly there is no need (and much less desire) for this to be the case. The holistic practitioner (whether phytotherapist or not) is able to work with the patient across a broad spectrum of activity and advice. Yet it may still be questioned to what extent any one practitioner can be qualified (with the legal implication here of 'certified') to deal with the vast scope of the themes, practices and perspectives we have just described. Here again we need to assert the value of the approach of the generalist and to question the dominant hierarchical position that the specialist currently occupies. Indeed, if the phytotherapist is to work simultaneously with the ancient multiplicity of the healer's roles (as philosopher, priest, teacher, trickster, etc.) and the potentials offered by the new approach to physiology (as psychoneuroendocrinoimmunology) then she need not, and in fact *cannot*, unduly restrict the cast of her therapeutic net.

A key query here concerns the extent to which a practitioner can work holistically without possession of a set of values and a broad range of perspectives informing appreciation of such vital questions as: What is life for? What is death? How can we be happy?

## THE PRACTITIONER AS TEACHER

Doctor from the Latin *docere*, to teach.

Dixon et al. (1999) consider that:

> *Inspirational doctors are as important as inspirational teachers, and a skilled physician healer may change a patient's perception of his disease ... and thereby improve symptoms in the short-term and possibly affect physiological processes in the longer term ... Another long-term skill is the ability to induce a positive illness attitude and coping style, which may change the course of a patient's life as well as his illness.*

When the practitioner facilitates the patient in reflecting on the nature of their predicament and provides suggestions on how to positively modulate their attitudes and behaviours to improve their situation, then the practitioner is acting as a teacher–healer. Teaching may also extend to specific activities, where the practitioner may provide instruction as well as reflection on, for example, how to:

- Eat
- Breathe
- Move
- Sleep
- Laugh
- Meditate.

These core activities are fundamental to health and wellbeing and improvements in their practice can be taught. Practitioners may give classes to focus on particular learning needs common to their patient group. For a phytotherapist this may include classes teaching:

- Self-care with herbal medicine
- Meditation techniques
- How to cook wholefoods
- Relaxation techniques
- Methods for stress-management
- How to grow culinary and medicinal herbs
- Ways to promote sound sleep
- Enabling personal growth and development
- Finding a new perspective on health and illness.

## THE SETTING FOR THE CONSULTATION

The consultation is an exercise in time travel wherein the patient may visit the past ('previous medical history') and imagine the future (health aims, hopes, wishes, choices) as well as exploring their present symptoms and situation. This exploration is limited in space however. In phytotherapy, as in mainstream general practice, the consultation usually occurs in a clinic setting; a territory that might be classified as 'neutral' but which is in fact a medicalized space to some degree and which is the 'home' of the practitioner and not the patient. The clinic space can hardly be credibly defended as a neutral space. Visits to the patient's home may occur but are not the norm in phytotherapy practice. Nonetheless, consultations at patients' homes may have the benefit of furnishing helpful details with regard to such areas as:

- Living circumstances
- Local environment
- Interactions with others at home
- Facilities available, e.g. for cooking
- Food types kept at home
- Factors such as noise, light, heat, dust, airiness, etc.
- Presence of animals
- Extent to which home is a pleasant place to be
- Order or disorder of the home
- Access to outdoor space.

Despite these potential advantages, an interview in the home environment may restrict the patient in being able to relax and explore issues outside of their day-to-day thoughts. The ability to move beyond familiar thought processes and reasoning may potentially be facilitated by being interviewed outside of familiar surroundings.

In the 1930s, the American physician and medical educator George Canby Robinson (1878–1960), author of *The Patient as a Person* (Robinson 1939), emphasized the importance of getting to know the patient in their home and work environments as well as in the clinic in order that they might be appreciated as 'total individuals'. His efforts led to the institution, in several medical schools, of programmes where medical students routinely interviewed patients at home and in workplace settings and focussed on counselling them in health promotion and illness prevention strategies. This approach became known as the 'biopsychosocial' model. It declined in popularity in the 1950s however, partly due to a lack of enthusiasm for the approach on the part of medical students, as Brown (1998) reports: '… students grew frustrated when families had little or no disease and found their health-counselling roles disappointing. They wanted to 'learn medicine', which for them meant learning the latest in the diagnosis and treatment of organic disease … They regularly sabotaged case conferences by claiming that social and psychological problems were unimportant and by trying to restrict discussion to purely medical issues'. The students preferred that their interactions with patients were both contained with regards to location (within a clinical rather than a domestic setting) and limited with regard to content (to 'medical' matters, which excludes psychosocial phenomena). This containment and limitation reduces boredom, heightens drama and bolsters status. Working with patients holistically exposes us to the mundane and requires the generation of a taste for subtlety and complexity on the part of the practitioner. There also needs to be a degree of humility in the face of the low impact that the practitioner's contribution may frequently have and patience in seeing results accrue over long periods of time. Subtlety, humility and patience are among the hard-won fruits of an experienced practitioner's labours and require a slow maturation process in order to be fully relished. These are qualities that are not easy to instil in students and are more difficult still to sell to them.

The consulting room is a theatrical space in which a play is enacted – part-scripted, part-improvised. The Acts of the play are known as:

- Entrance
- Introductions
- Case history
- Physical examination
- Summary/Conclusion
- Exit.

Some of the lines are prepared in advance:

*'So, tell me what you would like help with'.*

If the practitioner asserts herself as chief actor, directing the patient to provide stock answers to leading questions drawn from a narrow repertoire, then little of novelty or artistic merit (clinical insight) is likely to emerge. However, when the practitioner is subtle and skilful and has a broad scope then the performers might be transported to far distant realms – all without leaving a small, fixed stage. Thus, careful questioning about home and work factors may go a long way to compensating for lack of physical exposure to those environments. (We will discuss the detail of such questioning later, in Ch. 6.) Even so, there are limitations as to how far this is able to provide an adequate replacement for a site-specific consultation in some cases.

During the consultation, the patient and practitioner traverse a landscape in companionship, telling each other stories as they do so. This landscape is imaginary and is constructed by moving back and forth in time during the exploration of the case history in the consultation, and moving between places, events and life-stages that the patient has inhabited. This journey is usually taken with the patient and practitioner sitting down together, with no physical motion occurring apart from slight adjustments in posture and, perhaps, changes in natural light or the movements of trees through a window. Carpiano (2009) has described a technique in qualitative research known as the 'go-along' interview, where the interview takes place while the interviewer and participant walk (or ride) through a pertinent physical landscape such as a local neighbourhood. Carpiano states that: 'because of its ability to examine a participant's interpretations of their contexts *while experiencing these contexts*, the go-along offers a number of potential benefits for studying how place may matter for people's health and well-being ...' [original italics]. This method raises intriguing questions about the potential value of conducting some consultations in this manner – if practical impediments can be overcome. In addition, one wonders about the benefits that might possibly be obtained from walking as opposed to sitting consultations, in broader terms. Would interviewing patients while walking in a park or herb garden lead to greater relaxation, enhanced connection-making and more poetic insight into the patient's predicament? Which other ways might there be for creatively shifting the standard clinic-room sit-down consultation?

## THE STRUCTURE OF THE CONSULTATION

The guide structure of the consultation in phytotherapy differs little from that used in many other medical modalities, including conventional medical practice. The map of the territory of the consultation in phytotherapy is not especially distinctive – the more crucial areas for us to focus on have to do with the way in which the terrain is navigated and what the phytotherapist is looking out for along the way. Let us begin with the cartography of the consultation in any case.

### OUTLINE FORMAT FOR AN INITIAL CONSULTATION

- Welcome
- Check personal details
- Introduce the consultation
- Presenting complaint
- History of the presenting complaint
- Previous medical history
- Family history
- Drug history
- Allergies/intolerances/sensitivities
- Social history
- Systems exploration
- Physical examination
- Summarize conclusions and discuss
- Treatment plan
- Arrange next visit.

### OUTLINE FORMAT FOR FOLLOW-UP CONSULTATIONS

- Welcome
- Check changes since last visit
- Review issues recorded at last visit
- Physical examination
- Summarize conclusions and discuss
- Treatment plan
- Arrange next visit.

Herbal practitioners tend to allot 1–1.5 h for initial consultations and 30 min to 1 h for follow-ups, in adults. For children, typical consult times are 45 min to 1 h for initial consultations and 30 min for follow-ups. These times are much longer than those allocated in conventional medical practice but are similar to those offered by many CAM practitioners such as osteopaths, acupuncturists and reflexologists. However, in CAM modalities such as the three just mentioned, the consultation itself occupies only part of the total appointment time since the treatment is also delivered within that time, e.g. in a 45 min follow-up appointment with an acupuncturist, 15 min might be spent on the interview and 30 min on applying the treatment. In the phytotherapy consultation, the entire appointment time is dedicated to interview, examination, advice giving and discussion – the treatment being taken at home, not in the consulting room. Very few other modalities devote so much time to the interview as phytotherapists, outside of the psychotherapies and homoeopathy.

The extended duration of phytotherapy consultations allows for a thorough exploration of the patient's history, concerns and wishes. It provides the patients with an opportunity to express themselves and to engage in reflection upon their predicament. It also gives adequate time for the practitioner to give advice and discuss its implementation with the patient. In my experience, it is common to find that patients have never been given so much room to explore their condition in such depth before and they frequently contrast the experience with previous conventional medical encounters – often expressing understanding of the institutional limits set on the doctor's time ('My doctor is very good but she doesn't have the time to look at things in detail'), although frequently critical of the perceived narrowness and shallowness of the conventional consultation: ('It's ridiculous, how can you treat someone without getting to know them properly and understanding what the problem really is?'.)

It is curious that time and the consultation, although commonly an issue identified by patients, is inadequately explored in the literature. Thompson et al. (2007) in their study of patient participation in consultations saw the issue of time as one of the gaps in knowledge pertaining to this area; they expressed the opinion that 'although lack of time is in itself insufficient explanation for restrictions on patient participation, it does play a part'. One issue that arises when beginning to consider time and the consultation is with regard to how the passing of time is perceived. Klitzman (2007) considers that:

> *Time is measured in not only objective, standardized units, but in sociocultural terms ... types of tasks and social structures affect how groups experience dimensions of time such as its 'flexibility, linearity, pace, punctuality, delay ... urgency, scarcity, and future and present time perspectives ...'. In general, the duration of time is also experienced subjectively ...*

Klitzman studied the perceptions of time as experienced by doctors who later became patients with a serious illness and proposed that three broadly differing perceptions of time arise in healthcare encounters: 'patient-time', 'doctor-time' and 'institution-time'. These relate to the patient's and doctor's sense of time and the time-framing set by, or occurring as a consequence of, institutional policies and processes with regard to, e.g. waiting times for and at appointments, and time-limits set on consultation length. Differences between the three perspectives occurred in defining concepts such as 'how long is "long"?' and with regard to terms such as 'soon', 'fast', 'slow', 'plenty' and 'quickly', e.g. one of Klitzman's doctor/patients commented:

> *'My doctor said that Hodgkin's doesn't spread "that quickly"; and the speed probably wasn't going to change what they did, or my outcome. But once you're told that you have cancer, it's very hard to have that overall perspective'.*

The initial phytotherapy consultation, particularly, can affect patients profoundly, especially if they are only used to conventional medical encounters that typically span only a few minutes. Representative comments from patients include reference to the extent of ground covered: 'Now you know more about me than anyone else!' And to the impact of being able to explore their situation in such depth: 'I feel like I'm going to be able to get on top of this thing now'. The impact may be especially pronounced when the phytotherapy consultation represents the first time the patient has had to explore a 'physical' condition in great detail. While it is culturally permissible to spend an extensive amount of time discussing a 'mental health problem' with a psychotherapist of some description, it is less acceptable to spend a large amount of time discussing physical conditions. The popular perception is that treatment of physical conditions requires action, not talk. The more time you spend talking about it the greater is the chance that your condition will lose its status as primarily physical in nature and start to be considered as something 'in the mind'. Patients with conditions that are accompanied by significant physical symptoms but for which there is no reliable quick-acting treatment available (such as chronic fatigue syndrome, irritable bowel syndrome and endometriosis) are particularly prone to this process. Being given time and permission to express and voice feelings and thoughts about one's predicament; being encouraged to test making new connections and to ponder different explanatory models; and examining new strategies to consider and practise in ameliorating or transforming one's condition – these are powerful facilitations *but* they require time to be done 'properly', meaning with adequate time to feel and to think and to process what arises to a point where the learning is embodied. The generation of insights during the consultation takes time and skill but further time is required for insights to be processed and fixed.

The consultation should be a fresh, nutritious, nurturing experience with time for its substance to be properly digested. The conventional medical consultation is analogous to having a fast food meal, whereas the phytotherapy consultation has the capacity to be a deeply satisfying slow-cooked wholefood banquet. The doctor is driven by corporate constraints to get as many customers in and out of the restaurant as fast as they can. The phytotherapist in the UK is usually self-employed and can set her own consultation times to allow enough space for a holistic consultation protocol to be applied and for maximum nourishment to be derived by the patient.

This is not to suggest that a long consultation time is always necessary. Some conditions are straightforward and some patients have already explored their situation in enough detail to be clear where they stand and to not currently need any further exegesis. In these circumstances, the necessary orientation and understanding required by both patient and practitioner may be achieved more rapidly. In a letter referring to research into patients' wants and the extent to which they are met in consultations in general practice Jenkins et al. (2002) stated that: 'our findings indicate that consultations do not have to be longer for patients to have good outcomes, and even the shortest of consultations can provide all that patients want. From the patient's perspective it seems that satisfactory consultations do not have to be long ones'. (*Note*: In the study referred to, consultation times varied between 2 and

21 min). The nature of how patient's wants are shaped and framed needs to be questioned here. Wants are influenced, in part, by previous experience and by expectancies of whether they can be met or not. For example, a CAM-disposed patient may visit a doctor to receive a medical diagnosis to inform their understanding of their predicament but they may neither want nor expect to receive any other insight into their condition or any treatment for it. In such a case, the 'want' of a conventional diagnosis may be met by the doctor with the patient fulfilling other 'wants' elsewhere.

Work into determining the quality of consultations in general practice settings has focussed on the extent to which the consultation 'enables' the patient, i.e. following the consultation, to what extent does the patient feel more able to do such things as to cope with their lives, understand their illness, help themselves and keep themselves healthy (Howie 2000). Another study by Howie et al. (1999) found that the two key factors resulting in improved enablement were longer consultations and 'how well the patient knows the doctor'. Among their major conclusions was that, as opposed to patients with more straightforward problems: 'patients with more complex problems require longer consultations to achieve equal enablement'. Mercer et al. (2007) found that patient enablement was significantly increased by longer consultation times for both complex and non-complex consultations. It is important to bear in mind that perceptions of what constitutes a 'long' consultation time will differ enormously between conventional and phytotherapy practitioners, e.g. 'long' in Mercer's just cited study was 'around 15 min', while we have previously said that phytotherapy follow-up consults commonly can last for an hour. The phytotherapy consultation provides an extended duration of consultation time and phytotherapists mostly operate single-phytotherapist practices so that the requirement of 'knowing the practitioner well' can also be accommodated. Freeman et al. (2002) found that longer consultation times yielded several benefits, including: 'more advice on lifestyle and other health promoting activities … better recognition and handling of psychosocial problems and … better patient enablement. Also (better) clinical care for some chronic illnesses …'. Although no studies are available to support the claim, this list of benefits is consistent with areas emphasized as key areas of practice by phytotherapists.

The phytotherapy consultation is potentially therapeutic in its own right since its extended and in-depth nature provides a cohering force that may power a renewed vitality on the part of the patient in re-engaging with their predicament from an enhanced perspective. Other possible therapeutic influences and outcomes of the consultation include:

- The sense of having been taken seriously
- The feeling of having been understood
- The forging of new connections in interpreting their situation
- Arriving at an enhanced level of meaning and self-perception
- Gaining new techniques and strategies for coping and developing.

## THE CONSULTATION AS LABYRINTH

We have established that the outline format for the consultation in phytotherapy (as listed above) is essentially the same as that used in many other therapeutic modalities, including conventional medicine. Students of herbal medicine generally learn to proceed through this list sequentially, hopefully spending plenty of time in each section to explore its dimensions fully but nonetheless steering a steady course through each successive category. Phytotherapy can be successfully practised in this way, with the key point of distinction from many other modalities using a similar step-by-step guide being, in this instance, the degree to which the herbal practitioner gathers detail and looks for connections.

A more potent method for traversing the landscape of the consultation is available, however. This method is more suitable for adoption by advanced practitioners (indeed it appears to spontaneously arise in such practitioners) but its principles can be taught to students. This is the 'non-linear path'. In the non-linear approach the practitioner has internalized the sections that comprise the outline format of the consultation but is not compelled to follow them sequentially. There is instead a freedom to follow the patient's lead and to go with what appears to be the most significant need in that particular consultation, while at all times being aware of the elements that might need to be drawn-in to ensure safety.

In this approach, the 'sections' of the classical consultation become unbounded and allowed to meld into each other. For example, if during the early stage of an initial consultation (classically the territory of the 'presenting complaint' or the 'history of the presenting complaint'), the patient mentions that they are taking *Seretide* for asthma, the practitioner may say: 'Since you mentioned that, can we take a pause here to check what other medications you might be taking?' In this way, the 'drug history' is contained within another classical section rather than outside of it.

Sections of the classical format may also be repeated several times rather than gathered together in one particular group, thereby ceasing to be 'sections' and instead merely being themes or strategies that can be employed as appropriate rather than waiting until their turn comes. For example, advice-giving does not have to wait until the end of the consultation – separate pieces of advice can be given as they come to mind or seem most relevant at various junctures in the consultation, perhaps being brought together and reiterated under the heading of 'advice' at the end of the consultation to help coherence. Another example: pieces of physical examination might be dispersed throughout the consult rather than being herded together into one section. This may not always be appropriate since it may be disruptive and cause the patient unnecessary inconvenience, particularly if they to have to undress and dress again several times over. Yet, if the patient mentions that they have a sore tongue or tingling in their hands or a click when opening their jaw it may feel more appropriate to look at those things as they arise rather than waiting to look at them in the 'physical examination section' later, when the examination will be divorced from the initial discussion of the phenomenon.

Simply asking the patient to: 'Tell me about your ... asthma/pain/sleep/skin/weight/breathlessness, etc.' tends to stimulate the patient to tell a story that crosses the boundaries of previous medical history, social history and drug history. Initiating an open approach to storytelling on the part of the patient in this way, and then following the patient's lead as they set off, naturally takes one into the labyrinth of the consultation. Recall that the labyrinth is *not* a maze – the centre of the labyrinth is reached by merely following the path, there are no dead ends or trick turns, rather every step is significant, purposeful. Yet the path to the centre of the labyrinth is non-linear – it meanders and twists. We approach things in the labyrinth sideways, obliquely, sometimes seeming to be moving further away from the centre until suddenly we turn a corner and move closer back to it. This is the way that patients tend to recount their narratives. The practitioner in the labyrinth must keep careful track of the patient's route and be able to respond spontaneously to new themes and ideas that arise as the course of the consultation is trod.

Students tend to find it difficult to work in this way since they feel themselves losing their place as they attempt to follow the patient. There is an attempt instead to impose order on the patient's narrative by steering it, and by disregarding information that they were not seeking. The student may stare blankly at intruders who do not belong in the section they are currently focussing on. It is only when the practitioner is experienced enough and has developed fluency and flexibility in accompanying the patient on their journey that she is able to relax and cede control, secure in the knowledge that she knows the highways and byways of the consultation territory well enough not to get lost.

As the consultation is unfolding, the practitioner is alert to particular cues, especially those conveying signals about:

- Abnormality
- Illness and disease
- Risk
- Corrective measures required
- Treatment potential.

Articulation of this information gives rise to discussion about diagnosis, the need for further investigation and appropriate advice and treatment. None of these areas are value-free – they all depend on the practitioner's own orientation, which is shaped by personal, educational and sociocultural influences, as we discussed earlier in this chapter. Thus, actions, attributes and behaviours that constitute normality/abnormality; health/disease; risk/safety; requiring treatment/to be left alone, in any practitioner's schema, are sensitive to a range of modulating factors. Two that need to be highlighted are:

1. The principles and dictates of the school of thought and practice into which the practitioner has been trained and inducted
2. The nature and potentials of the therapeutic options to which the practitioner has access.

Both these areas fundamentally direct what the practitioner is seeking in the consultation (and therefore what they are likely to find) and how she will respond to what she has found.

In phytotherapy we can posit the ways in which the physical process, and the internal processing, of the consultation are directed and limited/liberated by the particular beliefs and convictions that the phytotherapist holds about (1) the human body and (2) the healing plant. We have visited some of this area already in this chapter but it may still be worth bringing some of the themes previously discovered together again at this point.

1. Phytotherapist's view of the body:
   - The body is 'one' – within itself and with its environment
   - It has a four-fold nature: physical, emotional, mental and spiritual
   - These four aspects, like its organ systems, are integrated
   - The four aspects each require an appropriate balance of activity and rest
   - The body is animated by a vital force that can be modulated by the *vis medicatrix naturae* (healing power of nature)
   - It is self-organizing
   - It is self-healing
   - It is complex
   - It is subtle
   - It responds to gentle influences ('nudges')
   - It is adaptive and creative
   - It cannot be fully known or understood
   - Small changes in the body are important to note as they signify larger potentials
   - The body conveys messages to the person which the person can 'hear'
   - The body has an inner wisdom
   - It is both robust and sensitive
   - It is part of nature and is diminished when separated from nature or when exposed to agents that are unnatural
   - It is whole and is sustained by contact with other wholes – wholefood, whole plant remedies, other bodies
   - It is sentient and sensual – senses and feelings are as relevant as thoughts and ideas
   - It is social and requires interaction with other bodies, other species and nature
   - It delights in novel experiences and play
   - It possesses a profoundly developmental and transformative capacity mediated by the power of imagination
   - Disease and dying are natural elements in a body's history – they need not always be fought or feared
   - It is to be approached with awe and wonder.
2. Phytotherapist's views of the healing plant:
   - The plant is 'one' – within itself and with its environment
   - It is whole and has affinity for other wholes, such as the human body
   - It is a primary agent of the *vis medicatrix naturae* (healing power of nature)
   - It can potentiate self-healing in the human body
   - It is complex
   - It is subtle
   - It cannot be fully known or understood
   - It provides gentle influences ('nudges') that can trigger small changes in the human body that lead to larger enhancements

- Certain plants can also provide more aggressive stimuli and are to be used with caution
- It has a long and intimate history of entanglement with the human body and therefore is not alien or foreign
- It can educate or guide the human body towards normal/optimal physiological behaviour
- It can modulate a wide range of human bodily activity via adaptation of major control systems (e.g. circulation, immunity, hormonal and neurological activity)
- It usually has multi-system effects
- It can exert local effects at a cellular, tissue or organ level (e.g. at the mitochondria, mucous membranes, and organs such as the liver)
- Healing plants can treat pictures of both deficiency and excess
- Healing plants have some role to play in virtually every predicament of the human body – both in health and illness
- They tend to act quickly in acute conditions and gradually but cumulatively in chronic ones
- They are highly malleable in being transformed into a wide variety of preparations
- It is to be approached with awe and wonder.

These factors form the precepts by which the herbal practitioner conducts the consultation, both in terms of the process of the consultation itself and the internal processing that accompanies it. They shape the way that the phytotherapist looks at the patient and what she is looking for. These two views – how the body is and how the plant is – combine to give rise to a number of conclusions, attitudes, practices and behaviours on the part of the phytotherapist, which are implemented (consciously or unconsciously) during the consultation. They inform the enactment and navigation of the consultation and the nature of the advice and treatment given. These guiding principles/practices include:

- Being comfortable with uncertainty since the body and the plant, and their interactions, cannot be fully understood
- Allowing for mystery in the consultation
- Flexibility in responding to emergent properties arising from the interaction of two complex systems – body and plants. This means that the prescription will tend to change from consult to consult to mirror the change in the patient
- Paying attention to small details of the patient's awareness of themselves
- Considering the relevant involvement of activity at the level of major control systems, organs, tissues and cells
- Noting where excesses need to be calmed and deficiencies need to be replenished
- Reflecting on the need for balancing activity and rest across the four aspects of being – physical, emotional, mental, spiritual
- Patience and confidence in the face of gradual progress in chronic conditions
- Preference for using the gentlest remedies possible in any given situation

- Creativity in adapting the form of herbal preparation to meet the patient's needs
- Thoroughness in advising a suitable range of remedial strategies and concepts.

Application of these approaches will translate, in terms of the prescription, into designing a medicine that will include specific herbs providing appropriate actions to modulate the patient's physiology. For example:

- Adaptogens: used where vitality is low; immune resistance is diminished; stress is present
- Nervines: used to soothe, calm, promote sleep, reduce anxiety, strengthen in depleted and convalescent pictures
- Carminatives: to enhance digestive function; ease spasmodic abdominal pain
- Circulatory stimulants: to warm the peripheries; enhance the delivery of nutrients and oxygen to tissues; improve elimination of waste products
- Antioxidants: to stabilize and protect tissues; reduce inflammation; stimulate wound repair.

So a prescription is built and we arrive at a combination of herbs being compounded and given to the patient to take away as the most tangible fruit of the consultation – yet it is not necessarily the only one.

To conclude this chapter, a more detailed discussion of the nature of complexity and its relevance to the consultation is offered below.

## COMPLEXITY AND THE CONSULTATION

The concept of complexity is variously defined in the literature, substantiating Sole and Goodwin's (2000) assertion that: 'There are many possible definitions of complexity'. The search for a clear definition of complexity is made more difficult by the frequently encountered confusion or blurring of complexity and chaos theories. Camazine and co-workers (2001) broach this difficulty, first identifying that: 'The literature on nonlinear systems often mentions self-organization, emergent properties, and complexity as well as dissipative structures and chaos …' They go on to define complexity and complex systems by saying that these:

> … *generally refer to a system of interacting units that displays global properties not present at the lower level. These systems may show diverse responses that are often sensitively dependent on both the initial state of the system and nonlinear interactions amongst its components. Since these nonlinear interactions involve amplification or cooperativity, complex behaviours may emerge even though the system components may be similar and follow simple rules.*

Such a clarification is helpful but it shares many of the features that others apply to a definition of chaos! However, chaos theory does contribute to an understanding of complex systems, and vice versa. There is an overlap, indeed an *intertwining* between the two, but some authorities assert that there are important points of difference. Cilliers (1998) has observed that:

*When analysing complex systems, a sensitivity to initial conditions, for example, is not such an important issue. As a matter of fact, it is exactly the* robust *nature of complex systems, i.e. their capability to perform in the same way under different conditions, that ensures their survival.*

A further consideration is the differentiation between systems which are *complex* and those which are *complicated*. Cilliers, again, has summarized the position as follows:

*If a system – despite the fact that it may consist of a huge number of components – can be given a complete description in terms of its individual constituents, such a system is merely* complicated. *Things like jumbo jets ... are complicated. In a* complex *system ... the interaction among constituents of the system, and the interaction between the system and its environment, are of such a nature that the system as a whole cannot be fully understood simply by analysing its components. Moreover, these relationships are not fixed, but shift and change, often as a result of self-organization.*

This latter point seems crucial and means that complex systems are usually living ones. It also aids our appreciation of the difference between chaotic and complex systems, as Cilliers further explains:

*... the discussion of self-organization ... helps us to make the ... point that the behaviour of a system without a predetermined or fixed structure is not necessarily random or chaotic, in other words, that anything does not go.*

Before proceeding it is worth noting Strumia's (2007) reminder that much of the language used in the science of complexity and chaos is not really new, indeed many of the words: 'sound similar, even if not identical, to some (Latin) terms of ancient (Greek and Mediaeval) philosophy of nature, metaphysics and logic ...' For example: complexity/*complexio*, chaos/*quies*, dynamics/*motus*, self-similarity/*similitudo*, etc. The work around complexity can be seen as a re-engagement with an ancient project.

## THE CONSULTATION IS A COMPLEX PROCESS

The healthcare consultation may have several components, including:

- Case history-taking
- Physical examination
- Discussion of case management.

Overall, these components involve evidence gathering, storytelling and story interpreting, and advice giving.

From the perspective of complexity theory, we might describe the phytotherapy consultation process as: the interaction of complex living creatures (human beings), using a complex living system of meaning representation (language), and specific complex sense-making strategies (storytelling and story interpretation) to assess the emergent status of the patient and help facilitate self-organization, specifically through prescription of complex, systems-level medicines (plant remedies). In following this idea through it may be helpful to return to our earlier contrasting of homeostasis with homoeodynamism in questioning the concept of health care as focused on the re-establishment of homoeostasis (so that the internal milieu is stable and resistant to disruption). A homoeodynamic perspective fits more closely with the concept of health in a complex system and allows for therapy to facilitate change and enhancement of physiological functioning – not just a return to default settings. To put this into perspective let us cite Lloyd (2001) again:

> ... biological systems are homeodynamic because of their ability to dynamically self-organise at bifurcation points of their behaviour where they lose stability. Consequently, they exhibit diverse behaviour; in addition to monotonic stationery states, living systems display complex behaviour with all its emergent characteristics ... It is dynamic organisation under homeodynamic conditions that make possible the organised complexity of life.

## WORKING WITH COMPLEXITY IN THE CONSULTATION

As Cilliers (1998) has put it, complex systems: 'are not fixed, but shift and change, often as a result of self-organization'. The proposition in this section is that the consultation process itself may act as an agent of 'shift and change', having a therapeutic ('placebo') effect or negative ('nocebo') effect, depending on how skilfully it is conducted.

Drawing on the earlier stated differentiation between the *complex* and the *complicated* we might say that, while CAM therapists tend to approach the individual as a complex entity, the error of orthodox medicine has been to see the person as merely complicated. Where patients have complex conditions therefore, orthodox practitioners may have difficulties in furthering their progress. The process works both ways of course – the great success of orthodox medicine has been in treating those conditions which we might consider as complicated as opposed to complex (mechanical problems and those with an identifiable organic lesion which can be suppressed, removed or replaced). Even here though there are usually profound complex aspects that may be left unaddressed. A malignant tumour, for example, may be seen as merely complicated in terms of its physical substance but the situation becomes highly complex if we consider questions such as: how did the tumour arise and might it return again?

It follows from the above that a consultation style that appreciates and attempts to fully (that is to say, as fully as is possible) explore the complexity of the patient's predicament is: (a) more likely to arrive at a profound understanding of the person's situation and therapeutic needs, and (b) more likely to be therapeutic *in itself*.

Medicine has tended to emphasize the importance of a logical approach to the consultation, attempting to delineate clearly defined cause-and-effect relationships. Although we can assert that all practitioners additionally use intuition in understanding patients, this capacity has been little studied or appreciated. Greenhalgh (2002) has discussed how intuition might be developed and used by practitioners and describes one of the key features of intuitive thinking being that it: 'addresses, integrates, and makes sense of, multiple complex pieces of data'. Clearly a capacity that offers this potential seems ideally suited to working with the complex consultation. Greenhalgh goes on to further define intuition as:

> ... a decision-making method that is used unconsciously by experienced practitioners ... it is rapid, subtle, contextual ... [it] is not unscientific. It is a highly creative process ... [and] we can improve our intuitive powers through systematic critical reflection about intuitive judgements.

While the facility of intuition increases with experience, Greenhalgh presents evidence that intuitive skills can be developed using educational methods such as reflective discussion groups.

Traditional and complementary medicine approaches may be more congruent with the concept of complexity than orthodox approaches. Porkert and Ullmann (1988), for example, say this of Chinese medicine:

> ... it is functional (rather than somatic) and inductive and synthetic (rather than causal-analytic). It regards the human body as a system of function circles, or functional regions ... [it] is primarily concerned with functions and with movement, with the dynamic and the psychic.

This description fits well with our discussion of complexity so far.

## IMPLICATIONS OF WORKING WITH COMPLEXITY IN THE CONSULTATION

Some authors have attempted to link complexity, chaos and the consultation, such as Innes et al. (2005):

> ... metaphor from mathematical 'chaos' theory describes a state known as the 'edge of chaos' where a complex system is unstable and small changes within or external to the system may precipitate a radical change. Some consultations have this form of instability. Indeed, a doctor or patient may move a consultation to the 'edge of chaos' as a deliberate strategy to achieve greater creativity.

Many practitioners might view such a prospect with alarm – moving to the edge of chaos may present opportunities for creativity but some will be anxious that it also presents scope for litigation. A key challenge of working with complexity theory in the consultation is that of developing a sense of comfort with not knowing and with uncertainty. In a paper looking at how doctor's deal with uncertainty surrounding medical evidence, Griffiths et al. (2005) observed that: 'A dilemma for health professionals is creating a myth of certainty around what is inherently uncertain'. Much better to acknowledge, or even embrace, uncertainty and consider how best to work with it? Moscati, cited by Foucault (2007), has provided advice which seems particularly apt for phytotherapists:

> *Observe the sick, assist nature without violating it, and wait, admitting in all modesty that much knowledge is still lacking.*

Stacey (2001, 2002) has written about applying the principles of complexity and chaos in the business world, specifically in organizational management. Stacey's 'certainty-agreement' model is widely cited. This model describes three zones related to cases and decision making. These are – the simple zone where both certainty around the nature of the problem, and agreement between the parties on how to proceed are both high; the complex zone where both certainty and agreement are low and the chaotic zone where both are very low. Plesk and Greenhalgh (2001) assert that when we move out of the simple zone:

> *Our learnt instinct ... based on reductionist thinking, is to troubleshoot and fix things – in essence to break down the ambiguity, resolve any paradox, achieve more certainty and agreement, and move into the simple zone.*

There is an alternative however:

> *... complexity science suggests that it is often better to try multiple approaches and let direction arise by gradually shifting time and attention towards those things that seem to be working best.*

Herbs fit well here – also the idea of adapting the prescription at each consult to accommodate (or to dance with) the emergent properties of the patient.

Such a way of working calls for re-education, not only of practitioners, but also of patient's expectations. Many patients dwell in the zones of complexity and chaos, and these people may be better helped by a new type of relationship with their practitioners.

The zones of simplicity, complexity and chaos have some resonance with the three types of illness narratives identified by Frank (1995). These have been well described by Nettleton (2006):

> *[In] The* restitution narrative *... [the] person is ill, finds out what is wrong, seeks help and/or uses medication, and gets better ... [This model] fits social expectations, and is dominant in popular culture. It is the narrative that we are most comfortable with, and the one medicine can most comfortably bear.*

> *The* quest narrative *is 'defined by the ill person's belief that something is to be gained through experience ...' The illness may become a metaphorical journey from which the ill person may gain self-awareness, or the ability to help others ... The* chaos narrative *is the antithesis of the restitution narrative – in that there is no clear beginning and no actual or imagined end. There is no narrative 'structure' as such; no 'plot', no clear 'route map', and no 'metaphorical journey'. Consequently, chaos narratives are difficult to 'listen' to, and ... to 'hear', because they may invoke anxiety in that the very existence of an illness that cannot be 'cured' reminds the listener of their own vulnerability. Furthermore, chaos narratives remind practitioners of their limitations.*

The restitution model can only work within the simple zone. It also fits with the paternalistic medical approach and with the aims of reductive science – as such it is the default mode for both patients and practitioners interacting within the conventional biomedical framework. Patients engaged in the quest narrative will often feel best accommodated within complementary and alternative medicine settings, where their quest will generally be valued and supported. Those participating in chaos narratives, however, are unlikely to find an easy home with any practitioners – outside of the various psychological therapies. Such persons, particularly, need to be viewed with a more complex gaze by practitioners.

Even in the reductive world of pharmacology, a new movement towards recognizing the need for a more complex approach can be discerned (as mentioned in Ch. 1):

*In searching for new and effective therapeutics, it might be useful to use a systems-chemistry approach to modify integrated outcomes rather than targeting single molecules with the hope that the desired systematic effect might be generated. In other words, it is likely that creating a 'new homoeostasis' will require the modification of more than one target.*

Hotamisligil (2006)

Human beings are inherently complex. The biomedical project to find simple solutions ('magic bullets') in the face of the challenge presented by complexity has been partially successful – in the 'simple zone'. Yet, it leaves a large number of patients poorly served.

The American physiologist Walter Cannon coined the term 'homoeostasis' in 1926. It is easy to appreciate the broader significance/meaning of the notion of a 'steady state' articulated between the two World Wars. In the post-modern world (as in the ancient world of Heraclitus and Lao Tzu) the suggestion that maintaining a fixed state is the natural order of things is not supported by cutting edge science in fields such as quantum mechanics and cosmology. The nature of things lies in change, flux, movement, flow and dynamic shifts.

Ari Goldberger (2002) has observed that:

*According to classical concepts of physiologic control, healthy systems are self-regulated to reduce variability and maintain physiologic constancy. Contrary to the predictions of homoeostasis, however, the output of a wide variety of systems, such as the normal human heartbeat, fluctuates in a complex manner, even under resting conditions.*

Some authorities now consider that a lack of complexity, or 'too much order' as previously mentioned, is associated with ill-health. Martinez-Lavin et al. (2007) report the finding of decreased heart rate variability and monotonous circadian rhythm patterns in patients with fibromyalgia. They conclude that: 'These anomalies can be interpreted as a "decomplexification" of the autonomic nervous system …'.

We might suggest that the orthodox consultation presents an attempt at 'decomplexification' of the individual, in which case it can be said to be potentially contributing to the patient's ill health. Seen in this light, the case for developing better ways of working with complexity in the consultation becomes an urgent one and phytotherapists are well paced to provide an alternative model. The extended and comprehensive nature of the phytotherapy consultation allows for complex consideration of the patient. The properties and capacities of plant remedies provide treatment options that are not only consistent with the complex nature of the herbal practitioner's project, but which fundamentally shape it.

## Acknowledgements

The author gratefully acknowledges the influence on his thought in the section entitled 'Engendering Wellbeing' of Bob Duggan, Principal of Tai Sophia Institute for the Healing Arts, Maryland. Bob has been teaching many of the concepts and practices listed in this section in inspiring workshops for many years. A number of the strategies described derive from Bob's work though they represent the author's take and any crudities or errors of reasoning and expression are entirely the author's own. The reader might be interested to note that Ivan Illich was Bob's mentor for several decades.

## REFERENCES

Antonovsky A: *Unravelling the mystery of health: how people manage stress and stay well,* San Francisco, 1987, Jossey-Bass.

Barsky AJ: The paradox of health, *New England Journal of Medicine* 318(7):414–418, 1988.

Brown TM: George Canby Robinson and 'The patient as a person'. In Lawrence C, Weisz G, editors: *Greater than the parts: holism in biomedicine 1920–1950,* 1998, Oxford University Press.

Camazine S, Deneuborg JL, Franks NR, et al: *Self-organization in biological systems,* 2001, Princeton University Press.

Carpiano RM: Come take a walk with me: the 'go-along' interview as a novel method for studying the implications of place for health and well-being, *Health & Place* 15:263–272, 2009.

Cassell EJ: *The nature of suffering: and the goals of medicine,* ed 2, 2004, Oxford University Press.

Cilliers P: *Complexity and postmodernism: understanding complex systems,* London, 1998, Routledge.

Dixon M, Sweeney K, Pereira Gray D: The physician healer: ancient magic or modern science? *British Journal of General Practice* 49:309–312, 1999.

Dunbar R: The social role of touch in humans and primates: behavioural function and neurobiological mechanisms, *Neuroscience and Biobehavioural Reviews* 34(2):260–268, 2010.

Duggan RM: *Common sense for the healing arts: Essays by Robert M Duggan,* Laurel, 2003, Tai Sophia Press.

Egnew TR: The meaning of healing: transcending suffering, *Annals of Family Medicine* 3(3):255–262, 2005.

Emerson RW: *The essential writings of Ralph Waldo Emerson,* New York, 2000, Modern Library Classics.

Endler PC, Haug TM, Spranger H: Sense of coherence and physical health. A 'Copenhagen Interpretation' of Antonovsky's SOC concept, *Scientific World Journal* 8:451–453, 2008.

Feng, Gia-fu, English J: *Lao Tzu: Tao Te Ching,* London, 1973, Wildwood House.

Foucault M: *The birth of the clinic (first published 1963),* London, 2007, Routledge.

Fowler JH, Christakis NA: Dynamic spread of happiness in a large social network: longitudinal analysis over 20 years in the Framingham Heart Study, *British Medical Journal* 337:a2338, 2008.

Frank A: *1995 The wounded storyteller: body, illness and ethics,* 1995, University of Chicago Press.

Frankl VE: *Man's search for meaning: an introduction to logotherapy,* New York, 1963, Pocket Books.

Freeman GK, Horder JP, Howie JGR, et al: Evolving general practice consultation in Britain: issues of length and context, *British Medical Journal* 324:880–882, 2002.

Gesler W: Therapeutic landscapes: medical issues in light of the new medical geography, *Social Science & Medicine* 34(7):735–746, 1992.

Goldberger AL, Amaral LA, Hausdorff JM, et al: Fractal dynamics in physiology: alterations with disease and aging, *PNAS* 99(1):2466–2472, 2002.

Greenhalgh T: Intuition and evidence – uneasy bedfellows? *British Journal of General Practice* 52:395–400, 2002.

Greenhalgh T, Wessely S: 'Health for Me': a sociocultural analysis of healthism in the middle classes, *British Medical Bulletin* 69:197–213, 2004.

Greaves D: *Mystery in Western medicine,* Aldershot, 1996, Avebury.

Griffiths F, Green E, Tsouroufli M: The nature of medical evidence and its inherent uncertainty for the clinical consultation: qualitative study, *British Medical Journal* 330(7490):511, 2005.

Hatfield E, Cacioppo JT, Rapson RL: *Emotional contagion: studies in emotion and social interaction,* 1994, Cambridge University Press.

Herman J: The ethics of prevention: old twists and new, *British Journal of General Practice* 46:547–549, 1996.

Herzlich C: The individual, the way of life and the genesis of illness. In Bury M, Gabe J, editors: *The sociology of health and illness,* London, 2004, Routledge.

Holt T: *Complexity for clinicians*, Oxford, 2004, Radcliffe Publishing.

Hotamisligil GS: Inflammation and metabolic disorders, *Nature* 444(14): 860–867, 2006.

Howie JG, Heaney DJ, Maxwell M, et al: Quality at general practice consultations: cross sectional survey, *British Medical Journal* 319(7212):738–743, 1999.

Howie JG, Heaney DJ, Maxwell M, et al: Developing a 'consultation quality index' (CQI) for use in general practice, *Family Practice* 17(6):455–461, 2000.

Illich: *Limits to medicine*, London, 1976, Boyars.

Innes AD, Campion P, Griffiths FE: Complex consultations and the 'edge of chaos', *British Journal of General Practice* 55:47–52, 2005.

Jenkins L, Britten N, Barber N, et al: Letter: Consultations do not have to be longer, *British Medical Journal* 325:388, 2002.

'yotti' Kingsley J, Townsend M, Phillips R, et al: 'If the land is healthy … it makes the people healthy': The relationship between caring for Country and health for the Yorta Yorta Nation, Boonwurrung and Bangerang Tribes, *Health & Place* 15:291–299, 2009.

Kleinman A: *The illness narratives: suffering, healing and the human condition*, New York, 1988, Basic Books.

Klitzman R: 'Patient-time', 'doctor-time', and 'institution-time': perceptions and definitions of time among doctors who become patients, *Patient Education and Counseling* 66:147–155, 2007.

Lancet Editorial: The NHS: from religion to philosophy, *The Lancet* 373, 2009.

Layard R: *Happiness: lessons from a new science*, London, 2006, Penguin.

Lindstrom B, Eriksson M: Salutogenesis, *Journal of Epidemiology and Community Health* 59:440–442, 2005.

Lloyd D, Aon MA, Cortassa S: Why homeodynamics, not homeostasis? *Scientific World Journal* 1:133–145, 2001.

McEwen BS, Wingfield JC: The concept of allostasis in biology and biomedicine, *Hormones and Behaviour* 43:2–15, 2003.

McKenna: p.o.d. Details provided-on-demand.

McLuhan TC: *Touch the earth: a self-portrait of Indian existence*, London, 1982, Abacus.

Martinez-Lavin M, Infante O, Lerma C: Hypothesis: The chaos and complexity theory may help our understanding of fibromyalgia and similar maladies, *Seminars in Arthritis and Rheumatism* 37(4):260–264, 2008.

Mercer SW, Fitzpatrick B, Gourlay G, et al: More time for complex consultations in a high-deprivation practice is associated with increased patient enablement, *British Journal of General Practice* 57:960–966, 2007.

Milligan C, Gatrell A, Bingley A: 'Cultivating health': therapeutic landscapes and older people in northern England, *Social Science and Medicine* 58:1781–1793, 2004.

Needham J: *Time the refreshing river*, London, 1948, Allen & Unwin.

Nettleton S: *The sociology of health and illness*, Cambridge, 2006, Polity.

Nietzsche F: *The dawn/daybreak: thoughts on the prejudices of morality trans*, Cambridge, 1982, RJ Hollingdale.

Plesk PE, Greenhalgh T: The challenge of complexity in health care, *British Medical Journal* 323:625–628, 2001.

Plsek P, Sweeney K, Griffiths F: *Complexity and healthcare: an introduction*, Oxford, 2002, Radcliffe Publishing.

Porkert M, Ullmann C: *Chinese medicine*, New York, 1988, Morrow.

Richman J: 'Hospital' from the album 'The modern lovers', CA, 1976, Beserkley Records.

Robinson GC: *The patient as a person: a study of the social aspects of illness*, 1939, The Commonwealth Fund.

Rosenberg CE: Notes accompanying: Holism in twentieth-century medicine. In Lawrence C, Weisz G, editors: *Greater than the parts: holism in biomedicine 1920–1950*, 1998, Oxford University Press.

Selye HS: *The stress of life*, New York, 1978, McGraw-Hill.

Sole R, Goodwain B: *Signs of life*, New York, 2000, Basic Books.

Stacey RD: *Complex responsive processes in organizations: learning and knowledge creation*, London, 2001, Routledge.

Stacey RD: *Strategic management and organizational dynamics: the challenge of complexity*, London, 2002, Prentice Hall.

Strumia A: Complexity seems to open a way towards a new Aristotelian-Thomistic ontology, *Acta Biomedica* 78(1):32–38, 2007.

Sweeney K: *Complexity in primary care: understanding its value*, Oxford, 2006, Radcliffe Publishing Ltd.

Thompson A, Ruusuvuori J, Britten N, et al: An integrative approach to patient participation in consultations. In Collins S, Britten N, Ruusuvuori J, et al, editors: *Patient participation in health care consultations: qualitative perspectives*, New York, 2007, McGraw Hill/Open University Press.

Watts: p.o.d. Details provided-on-demand.

WHO: Preamble to the Constitution of the World Health Organization as adopted by the International Health Conference, New York, 19–22 June, 1946; signed on 22 July 1946 by the representatives of 61 States (Official Records of the World Health Organization, no. 2, p. 100) and entered into force on 7 April 1948.

# On profiling and diagnosis
Appreciating the patient's predicament

**4**

## CHAPTER CONTENTS

Introduction  133
Expectations and agendas: never assume  134
Weighing the three classic strategies  142
On convergence and divergence  144
Distinctive features of the phytotherapy approach  146
On diagnosis and assessment  149
Conceiving the self  158
Generalizing about individuals  166
On the nature of patients (and practitioners)  172
On the nature of conditions  187
    Public influence  195
    Public reception  195
    Public expression  196
Moving with the patient  200

## INTRODUCTION

The following chapters will explore the three basic, or classical, strategies used to assess the patient: case history-taking; physical examination and investigations. We will consider their relevance and application in phytotherapy. Before moving on to these, however, it will be useful to consider the general issues and challenges posed by, as well as the opportunities that may arise from, the process of attempting to understand patients and their predicaments and to assess and diagnose their conditions.

Foucault (1963) writes of: 'the endless task of understanding the individual'. The consultation provides a bounded space to pursue this quest – the attainment of which must always be limited but also, crucially, must always attempt to be sufficient. Before setting out on this journey of discovery, the practitioner needs to be equipped with a sense of the extent to which any person is knowable and any condition is diagnosable. It is a cliché beloved by many who speak about holistic medicine that the goal is to 'treat the whole person', the correlate association being that it is possible to first *know* the whole person; an assertion that stands in need of challenge. A further well-worn maxim is that the aim of holists is to treat the 'cause of disease, not its symptoms', again implying that causes can be commonly discovered. These blandishments are part of the hubris of some CAM proponents and practitioners and one looks askance at those who have actually spent much time with patients who continue to proffer them as attainable absolutes. Indeed, the uncritical reiteration of such statements proffered as mantras of holism has served to denigrate the notion of holism itself.

It makes for less exciting slogans but it reflects the reality of practice to state that the practitioner should attempt to:

- Appreciate the predicament of the patient, and the influences that have shaped and continue to adapt or contain that predicament, as broadly and deeply as is possible and practicable –
  We might add a rider to this instruction –
- In pursuit of the above goal the practitioner should temper her approach in the light of, and with respect for, the patients' agenda and the degree to which the patient either desires or is able to participate.

If the practitioner is to be successful in helping a wide range of patients – the goal of the phytotherapist as a generalist – she must be sensitive to the hopes, wishes, preferences and desires of individual patients and flexible and creative in adapting her approach in response. A base for proceeding in this way lies in the appreciation and exploration of the fact that both patients and practitioners bring their own expectations and agendas to the consultation. Much benefit will accrue if the practitioner seeks to perceive the patient's expectations and agenda and to critically reflect on her own.

## EXPECTATIONS AND AGENDAS: NEVER ASSUME

Practitioners may assume that they know what patients in general want from the clinical encounter but this, in actuality, varies between patients. Collins et al. (2007) observe that: 'there continue to be limits to, and uniqueness in, individuals' experiences of healthcare, for while some patients expect greater understanding and involvement, others want little'.

Not every patient is unhappy when their symptoms are superficially relieved (!) and not every patient has the orientation, temperament, will or capacity to engage in an in-depth exploration of their being. The phytotherapist may be disappointed when the patient shows no interest in, or even clearly voices their opposition to, partaking in a voyage to the outer and inner reaches of their existence. Patients are not always up for a profound experience, they may say things like: 'Look, I'm sorry, but have you just got something to stop this itching?'

Peck et al. (2004) distinguish between patient expectations and patient requests: 'An expectation refers to what a patient wants to happen or thinks will happen, while a request refers to what a patient asks of the clinician'. Expectations commonly remain unvoiced and therefore unknown unless the practitioner directly asks the patient to talk about them. Peck considers that: 'relatively little is known about the *specific* expectations patients bring to the clinical encounter' [original italics] but that: 'Patients' expectations are varied and often vague. Clinicians trying to implement the values of patient-centred care must be prepared to elicit, identify and address many expectations'.

Barry et al. (2000) studied unvoiced agendas in general practice consultations and their findings and conclusions warrant extended discussion here. While noting the difficulty in defining the notions of expectations and agendas, they consider patient agendas to include, yet constitute more than patient expectations so that patient agendas involve 'ideas, concerns and expectations'. One might additionally suggest that patient agendas include, or are moulded by, the patient's values, preferences, goals, aspirations, biases and personal influences (e.g. family opinions, pressures and commitments). Patients' agendas may be divided into particular areas of concern such as social agendas and emotional agendas. These can be combined into a concept of 'total agendas'. The extent to which practitioners are able to determine patient agendas is based on their beliefs and behaviours:

*What doctors both believe and do influences the expression of patients' agendas. Doctors may overestimate the extent to which patients are primarily concerned with medical treatment rather than with gaining information and support. Unless patients are overtly distressed doctors may have trouble in recognising those who are seeking support.*

The agenda items that were most commonly voiced in this study had to do with presentation of symptoms and making requests for diagnosis and treatment – the ordinary business of the consultation seen from a stereotyped view. The agenda items left unvoiced included:

*… worries about possible diagnosis and what the future holds; … ideas about what is wrong; side effects; not wanting a prescription; and information relating to social context.*

These themes have to do with subtleties and complexities that may not be considered by the patient to be allowable in the consultation format, and issues which, if voiced, might be the source of challenge to the practitioner and possibly lead to conflict. The authors ponder whether: 'Maybe patients are behaving as they believe they are expected to rather than as they would like'. The study also contrasted the agendas patients revealed to the researchers with those revealed to practitioners, concluding that:

*In consultations patients seem only partially present, with only limited autonomy – that is, to make requests but not to suggest solutions. Outside consultations patients are more fully present: as socially and contextually situated, thinking, feeling, people, with their own ideas on their medical condition and opinions and possible criticisms of medical treatments.*

Phytotherapists may contest that patients in herbal medicine consultations are empowered to be more themselves and therefore more forthcoming. Certainly the extended and in-depth nature of the phytotherapy consultation, coupled with the possibility that patients may feel less inhibited (and intimidated) when seeing a non-conventional practitioner, may be beneficial in facilitating greater expression on the part of patients. Yet phytotherapy practitioners still impose their own beliefs on the consultation and patients may similarly be wary of entering into areas of challenge and potential conflict regarding the practice of phytotherapy itself.

Overcoming obstructions that prevent the free and full expression of the patient's agenda is vitally important since: 'Patients have many needs and when these are not voiced they can not be addressed ... This suggests that when patients and their needs are more fully articulated in the consultation better healthcare may be effected'.

So what should practitioners 'believe and do' to enable the patient to be fully present and fully expressive of their total agenda in the consultation? Barry et al. (2000) note that:

> *A more complete view of the patient's agenda was only possible through a methodology that asked patients to present their full selves. When research methods are structured closer to the lifeworld – qualitative, loosely structured, open ended, people centred – a fuller more complex situated view of people and their agenda is gained.*

The practitioner needs first to be aware of the potential scope of the patient's agenda and the range of specific items it may contain. They then need to be open to receiving and attending to this broad array of factors and prepared to deal with the implications of doing so. A major implication for conventional practitioners will be the need for more time in the consultation – this is not an issue for most phytotherapists. A fundamental implication for *all* practitioners however, is exposure of the practitioner herself to risk, particularly the risk of hearing things that are personally difficult and challenging and which may cause one to question deeply and dearly held beliefs about the nature of practice. The practitioner may therefore feel resistance to engaging with the patient's full agenda. One example of risk in phytotherapy would be to invite the patient to express their full agenda regarding the herbal prescription itself. Although this may initially sound straightforward, it can actually strike at the heart of the phytotherapist's core beliefs and self-image as a practitioner – for if the patient is ambivalent or negative about the prescription where does that leave the practitioner?

In order to facilitate the patient in fully expressing their agenda about the herbal prescription, the phytotherapist may ask questions along the lines of:

- So what do you think of the herbal medicine?
- What do you think it is doing for you?
- Do you think it is doing anything?
- Do you think it is causing any problems?
- Is there anything you would change about it?
- What would you like it to do that it isn't currently doing?
- Are you taking the medicine?

Some of these questions provide the patient with an opportunity to say that the medicine does not appear to be helping or may be causing detrimental effects or is not actually being taken! Findings of this type are not what the practitioner ideally wants to hear and therefore may not usually be open to hearing. Working in this way does not mean that the patient's perception should be uncritically accepted or go unchallenged – it simply gives a clearer picture of what the patient is actually thinking and feeling. It is very common, for example, when asking patients the type of questions above to have an exchange along the following lines:

Phytotherapist: 'So do you think the herbs are having any benefits?'

Patient: 'Well, it's hard to tell. I'm not sure that there's much of a difference'.

Phytotherapist: 'Well I think, um, you know herbs can work quite subtly, and, er, for instance do you remember that when I first saw you, you were having headaches twice a week and you've just told me that you haven't had any headaches for the last 6 weeks? And I have been trying to treat that with the herbs'.

Patient: 'Oh that's true – I'd forgotten about that'.

Of course this is only one possible scenario, others may lead the practitioner to question how effective she is being as a phytotherapist. Such questions, squarely faced, generally lead not to abandonment of the modality but to increased appreciation of how to effectively apply it. Nonetheless, practitioners seem to intuit that there is danger in asking patients to express themselves in areas relating to the practitioner's core beliefs and practices, and they may shy away from encouraging this, lest the power of these is diminished as a consequence. There is an important correlate here, however, which, when appreciated, may encourage the practitioner to be bold in exposing herself to the risk of personal challenge. It is this – that the more open the practitioner is in hearing the patient's total agenda, the more powerful she becomes as a catalyst to the patient's self-discovery and self-healing. If the opening-up of the consultation to the full breadth of the patient's thoughts, ideas and expectations diminishes the place or power of the 'remedy', it will be compensated by an increase in the potency of the practitioner as a remedy in and of herself.

In exploring the patient's expectations and agenda, the practitioner must inevitably arrive at a point of critical reflection on her own expectations and agenda – regarding the patient, the consultation and her modality. A crucial development is for the practitioner to cease to identify her healing identity primarily with her tools (e.g. herbs) but rather with her *self*, in tune with Gordon's (1982) definition of holistic medicine as: 'an attitudinal approach to healthcare rather than a particular set of techniques'.

To bring things together: practitioner and patient both approach the consultation with their own expectations of what might, or should, come of it and with their own agenda around this. Each may make assumptions about the expectations and agenda of the other and in doing so, each is likely to reach some conclusions that are erroneous. Additionally, each will be ignorant of many of the specific expectations and agenda items the other holds. Matters are compounded by the fact that many expectations are poorly formed, vague or existing on the peripheries of consciousness – for both patient and practitioner. While we have discussed the usefulness of practitioners questioning patients regarding their expectations/agenda for the consultation, the patient would also be justified in asking the practitioner the same thing.

Usherwood (1999) refers to Levenstein and colleagues' (1986) discussion of the two agendas of patient and practitioner and summarizes thus:

*The patient's agenda reflects her ideas and questions about her illness, her hopes and expectations of the doctor, her feelings, her fears and her problems of living.*

*The doctor's agenda is concerned with correct diagnosis of the patient's complaints. It is the doctor's responsibility to respect the patient's agenda and to reconcile this with his own.*

This represents a questionably narrow, passive and acquiescent view of the practitioner. A different take on considering the practitioner's agenda would be to consider what the practitioner personally hopes to get out of the consultation process since agendas are based on goals. Daghio et al. (2003) and Fairhurst and May (2006) have looked at the elements that general practitioners felt as satisfying in their work. Daghio et al. found that:

*Professional skills and quality of the human/interpersonal interactions are major determinants of GPs' satisfaction in their professional activities.*

Fairhurst and May discovered evidence to support this, emphasizing the human/interpersonal elements of practice:

*Doctors' reports of satisfying and unsatisfying experiences during consultations were primarily concerned with developing and maintaining relationships rather than with technical aspects of diagnosis and treatment.*

It seems likely that this statement would hold true for practitioners in other fields and modalities, certainly it would seem to apply to phytotherapists. Fairhurst and May further discovered that personal aspects pertaining to the doctor were most highly associated with feelings of satisfaction:

*… greatest satisfaction seemed to derive from consultations in which doctors perceived they personally had contributed to a successful outcome by deploying personal attributes in addition to formal medical knowledge and technical skills.*

More than this, the consultation seemed to have its most pleasing outcome as a form of self-development and self-affirmation for the practitioner:

*The consultation experience appeared to open the doctors' identity to scrutiny and potential maintenance, challenge or modification. Mostly the consultation experience allowed doctors to maintain a coherent sense of themselves as doctors, and generally these consultations were satisfying.*

So it appears that part of a practitioner's agenda in the consultation is to facilitate and experience satisfying relationships and to conduct work on the self as well as on the patient. We might restate and posit this last remark as representing the practitioner's two agendas in the consultation: work on the patient and work on the self. The two agendas are likely to have synergistic positive effects if both are attended to and, conversely, each is likely to suffer if the other one is neglected. Returning to Barry et al.'s findings we might suggest that the patient can only be fully present in the consultation if the practitioner is also fully present. Being 'fully present' entails being fully alive to and engaged with the totality of the patient's predicament and agenda while dynamically applying one's whole self to the moment in a spirit of openness and mutual discovery. At this point let us attempt to summarize some of the implications of the foregoing discussion for the consultation in more detail.

At the outset of the consultation, and/or at other relevant points, it is crucial to ask patients about their expectations and explore the full extent of their total agenda. Some aspects of these (i.e. expectations/agendas) may not be accessible to patients early in the consultation but may emerge as an outcome of the consultation process or between or during subsequent consultations. Since expectations/agendas evolve, it is important to return to check this ground repeatedly over time. Expectations/agendas should always be respected but not passively accepted. If the patient's expectations are vague, then some exploration to achieve greater clarity is required. If the patient's expectations appear to the practitioner to be unreasonable, inappropriate or unachievable, they will need to be queried or challenged. The practitioner may take the role of teacher in order to transform a patient expectation that she considers to stand in need of revision or modification.

Simple questions can be posed at the outset of the consultation to check what the patient would like to attain from the encounter. Possible forms of this question include:

- So could you tell me what you would like, ideally, to get from this consultation?
- Is there something, particularly, that you would like to get from this consultation?
- What would you like to achieve from this consultation?
- What would you like to get out of this consultation?

In my experience, the replies to this type of question are diverse, and sometimes surprising. Examples include:

- I'd really like to get a better perspective on things.
- I want to know what's really going on.
- I want to understand what's happening to me.
- I want to know if you think he (referring to a child patient) really does have asthma because I don't think it is.
- I just want to be able to get to sleep!
- I just want this to go away.
- Well, if you've got something to take the pain down by even 10%, I'll settle for that.
- Well, I want a baby. I mean – not right at the end of this consultation!
- I don't want to take drugs for this. I don't want to be on something for the next 40 years.
- I just want to get my life back.
- Well just … you know … everything!
- Well the flushes really, if we could stop that then I can get on with things again.
- Peace of mind really … um …
- I don't know … I'm just ready to move on now.
- I just need something to help me cope.
- I need some ideas about what to do next.
- I just want a different viewpoint because I'm not happy with what I've got so far.
- Oh hell … I don't know … can we come back to that one?
- I need somebody to actually tell me what's going on.
- Well I don't want anything that will affect my medication.

- Well, yes ... I know what I don't want ...
- I don't know really ... to be honest I'm not even sure why I'm here.
- Now, I'm very sceptical about herbal medicine but my friend said you might be able to help so I'm willing to see what you have to offer.
- Well, I'm seeing a homoeopath who is clearing things at a very deep level but in the meantime I'm getting all these symptoms that I'd like you to sort out.

A linked question would query what result the patient wanted to achieve by means of the herbal prescription specifically. Possible forms for this question include:

- So, what, if possible, would you like the herbal medicine to do for you?
- How would you like the herbs to change your health?
- What one thing, particularly, would you like the herbs to do for you?

My experience has been that the response to this type of question is typically both appropriate and realistic. Patients rarely expect or ask for the earth and it may often be possible for the practitioner to exceed the patient's wishes. If such a question is left unposed, however, the practitioner may burden themselves with the assumption that the patient is looking for much greater results than is actually the case and the patient may be left uncertain as to whether the practitioner understood what they wanted.

Other questions can be used to clarify expectations/agendas during, or towards the end of the consultation, such as:

- So can I check in and see where we are at now? What are you thinking?
- Having got to this point, is it worth us pausing a moment to consider what you would like to do next?
- So tell me more about what you'd like to come out of what we're doing here.
- So before we move towards finishing for today – is there anything you wanted to talk about or know more about that we haven't covered?

Practitioners may be wary of asking many of the questions given in this section for fear of 'opening up the floodgates'. There is a fear of being 'swamped' or overwhelmed by a 'deluge' of comment or information. Yet it is the job of the practitioner to 'immerse' themselves in the patients' world.

From Barry et al. (2000) above, we have some hints as to how we might adapt the consultation structure, techniques and style to enable the patient to be more fully present in the consultation. Elements include:

- Ask patients to present their full selves
- Move the structure closer to the lifeworld and away from biomedical abstraction
- Make the structure looser
- Keep things open ended
- Aim for a fuller, more complex, situated view of the patient and her agenda.

We might add to this:

- Be open to questioning your own expectations and agenda as a practitioner
- Focus on working on the patient but do not neglect work on the self
- See the consultation as an opportunity for mutual self-discovery and learning
- Be open to having your beliefs and behaviours challenged
- Relish the opportunity for self-development that each consultation offers.

The more tightly constrained the consultation is (including time constraints and rigid questioning routines) and the more practitioner-directed it is, the less chance there will be of allowing the patient to be fully present in the consultation. For many patients it will be helpful for the consultation to possess a certain fuzziness as regards structure and explicit aims, since this will help the patient feel liberated in expressing themselves – indeed, so that they may behave as they would like to rather than as they are expected to.

There is not only room for, but also a clear and urgent need for, innovation in consultation methodology and patient profiling in order to greater appreciate patient expectations and total agendas. Middleton et al. (2006) has demonstrated two methods that have yielded encouraging results: practitioner education and the use of agenda forms for patients to complete themselves. Their study found that:

*If patients are encouraged to make their agenda explicit in consultations, doctors identify more problems although consultations last longer. Patients who completed an agenda form were more satisfied with the depth of the doctor–patient relationship. Similar changes were observed in the number of problems identified and the duration of consultations if doctors were taught to explicitly deal with the patients' agenda.*

As previously observed, the issue of time is not currently problematic for most phytotherapists in the UK. The phytotherapist is ideally placed to engage profoundly with the patient's expectations and agenda, yet it is unclear (since there are few studies) whether this potential is being realized (though see Little for an interesting introduction to this area). Individual practitioners can raise their own awareness of this issue through directed reading and critical reflection and herbal medicine students should be trained to elicit patient expectations/agendas as a core element of practice.

Katz (1986) underlines the centrality of reflection in enabling patient autonomy:

*… the right to self-determination about ultimate choices cannot be properly exercised without first attending to the processes of self-reflection and reflection with others. This holds true for patients as well as physicians.*

He goes on to put this principle into perspective, touching on the issues discussed in this section:

*I am not suggesting, however, that the conversations between physicians and patients be converted into an exploration of the psychological roots of patients' and physicians' motivations and expectations. This is neither warranted nor possible. I have in mind only a bona fide attempt by physicians and patients to explain what* they wish from one another and what they can do for and with one another, and to clarify, to the extent possible, any misconceptions they may have of each others' wishes and expectations. In the end, irreconcilable differences may persist. If they then realize that they must part company, at least they will do so with a greater appreciation of their respective position.

## WEIGHING THE THREE CLASSIC STRATEGIES

Although the strategies of case history-taking, physical examination and investigation are usually presented as three discrete yet complementary methods for exploring the patient's condition, which can be deployed in an orderly manner to inform each other, the reality in practice is that they tend to have a messy and tense relationship that is frequently dysfunctional. Their professed relationship is that of a tripartite approach to diagnosis, yet definitive diagnosis is commonly unattainable in practice. The classic sequential procession from case history (generating hypotheses) to physical examination (clarifying the differential diagnosis) to investigation (confirming diagnosis) is rarely a straightforward one and often does not occur in this order, e.g. an abnormality found on routine screening physical examination or investigation may lead to a case history being taken.

In phytotherapy, as in other medical modalities, the case history is by far the most generally important of the three strategies. The vast majority of the consultation time is spent on the consultation with most phytotherapists, like most doctors, paying scant regard to physical examination. Not that physical examination is without merit, just that it tends in practice to be given a minor role and is frequently overlooked. Investigations take place outside of the consultation so cannot properly be regarded as part of the consultation, although they provide information that may, indeed, inform it.

Although phytotherapists can refer patients to private laboratories and specialist clinics for investigations to be undertaken, this rarely occurs. It is generally more convenient and economic to advise the patient to visit their GP and request the relevant test/s or to contact the GP on the patients' behalf. In either case, phytotherapists will not normally receive a statement of the results unless the patient has obtained them and brings a copy. The lack of direct access to tests and their results distances the phytotherapist from this source of information, although it remains essential for herbal practitioners to recommend tests when appropriate and to take steps to access results when necessary.

Tensions arise in the relationship between history, examination and investigation as an effect of the types of knowledge they are considered to represent. The history and most examinations are considered to provide subjective findings, whereas investigations are designated objective. Objectivity is associated with 'real', whereas the subjective is considered suspect, debatable, open to question. Since medical science prioritizes objective information, the status of investigation as prime arbiter of diagnostic veracity has now been assumed. Although investigations do, of course, contribute to the understanding of patient's situations (significantly and crucially in some cases), they remain an extremely limited means of knowing the patient. Despite this, such value has been placed on investigations that the phrase 'treating the test results not the patient' as an attack on over-reliance on tests is now in popular use. Numerous factors (individual, procedural, environmental) can lead to erroneous or misleading test results being given – investigations are not fault-free, nor are they all-encompassing. Investigations are rarely pathognomonic – they require interpretation and/or hypothesis-testing in practice. Concern has been expressed that the move to conduct routine screening investigations to test for the presence of pathologies in apparently healthy people may often be useless at best and sometimes harmful (Hadler 2004). It also remains the case that the vast majority of conditions presenting in general practice, as in phytotherapy, are diagnosed (or remain un-diagnosed) on the case history alone. Excessive, non-contextualized or unquestioning reliance on data derived from investigations can critically undermine the purposes of the consultation.

The consultation still tends to be taught to students of medicine and of phytotherapy as an orderly movement through history, examination and investigation. This is a grossly misleading preparation for the realities of practice and one of the great early challenges of fledgling practitioners is to adapt inadequate theory to the demands of unsupervised practice. We have already noted that investigation is not part of the consultation at all, since it is generally conducted: at a separate time to the consultation; in a different location; with another person! Additionally, investigation is normally employed infrequently, if at all, in chronic conditions. We have also said that physical examination is commonly neglected but even when it is fully utilized, it is rarely the most significant part of the consultation. That position falls consistently, and correctly, to the case history.

The consultation also tends to be taught as if the only encounter that practitioner and patient ever have is that of a first visit. In chronic conditions, where the patient sees the same practitioner over a long period of time (this is the norm in phytotherapy but has become less common for doctors), the greater challenge and skill lies in successfully using the potential of the follow-up visit to provide support and further advance healing. (We will explore this idea further in Chapter 5.)

The classical model of tightly structured case-taking, followed by physical examination and investigation is inappropriate to most patients' predicaments and hence is quickly dispensed with by practitioners once they enter unsupervised practice. Rather, these three territories represent resources that the skilled practitioner combines and deploys as necessary. The case history remains the pre-eminent means of knowing the patient – and even that is badly named; perhaps we should just call it 'the clinical conversation'.

Thus, the subjective domain of talking about, and listening to, the patients' narrative and its contained hopes, wishes, desires, fears, impressions, concerns, insights, and so forth, provides not only the bedrock of the consultation but also most of its substance. We do not live or experience our lives objectively, nor can we get to know and understand people objectively. Objectivity is a method of abstraction and is valued in cultures where abstraction has assumed a dominating force. The origin of the word abstraction lies with the Latin for 'to draw away'. Practitioners are exhorted to maintain a 'clinical distance' from patients when in fact the best practitioners draw close, carefully and appropriately to be sure, but close. Contemporary western culture has drawn away from nature, allowing it to be exploited to the point where the viability of human life on this planet is now at risk. The objective assessment of patients, when unchecked, leads to a consequent *objectification of the person* and is connected with the same trajectory of abstraction that has its origins in the western commitment to an unhealthy emphasis on science to the exclusion of other explanatory models. Although many commentators have criticized the medicalization of life it is important to recognize its origins in the scientization of life. Placing the subjective elements of the consultation at the centre of the consultation is a means of re-emphasizing the humanistic nature of medicine.

## ON CONVERGENCE AND DIVERGENCE

Since the mid-1990s, in the UK, herbal medicine practitioner education has moved out of the independent sector and into academic institutions of the state, i.e. universities. Many herbal practitioners have seen this as a sign of the success of the discipline and as a marker of its legitimization. Some other CAM disciplines have also made this transition. Opponents of CAM have railed against this development precisely because they too consider that incorporation of CAM courses into state institutions provides tacit legitimatization – a step that they consider unwarranted and which they invariably criticize vehemently. An editorial in *Times Higher Education* (2008) presented the usual litany pertaining to this issue – and a case study: 'Opponents have derided CAM as 'mumbo-jumbo' that 'no respectable university should provide', 'bogus' and 'the denial of rationality' – and these are all criticisms that must be taken seriously … the University of Central Lancashire faced a revolt from its own staff, who claimed it was promoting 'quackery' by offering courses in homeopathy, acupuncture and herbal medicine'.

The reality is that when CAM courses are offered by universities, they are inevitably attenuated in some regard, although perhaps enhanced in others. When a CAM programme is poured into a university, it must necessarily fit the shape of the vessel that contains it. While independent educational courses in CAM are generally bespoke, tailored (more or less successfully) to fit the needs of specific groups of students, university courses usually introduce off-the-peg elements into the syllabus and its delivery: an existing anatomy module here, a generic ethics module there, and let's throw in an existing research module or two. It is possible to cobble a CAM programme together quickly by adding the new students on to existing classes (in subject areas such as anatomy and physiology) and introducing a few new modules to account for the specific elements of the particular modality. Such courses tend to lead to a fragmented education and training that is lacking in a coherent ethos embodied in each module or element and which may, subsequently, compromise the integrity of the modality. If this is the case then the revolting staff at CAM-incorporating universities need not lose too much sleep – the straight-science rigor of the institution (if indeed it possesses such a thing) is likely to shape and pervade the CAM course. One risk is that students are rendered ambivalent, being partially exposed to two non-integrated approaches – that of biomedical science and that of the CAM modality.

Of course, delivery by conventional academic institutions *may* improve some aspects of CAM courses. Perhaps, for example, there will be improved criticality, greater insight through research, improved interprofessional activity (the usual claims to enhancement made by universities) but this is not a given, and they may not come without a cost. In any case pressure will come to bear on the approach, in our case phytotherapy, to fit, to some degree, the dominant biomedical model (since state institutions are usually not only imbued with the values of the dominant culture but also required to inculcate them). A process of appropriation of the CAM modality may then occur where it is gradually sculpted (by means of the application of various types of instrument such as staff changes, curriculum reviews, implementation of internal and national policy changes, accrediting and regulatory body edicts, etc.) to more and more closely resemble the icon revered by the revolting staff – re-made as a new, scientifically approved (and improved) product ('Now with 20% Extra EBM!').

State academic institutions will tend, then, to normalize CAM courses, which means to biomedicalize them. Although CAM therapists involved in running and teaching on such courses will try to protect the identity of their profession, this is only likely to remain in corners of the course, that is to say in certain specific modules where a reasonable degree of content and management control can be exerted.

The process of biomedicalization of herbal medicine had begun long before the incorporation of herbal education and training into universities in any case. Independent herbal practitioner courses have, for decades, taught conventional medical subjects such as anatomy, physiology, histology and microbiology. Yet they have always had the opportunity to tailor these subject areas to the particular needs, interests and perspectives of phytotherapists. When phytotherapy students are in the position of merely sitting-in on generic modules addressing these topics the scope for appropriate modulation, emphasis-placing and setting the locus of critique is much narrower. Phytotherapy has long incorporated biomedical subjects into the traditional herbal model but independent courses have been at liberty to do this on their own terms. The move to universities has reversed this position so that the control now lies outside of the herbal professions' hands – biomedicine-based (and inevitably biased) university departments are now in the position of determining which elements of herbal medicine should be included in new biomedically-oriented herbal medicine courses.

There is a danger that herbal practice could now develop as a quasi-biomedical discipline where its practitioners ape general practitioners except providing a vegetable remedy in place of a synthetic chemical one. Many herbalists would accuse that this is actually a pretty accurate description of phytotherapy in its current state already. I continue to argue the case for a different perspective on phytotherapy, however as one which denotes (as discussed in Ch. 2) an approach to herbal medicine that engages with science and biomedicine while continuing the herbal tradition – but which is able to deal with all of these strands critically. Traditions of medicine should not be fixed – they must adapt and evolve or be consigned to the history books. Certainly there are perennial values and perspectives, which will remain as touchstones that define the herbal profession – these are the very aspects that should be defended and promoted – but much of value will be gained by keeping the doors of innovation and creativity open. The challenge for herbal medicine, in education, research, promotion and practice, is to make the case for, and to proselytize, its core principles and tenets while embracing and applying new information and techniques that increase its ability to benefit patients.

## DISTINCTIVE FEATURES OF THE PHYTOTHERAPY APPROACH

Herbal medicine can be practised in a manner that uses the consultation to arrive at or confirm a conventional medical diagnosis before treating it with an unconventional (i.e. herbal) remedy that nonetheless replicates conventional treatment, e.g. using a herbal anti-inflammatory in place of a pharmaceutical antiinflammatory. This is no bad thing as far as it goes – and if it means that the patient receives a treatment that is more effective and/or less toxic, then it will go a very long way indeed. Yet, herbal medicine offers much more than this – an alternative way of viewing the patient and her predicament, and therefore of helping her to adapt it, that includes a conventional diagnosis as merely one aspect of information and not necessarily the most significant one.

We have already suggested (in the preceding chapter) that the distinctive features of herbal medicine in this regard are shaped to a large extent by the characteristics and capacities of herbal medicines themselves. It might be useful to summarize and reiterate some of the features that arise from this view with regard to what is distinctive about herbal practice in profiling the patient and coming to conclusions about the nature and detail of her predicament. The herbal practitioner will:

- Aim to take a very broad view of the patient
- Pay attention to subtle detail that might be interpreted as bodily messages that the patient needs to hear but which would conventionally be considered of little or no significance
- Be concerned with the milieu intérieur, or terrain, of the patient
- Seek opportunities to enable the patients' self-healing
- Identify factors that are disruptive or unsustainable in terms of the body when viewed as a balanced ecosystem
- Be more concerned with assessing general systems performance than seeking specific sites of lesions
- View the appreciation of the patients' nature and personality as pivotal in determining the course of treatment
- Be generally more fixated on the macroscopic as opposed to the microscopic features of health and illness
- Seek to integrate features into distinctive but diffuse general patterns rather than separate them into precise and separate phenomena
- Be concerned with such features as the thermal and hydration features of the patients' condition – the combination of factors such as heat, cold, moisture and dryness
- Be concerned with the extent to which a particular aspect or pattern is a sign of an excess or deficiency picture

- Consider the degree to which the patients' picture can be said to represent an imbalance in pairings such as stimulation-depression and contraction-relaxation
- Pay particular attention to bodily systems and functions that are considered to be of fundamental importance in maintaining the integrity of the body, such as: digestion, elimination, immunity, nervous function, hormonal function
- Seek to determine which organs, systems or functions need to be modulated using such terms as: support, strengthen, tonify, nurture, calm, drain, cool, warm, moisten, etc.
- Place high priority on psychoemotional influences
- Be concerned to determine the patients' attitudes and beliefs about their own condition and to life issues in general
- Place high value on the patients' own evaluation of their condition and its causative influences
- Have confidence in her ability to address a wide range of conditions and features due to the huge scope of herbal medicines and their flexibility in being applied in numerous types of preparations to suit almost any eventuality
- Be alert to subtle changes in treating chronic conditions in the awareness that herbal medicine tends to gradually accrete changes.

To further discuss what is distinctive about phytotherapy we need to name the relation that it can be distinguished from – this has to be the dominant medical form, biomedicine. In comparison with biomedicine then:

- Phytotherapists may place emphasis on some concepts and practices that are now considered outmoded, or which have been neglected by conventional medicine, such as convalescence.
- The majority of herbal medicines possess a wide therapeutic window – meaning that any toxic dose is distant from the therapeutic amount and consequently a broad range of dosages are recommended by various herbal authorities. Pharmaceutical drugs have a narrower window – meaning that the toxic dose is relatively close to the therapeutic dose and therefore great precision is required in prescribing. The size of the safety zone for most herbal medicines means that the phytotherapist may take a more relaxed, looser, attitude to prescribing and be more willing to consider a degree of experimentation or trial in formulating and applying prescriptions to be not only ethical but essential to remedial success. This capacity, afforded by the plants themselves, may be reflected in a looser, more experimental approach to the consultation in general.
- Due to the close proximity of the therapeutic and the toxic dose the application of conventional drugs is closely associated with notions of risk and danger and their accompanying emotions – anxiety and fear. Since the greater percentage of herbal medicines are relatively benign the phytotherapist will tend to view her materia medica as a collection of subtle, safe and trustworthy entities that the patient should be able to entertain with confidence. While conventional medicines tend to be viewed by doctors as precision tools working on specific receptors,

phytotherapists look upon their herbs as general systems adaptors. (This notwithstanding the fact that drugs can exert general effects and herbal constituents do bind to specific cell receptors.) If the classical concept of efficacious drug treatment in biomedicine can be illustrated as a magic bullet hitting the centre of a target within a terrified body then the herbal counterpart image is that of laying a healing blanket over a relaxed and resting body. The cartoon conventional drug is an incendiary device strategically deployed as part of the war being waged in the body during disease versus the equivalent herbal caricature of the mother embracing us and kissing away the hurt.

- Since herbs can do things that conventional drugs cannot, phytotherapists will look for things in the consultation that doctors do not. The propensities (seen in terms of actions here) of herbs which give rise to different ways of looking and acting include: the trophorestoratives, the adaptogens, the immunostimulants and modulators, the antioxidants, the nourishing nervines, the bitters, the circulatory stimulants, the aromatic digestives, etc.

We might formulate a list of words (Table 4.1) and their pairings that roughly distinguish the differences between conventional and herbal medicines with regard to their relative qualities and behaviours.

These characteristics and properties are not confined to the remedy itself but they extend to mould the practitioner's attitude and behaviour, her notions of what can (and cannot) be done with medicine, and *how* medicine should or must be done. These beliefs translate into forces that are played out in the consultation.

While the list of words in Table 4.1 is indicative of the nature of the two types of remedies they are also suggestive of the manner in which the consultation is constructed and conducted.

**Table 4.1** A list of words and their pairings

| Herbal medicine | Pharmaceutical drug |
| --- | --- |
| Slow | Rapid |
| Subtle | Crude |
| Gentle | Aggressive |
| Familiar | Alien |
| Complex | Simple |
| Food-like | 'Un-like' |
| General | Precise |
| Total | Partial |
| Diffuse | Targeted |
| Natural | Synthetic |
| Messy | Tidy |
| Dirty | Sterile |
| Chaotic | Ordered |
| Attractive | Repulsive |
| From-life | Non-life |
| Feminine | Masculine |

## ON DIAGNOSIS AND ASSESSMENT

Medical textbooks on 'clinical examination' – a term that implies, and stands-in for 'the consultation' – typically follow the same format. 'Clinical examination' means 'case-taking and physical examination' and most books begin with a single chapter on case-taking (nowadays usually referred to as 'the interview') followed by 10 or 12 chapters dedicated to the physical examination of each bodily system (i.e. the cardiovascular system, the respiratory system, etc.). Within the (usually) solitary chapter dedicated to the interview, it is frequently stated that the interview alone accounts for 60–80% of diagnoses, which may seem odd given that most of the books allot less than 10% of their content to the study of this area. The meagre content that is dedicated to case-taking normally only covers the initial consultation, with only scant reference paid (if indeed any is given at all) to the purposes and techniques associated with follow-up consultations. Such textbooks are also almost entirely taken up (throughout their discussion of the interview and physical examination techniques) with considerations relating to diagnosis. Students learning from these texts could be entirely forgiven for coming to the following conclusions about the consultation:

- Its primary goal is reaching a diagnosis
- Its secondary goals are unclear, but in any case are of little importance
- Although the interview is said to be extremely important nobody seems to know much about how it works
- But an awful lot is known about physical examination
- A typical consultation would consist of about 10% case-taking and 90% physical examination
- Attainment of a definitive diagnosis is possible in most cases
- Patients normally fit general diagnostic pictures
- Conditions are generally acute
- Patients are normally only seen once.

Herbal medicine students generally learn about the consultation process from these same books, with additional insights (and, hopefully, critiques) provided by clinical tutors.

This emphasis on diagnosis belies the reality of herbal practice (and, indeed, that of every other therapeutic modality). While diagnosis is an important factor in phytotherapy, it is only one among a number of other significant areas of exploration and work. Effort applied to discovering diagnosis is normally a high priority in the initial consultation but declines or disappears in subsequent ones unless substantially different symptoms arise. Over time then, in chronic cases, diagnostic considerations become of only minor importance. The areas that are more pertinent include:

- Providing a space for reflection, review and re-orientation
- Assessment of change and degree of progression or regression towards or away from therapeutic goals and the patients' own targets
- Work on understanding and making sense of the patients' predicament; and on finding meaning
- Finding new ways of giving relief, support and care.

Greaves (1996) locates the emphasis on diagnosis in the consultation with the primacy accorded to the treatment of acute cases and to hospital medicine:

> *The traditional account of medical decision-making ... focuses on acute rather than chronic medical conditions and on hospital medicine rather than primary care. In doing so it detracts from medical work carried out with those suffering from chronic conditions, where establishing a diagnosis is only an initial and small part of the whole medical task, with assessment of progress, prognosis and amelioration of the condition being of far greater importance.*

Summerton (2004) has underlined the elusive nature of classical organic diagnoses in general practice:

> *One particular problem for those of us working in primary care settings is that the vast majority of symptoms seem to defy a clear-cut organic explanation.*

There are other problems associated with the act of making a diagnosis and the consequences and repercussions of this act. The stated agenda that underlies the pursuit of a medical diagnosis typically masks a number of hidden agendas with social and political import. Patients whose presenting picture does not match a classical diagnostic pattern may be negatively labelled, or indeed left un-labelled, in such a way as to effectively designate their suffering as invalid. Even when a diagnosis is attempted in such cases the particular label used may be one that is considered to be lacking in credibility, e.g. irritable bowel syndrome, chronic fatigue syndrome and fibromyalgia. These diagnostic constructs are sometimes referred to by clinicians as 'dustbin diagnoses', which is to say that they are repositories into which botched attempts at a proper diagnosis can be tossed.

The provision of a credible medical diagnosis validates the patient's predicament as a sick-person and legitimizes their entitlement not only to statutory care and the consumption of related resources, and to exemption from work and family duties and other commitments but also to the sympathy and support of family, friends and the wider society. Conversely, the un-labelled (or unconvincingly labelled) patient is either barred from these privileges or granted only limited, and in which case probably grudging, access to them. Parsons (1951) described the valid patient as one who fits the socially defined 'sick-role' – the ultimate arbiter of this is the doctor and his primal act of power in conferring this role lies in the making of the diagnosis. A patient in possession of a credible diagnosis is said by Parsons to have both rights and obligations:

- The right to exemption from normal social roles and the right to be considered innocent in generating his condition (i.e. the patient is not personally responsible for his predicament and therefore should not be held liable for it)
- The obligation to do all he can to get well, including following the advice and taking the treatment provided by the doctor.

The degree of entitlement to rights increases with the degree of severity of disease and the extent to which obligations are required to be met in order to retain access to rights diminishes with reference to how incurable the condition is said to be.

Patients who are not provided with a medically legitimate diagnosis may then be considered to be conducting themselves in a manner that is socially illegitimate and therefore socially deviant. Such patients will have none of the rights of the sick-person but, in order to attain a state of social conformity and thence potential social acceptance they must make extra efforts to attend to the obligations of the sick-person. Such attention may not be possible however, since, in the absence of a diagnosis, the doctor may be unable to provide the means for the patient to meet his social obligations – meaning that they may not be in a position to provide advice or treatment.

Arising out of this latter point, a further crucial relationship in the determination of the pivotal significance of diagnosis in the consultation needs to be emphasized. This is the relationship between diagnosis and treatment with regard to the curious fact that the one rarely exists without the other. Credible diagnoses are normally entities for which a treatment is available, regardless of whether the treatment actually works with any degree of reliability (consider cancer and its treatment). At least in conventional medicine, a condition that cannot be treated cannot be diagnostically conceived. New treatments may lead to the invention of a diagnosis or the substantial revision of an earlier diagnostic picture. Consider the manner in which the menopause was repackaged as a new zone of diagnostic possibilities with the introduction of hormone replacement therapy. HRT pathologized phenomena which were previously considered to be part of normal and non-medical life experience into symptom pictures which led to a medical diagnosis. In this case, the construction of the menopause as a disease to be diagnosed and treated was driven by corporate players (pharmaceutical companies) abetted by public demand – the locus of origination of the diagnosis was not within the medical profession but rather was imposed upon it. This illustrates that the notion of clinical diagnosis identifying a clinical need that eventually leads to the development of a treatment is not necessarily a reliable one. The process can, and does, happen in reverse.

A diagnosis only tends to be considered biomedically valid in the absence of the existence of a treatment when considerable organic lesions or morbid phenomena can be demonstrated, e.g. in motor neurone disease. Conditions that are lacking in consistently demonstrable organic lesions; where the morbid phenomena are relatively subtle or un-dramatic; and where no effective pharmaceutical treatment pertains (i.e. the vast majority of the human experience of illness) do not receive specific medical diagnosis and instead reside in the vast territory designated variously as 'stress-induced', 'idiosyncratic', 'one of those things', 'hypochondriacal', 'all in the mind', 'self-limiting'. This position obtains to the extent that even when a patient exhibits extreme morbid phenomena (as for instance can occur in some severe cases of 'chronic fatigue syndrome' where patients may be bed-ridden and incapacitated for years) if there is no organic lesion and no treatment there will be no diagnosis and, consequently, no entitlement to statutory care or public sympathy.

Diagnosis may be misused by practitioners (usually unawares) as a tool of political control, facilitation or expiation. Illich (1976) alerts us to this:

*If it were recognized that diagnosis often serves as a means of turning political complaints against the stress of growth into demands for more therapies that are just more of its costly and stressful outputs, the industrial system would lose one of its major defences.*

In the last few decades, Illich's use of the phrase 'industrial system' has seemed increasingly incongruous and dated to readers in the developed world as the phrase itself has declined in use. This decline may reflect several developments and agendas, including:

- The decline in 'heavy industry' in developed-world countries in favour of the rise of the 'service economy' (notwithstanding the fact that the term 'service-industry' is in use)
- The intentional identification, and disguising, of 'the industrial system' as belonging to a historical era that has now passed to admit a more benign age (when in reality the physical labour demands of the past have merely been replaced by an equivalent set of excessively depleting integrated physical-emotional-mental work demands: the call centre overtaking the factory).

We might therefore update Illich's use of 'industrial system' with 'economic system' or 'corporate interest'. In any case, the accusation remains that in uncritically diagnosing and treating conditions that arise as a consequence of unjust and inhumane economic agendas, the healthcare practitioner is complicit in enabling and maintaining those agendas. The correlate challenge is that healthcare practitioners should be both politically aware and politically active – *politically aware* in the act of diagnosing, and *politically active* in resisting providing a diagnosis that masks the politically derived aetiology of the condition.

One stunning example of how diagnosis can be formulated to accurately reflect the sociopolitical aetiology of a condition and to point up rather than mask the political nature and challenge of the phenomena is provided by the concept of *karoshi* used in Japan. *Karoshi* may be translated as 'death from overwork' and has been applied as a 'socio-medical term in relation to workers' compensation' (Iwasaki et al. 2006) when it may also be taken to refer to disability arising from overwork. In the first few years of the twenty-first century, the Japanese Ministry of Health, Labour and Welfare, reinterpreted hundreds of cases of cerebrovascular and ischaemic heart disease as 'labour accidents resulting from overwork (*karoshi*) …' (Iwasaki et al. 2006). However, this was a development with a long history, since the relationship between sudden death and the Japanese production management (JPM) model had been noted and discussed since the 1970s (Nishiyama & Johnson 1997).

The designation of *karoshi* enables the causative factors that are absent in diagnoses such as 'cerebrovascular accident' and 'myocardial infarction' to be clearly stated. The genesis of the concept of *karoshi* lies in the extraordinary degree to which Japanese workers have been pushed to enable economic development. Iwasaki (2006) reports that: 'in 2001, 28.1% of Japanese employees were working for 50 hours or more per week … much higher than those in European countries such as Netherlands (1.4%), Sweden (1.9%), Finland

(4.5%), and Germany (5.3%)'. The eventual Japanese government recognition of overwork as the key aetiological factor in specific cases of cardiovascular disease was not a move of enlightened benevolence to the populace but rather one of economic pragmatism. The limit of overwork had been pushed so far that it was threatening to fundamentally destabilize the economy – a programme of compensation matched with measures to limit overwork was a necessary means of maintaining the economy. This case study illustrates how far a malign economic practice has to go before it is acknowledged by the state (it has, in fact, to become a threat to the maintenance of the state) and some degree of remedial political action is taken.

Seen in the light of the example set by *karoshi*, any diagnosis which omits to nail the key social, political or/and personal aetiological factor/s can be viewed as fudging the issue. While purporting to provide an insight into the patient's condition the diagnosis then also typically conceals the true nature of the situation in:

- Every relevant asthma diagnosis that is not accompanied by a word denoting 'exposure to pollution and lack of safe town planning'
- Every relevant depression diagnosis that is not accompanied by a word denoting 'absence of a satisfactory sense of personal meaning due to alienating factors in society'
- Every relevant attention-deficit hyperactivity disorder diagnosis that is not accompanied by a word denoting 'poor diet and parental absence due to lack of time deriving from economic pressures'.

Each of these is an example of a failure to *accurately* diagnose that will result in a failure to *effectively* treat.

The act of making a diagnosis is therefore not value-free and it has social and political associations and implications. *Karoshi* was above referred to as a 'socio-medical' term. We can suggest that diagnoses are always socio-medical terms and that the process of diagnosing is a politico-medical act. Practitioners may wish to avoid or deny these associations as a means of avoiding the consequent responsibility that comes with their acceptance but this represents a form of denial that is unacceptable given the duty of care owed to patients – because such denial crucially undermines the practitioners' ability to cut to the quick of the patients' predicament and to provide the deepest level of insight and stimulus to profound, transformative healing.

In phytotherapy practice, the patient has commonly (but by no means always) received a conventional medical diagnosis before attending, or is in the process of awaiting tests to achieve one. In such cases there is potential for the phytotherapist, as appropriate, to:

- Seek the patients' views and perspective on the diagnosis
- Question the conventional diagnosis – does it appear to be accurate?
- Provide supplemental information and interpretation of the diagnosis
- Offer an alternative perspective.

In seeking the patients' views and perspective on the diagnosis, the phytotherapist is aiming to assess the degree to which the diagnosis is acceptable to the patient or not, and the extent to which she understands it. It is also crucial to gain the patients' self-diagnosis and views on aetiology since insights provided here may lead the phytotherapist to suggest an alternative diagnosis based on the patients' evidence.

In routinely questioning the conventional diagnosis it is not suggested that biomedical diagnoses are routinely wrong in terms of their own frame of reference, rather that they may occasionally be inaccurate or incomplete. The views of any fellow clinician should be respected but never uncritically accepted. Should the reliability of a conventional diagnosis be substantially challenged, it may be desirable for the phytotherapist to communicate with the physician concerned – such a situation is discussed in Appendix 3.

In providing supplemental information or interpretation relating to the biomedical diagnosis the phytotherapist may comment on such matters as:

- The meaning of the diagnosis and details such as the significance of test findings
- Complicating and confounding factors
- Prognostic considerations
- Implications for treatment – conventional, phytotherapeutic and otherwise.

In assessing the patient, an alternative perspective on diagnosis and aetiology may have formed or presented itself to the phytotherapist. This may need referral for investigation to be further explored but might also, and more commonly, derive from a different take on the nature and processes of illness. This orientation will frequently leave the conventional diagnosis intact but speak to an alternative worldview that can co-exist with it. For example, in a patient with a diagnosis of hypertension a question along the following lines might be composed:

*Hypertension represents a constriction of the heart and the arteries. This might relate to something – an issue, an experience, a worry or a fear – that you are tightly holding on to and that you need to open up and let go. Can you think of anything that feels like this for you?*

In a case like this, the locus of the alternative perspective relates to causality and is not incompatible with the conventional diagnosis although, if the alternative aetiological view is valid it will tend to subvert the diagnosis or reveal it as inadequate. For example, *if* a case of 'hypertension' is due to fear, or holding on to a hurt that needs to be processed and released, then a more accurate, or more insight-rich, diagnosis might be framed as something like 'cardiovascular fear response' or 'arterial hurt-holding phenomenon'.

Although phytotherapy students in the UK usually learn conventional medical examination techniques only, many practitioners later add study and training in alternative techniques to their repertoire – such as aspects of traditional Chinese tongue and pulse diagnosis. If these are present, then they will be an additional factor that might enable and inform the phytotherapist in offering an alternative diagnostic perspective.

Patients do frequently present to phytotherapists as primary carers, having had no assessment or diagnosis from any other type of practitioner. In such instances the phytotherapist should be simultaneously confident in her own capacity to assess and advise and be keenly aware of her limits to competence and the importance of appropriate referral to other practitioners.

Patients may also present with a firmly held self-diagnosis or they might be in possession of a diagnosis from another CAM practitioner or alternative diagnostician such as a vega-tester or iridologist. Wherever the diagnostic opinion arises from (the doctor, the patient, another practitioner or alternative diagnostician) the phytotherapist may find herself in accord or conflict, to varying degrees, with that opinion. Her personal beliefs, education, training, research and biases will colour her views and these should always be identified and questioned. The phytotherapist *will* hold general views that influence her perspective and these especially should be sought out and held up to the light for scrutiny. We might express such views and biases in the form of statements such as:

- The doctor is usually right
- Iridology is never reliable
- Patients always have a good insight into their condition.

The phytotherapist might ask herself whether such statements are justifiable and to what extent they might colour her judgement or influence her relationship with patients.

In summary, a number of diagnostic scenarios or issues might be encountered by a phytotherapist, including:

- The patient has self-diagnosed
- The patient has no prior diagnosis
- A conventional diagnosis has been given by a doctor
- A conventional diagnosis is currently being sought (e.g. the patient is awaiting investigation or the arrival of test results)
- A diagnosis has been given by a non-conventional practitioner (e.g. an acupuncturist or osteopath)
- A non-conventional diagnostic technique has been used (e.g. iridology, vega, reflexology, hair mineral analysis)
- A diagnosis has been provided by a health-screening service.

Each of these situations or factors presents a number of possible challenges for the practitioner. The phytotherapist will be best equipped to meet such challenges and consequently most able to assist the patient if she reflects on the dimensions and potentials of these situations and factors and questions her own beliefs, practices, behaviours and biases.

The phytotherapist will attempt to diagnose the patients' condition and assess their predicament. Diagnosis and assessment may be contrasted as follows:

*Diagnosis*: an attempt to define, as precisely and definitively as possible, the patient's medical condition.

*Assessment*: a broad survey and gathering together of factors initiating, modulating and sustaining the patients' predicament that is as full as possible.

While diagnosis is classically related to an appreciation of symptoms and signs, the assessment will include the patients' feelings, thoughts, behaviours, attitudes, aspirations and commitments. The diagnosis might be considered as providing a point of focus on which a prescription and management or development plan can be based while the assessment keeps in play all of the issues for more general or less immediate attention and which represent problems and potentials for future work.

In working with these two dimensions – both centre stage and behind the scenes – it is necessary to keep all factors continually or repeatedly in sight. The nature of the diagnostic-related working processes should match those that underpin the consultation as a whole, namely: holistic (taking a broad and inclusive view) and integrated (recognizing patterns and making connections).

A holistic and integrated approach must be able to accommodate and interpret a wide range of patient experiences, including those facets that do not fit classical diagnostic pictures. Such facets are sometimes referred to as 'medically unexplained symptoms' (MUS). Epstein et al. (2006) have researched and discussed the ways in which ambiguity generated by MUS impacts the consultation. They state that: 'Dealing with ambiguity … increases the cognitive complexity of the encounter and physician anxiety …' and suggest that: 'In an effort to manage their own anxiety, physicians … either reject the patient's symptoms (or ideas about causation) as not legitimate or collude with the patient's proposed explanations and requests in an attempt to please the patient'. Each of these coping methods is problematic, with collusion proving little better than rejection, since it: '… may limit consideration of a wider range of diagnostic alternatives, whereas premature reassurance may paradoxically raise patients' anxieties'. The authors further describe two varieties of communication style that are commonly employed in response to ambiguity in the patients' case, these are: 'usual care, in which ambiguity is denied and closure sought' and: 'a "partnering" approach in which the patient's experience is understood, ambiguity is acknowledged, and patient input is sought'. This latter style is referred to as an example of patient-centred communication and it is suggested that additional patient-centred strategies will complement this manner of response, such as: '… coming to agreement on a name for the illness and a plan for follow-up visits, diagnostic testing, and treatment, recognizing that ambiguity about the nature of some symptoms may persist for months or years'. These various strategies are worth summarizing and elaborating as guidelines in dealing with situations wherein a concrete diagnosis cannot be given:

- Acknowledge that there is uncertainty regarding the diagnosis
- Seek, nonetheless, to appreciate and understand the patient's predicament as fully as possible in the absence of a diagnosis
- Reflect on the patient's interpretation and explanations
- Negotiate a working description (or 'name') for the predicament in lieu of a diagnosis
- Develop a plan to address the situation over subsequent visits
- Consider whether further investigation may be helpful
- Construct a treatment plan to address the working hypothesis regarding the patient's condition

- Be able to continue caring in this way should a more concrete diagnosis fail to be arrived at over time.

Such a formulation should present no conceptual challenge to phytotherapists since ambiguity is a commonplace result of applying the holistic approach and the act of acknowledging complexity. Many patients present with pictures that do not fit, or which only partially fit, conventional diagnostic pictures, since these tend to be narrowly framed. In fact, in order to precisely match a conventional diagnosis, the patient's experience must be sifted and delimited and such a process runs contrary to holism. This does not mean to say that conventional diagnoses are never derived from the holistic assessment but rather that the yield of such an assessment is typically greater than this. The holistic net typically gathers a large catch that may include one or more conventional diagnoses as well as other perspectives derived, e.g. from MUS.

Butler et al. (2004) argue that strategies related to the patient-centred model remain inadequate in the face of MUS since the patient-centred approach continues to be essentially situated within an analytical philosophical tradition which is constrained in its capacity to understand and make sense of the patient's predicament. The authors discuss the development of the biopsychosocial medical model, arising out of criticisms of the biomedical model. They relate the biopsychosocial model to the patient-centred approach and describe: '... the concept of triple diagnosis, whereby clinicians make diagnoses at three levels, the biological or physical, the personal or psychological and the social or contextual'. This combination may fail to attain a satisfactory appreciation of the patient's situation however, since its analytical underpinning will still tend to lead the practitioner to: 'break down complex phenomena in the hope of finding meaning in the simpler constituents (reductionism)'. Typically, this will result in the rationalization of medically-unexplained symptoms as examples of somatization. Butler et al. argue that there is a need to move beyond this type of conclusion arising from analytical philosophy by applying an 'interpretivist' philosophical approach whose goal is to: 'understand the whole experience as a complex unity, embedded in (and hence partly characterized by) a specific context or frame of reference'. While the notion of somatization may appear to represent progress in connecting the mind and body, it continues in fact to maintain and reinforce the dualistic-mechanistic view of the body by asserting that psychological phenomena can manifest physically and vice-versa. Mind and body may interact but they still represent distinctly separate poles of being. McWhinney et al. (1997) explain that: 'Somatization is a product of western medicine's dualistic ontology. The assumption is that emotions, instead of being expressed symbolically in words, are transduced to bodily events. A further assumption is that our emotions are not embodied in the first place'. In the interpretivist view, the body and the mind are one so that: *'the psychological now becomes an essential mode and expression of the somatic'* [original italics], e.g.: 'Just as nausea may accompany the interpretation of something as disgusting, so back pain is an inherent part of some people's response to their life situation'. The key to working in this way lies in helping patients to: 'consider the meaning of (their) symptoms in their own lives'. The application of interpretivist philosophy will tend therefore to lead to explanations and to sense-making and thereby remove ambiguity from medically unexplained symptoms. Butler et al. (2000) suggest that adoption of the interpretivist model to replace the analytical one will facilitate the further development of the patient-centred approach.

It may be worth our while to linger in the realm of somatization for a moment longer in order to further explore its relevance in reflecting on diagnosis. McWhinney et al. (1997) remind us that the notion of somatization originates from the concept of conversion in psychoanalysis whereby psychological conflict manifests in physical symptoms. In this original view the symptoms of conversion were: 'considered to be forms of communication rather than physiologic disturbances'. This returns us to interpretivism and the notion that so-called somatic phenomena (which are frequently synonymous with MUS) are there to be listened to and decoded rather than to be classified and treated. Interpretation of course implies a subjective reading of the patient's situation. Malterud (2001) points out that: 'The task of the physician is two-fold: to understand the patient and to understand the disease'. Understanding disease (i.e. diagnosis) has come to be prioritized over understanding the patient, since the former is seen (erroneously) to be a generally objective pursuit while the latter implies a high-degree of subjectivity such that it is not deemed compatible with a positivist medical approach. Malterud mentions Leder's (1990) observation in this connection, that: 'In seeking to escape all interpretive subjectivity, medicine has threatened to expunge its primary subject – the living, experiencing patient'. The insistence on analytical as opposed to interpretive philosophy therefore negates the person of the patient.

All of the foregoing serves not to reject the business of diagnosis-making but to put it in its proper place. Diagnosis should be sought, but not to the exclusion or negation of the patient. Achieving a diagnosis is only one of the aims of the consultation – and frequently not a major one. In many cases in phytotherapy practice it will not be possible, and in some cases not desirable, to accord the patient a classical diagnosis. The primary focus of the phytotherapist will be to assess the patient, to appreciate her predicament and to help her locate, interpret, understand and discern the meaning of her symptoms. Such a process will not only help to determine appropriate advice and treatment but act as a therapeutic intervention in its own right.

## CONCEIVING THE SELF

In attempting to assess the patient, the practitioner uses her own self as a means of appreciating the patient's self. The sense of 'self' that each brings to the clinical encounter will shape its content and outcome/s. Perceptions of 'self' are not necessarily fixed or consistent within any one person or when considered from such angles as those pertaining to history and culture. Rather the notion of 'self' is fluid and mutable, played upon by changing influences in society and personal life events. Schilling (1993) contends that: 'In traditional societies, identities were received automatically through ritual practices which connected people and their bodies to the reproduction of long established social positions'. In more rapidly changing and diverse cultures the notion of self is called into question: 'By undermining traditional meaning systems, the conditions of high modernity stimulate within people a heightened reflexivity about life, meaning and death. In this context, the formation of self-identity becomes a particular problem for modern people'. Cultural revision and societal uncertainty are mirrored in adaptation and uncertainty within, and about, the self:

> The self is no longer seen as a homogenous, stable core which resides within the individual. Instead, identities are formed reflexively through the asking of questions and the continual re-ordering of self-narratives which have at their centre a concern with the body. Self-identity and the body become 'reflexively organized projects' which have to be sculpted from the complex plurality of choices offered by high modernity without moral guidance as to which should be selected.

The consultation then may be considered as providing an extraordinary and rare opportunity for the ordering or modulating of self-identity. It offers a context in which questions regarding the self can be formulated and posed; where self-narratives can be articulated and contrasted and where choices can emerge or be laid out. In acting as a guide in this territory, the practitioner is inevitably drawn into scenarios where moral questions arise and where she may consequently move into a pastoral role. We have previously discussed the importance of aiding the patient in finding meaning in their predicament and we can now make clear that this process can be conflated with that of the discovery or formulation of the self. In facilitating the patient's self-discovery the practitioner simultaneously inhabits, or shifts between, a number of ancient and sacred roles: spiritual adviser, moral authority, elder, parent, teacher, 'one-who-knows'. The extent to which the practitioner is able to appropriately perform these roles and their associated rites will determine her effectiveness in acting as an agent facilitating self-actualization in the patient. Effects towards such an eventuality might be achieved by the bringing-into-consciousness of issues that stand in need of reflection by the patient and in aiding the clarification or even resolution of perturbing or apparently conflicting thoughts and ideas concerning the self. Maslow (1968) has described how: 'Resolving a dichotomy into a higher, more inclusive, unity amounts to healing a split in the person and making him more unified'. Maslow describes personal integration as 'self-consistency, unity, wholeness', the practitioner can assist the patient's integration of the self by enabling reflection and work on these aspects of being.

Sorabji (2006) points out that analytic philosophy – the approach underlying the practice of biomedicine – has often denied that there is such a thing as the self. Interpretive philosophy, on the other hand, is primarily occupied with elucidation of the self. In outlining his exploration of the self Sorabji says that:

> I believe Plato sowed the seeds of a problem when he made reason the true self ... I discuss whether this did not make the true self rather impersonal and whether, consequently, it leaves sufficient room for individuality.

In the western rationalist tradition, the real self is identified with the reasoning *part* of the person, the scientific man, an objectified and universal self set-apart from nature and placed outside of the body. This is an abstracted, formless, disembodied, self-denying 'self'. The humanist medical practitioner naturally stands in opposition to this non-human notion of the self. More than this – the practice of humanistic, person-centred, holistic, integrative medicine provides a remedial means of bringing the separated self back into the body and back into communion with the additional aspects of personhood that it had been parted from. In order to work in this way, the practitioner must perpetually seek to integrate her own self. We can note here the earlier discussion in this chapter of practitioner satisfaction in the consultation deriving from two sorts of complementary work – work on the self and work on the patient. This is the very core of humanistic medical practice – enablement of the selves of practitioner and patient.

The concept of 'the self' today includes a sense of its plasticity. We are no longer stuck with one self for life – the self can be changed physically and psychologically; with a little expert help one can be 'made-over' into a more attractive and higher achieving person. Alternatively, we may apply 'self-help' methods to adapt, enhance and remodel ourselves. The body can be changed quickly and radically with cosmetic surgery, which has attained an increased degree of public acceptance alongside a heightened media presence. Numerous diet (Shapin 2004: 'Dietetics is a good place to look if you want to document recent changes in conceptions of the self') and exercise regimes promise to shape the body in non-surgical ways and a vast array of psychological and spiritual systems and techniques for emotional, mental and spiritual improvement are laid before us. Personal liberation is associated with access to, and the exercising of, *choice* in capitalist cultures and no limit can be set on this (at least not for the privileged elite) in free-market capitalism especially. The ability to make choices about the self then, and to consume products and services related to our choices, must be allowed and encouraged – for matters to be otherwise would be to call the political-economic system into question. Patients may approach practitioners to play a specific role in helping them to complete their changing-the-self projects. Problems may arise for the phytotherapist here in relation to – whether the project can be considered valid or achievable by the practitioner and, if it is, whether the patient will accept subtle change over a reasonable course of time when popular media has suggested that radical and rapid change is generally both possible and desirable.

Patients may be excused for being confused by exposure to dissonant messages blowing in the noise of popular culture. Authorities, experts, opinion-givers, journalists, celebrities, corporations, campaigners, elected and unelected officials and 'ordinary' people, magnified and edited by various media, combine to exhort the individual to consume and abstain, to relax and exert, to take control and to let themselves go. It may be difficult to perceive a sense of self, or to work out who the self should be, or how the self should behave in this cacophony – especially if one lacks a coherent sense of self to start with. In other times and in other places maintaining a sense of self was easier. Until very recent times, one of the first things that the son of a farmer would have known was that he was to be a farmer too. People have not always enjoyed career choices, or choices in many other critical areas of life. The modern mind rebels at such a state of affairs – surely these were repressed times, when people were not free to 'be themselves'. Certainly this is true; untold suffering has arisen in cultures where people have been prevented from being themselves due to unjust suppression and coercion being exerted around areas such as gender and sexuality. Yet some people, perhaps many, and not limited to the elite, may have enjoyed the security and sense of belonging that might sometimes have accompanied less choice around the question of self. Faced with the modern illusion of limitless choice the authentic self fails to develop or to thrive; or it contracts and is diminished. We are told that in a 'free society' we can 'be anything' we want to be – if we can find the appropriate inner resources of will and application. However, the unarticulated message is that if we can be *any* thing then we will have failed unless we become *every* thing – otherwise the self remains unattained and is at best only a partial *some* thing or, at worst, it is *no* thing.

A defining feature of the turn of the millennium, coming to prominence in the very late twentieth century and expanding considerably in the early twenty-first century, has been the laying-bare of the self. The self has become exposed in a number of ways and under a number of influences, including:

- Extended communication technology including the internet and mobile phones and mass consumption of these products and services
- Application of information technology to increase dissemination of data pertaining to the person and to increase public surveillance.

It has become difficult to keep the self private in the face of such developments and greater revelation of aspects of the self has, paradoxically, evolved as a coping strategy in this new world. Increased self-revelation is a means of limiting risk and disturbance from the intrusion upon the self – if such intrusion is inevitable, then why not pre-empt it and thereby reduce its threats? Some have exploited the opportunity that increased self-disclosure provides – if increased rendering-up of the self is to become the norm then publicly discussing what were previously considered private matters is a strategy of the savvy early-adopter. It can be argued that good may arise from this development – issues that were previously considered taboo may be aired and their stigma removed; people who do bad things will find it harder to hide. Counter questions can be posed – what impacts might increased surveillance and disclosure have on civil liberties? Is it not the case that increased public venting of formerly private matters merely fuel a voyeuristic culture that is morally illiterate?

In conducting practice, the practitioner needs to have a feel for the influences that play upon us all and that can adapt our attitudes and behaviours; to be in touch with the themes and features of the times that may alter our sense of self and how we see our place in the world. Who are we now? What do we do and how do we think? Is there anything here that is really significantly new or different; and, if there is, do we need to change anything in the way we think and act as practitioners? What kinds of care, support and healing are needed today? Do we need to change our attitudes, behaviours and practices to remain relevant and, moreover, be helpful?

Developments in information technology have enabled many of the forms of novelty that characterize life in developed countries in the early twenty-first century, e.g. providing us with the capacity to:

- Use our mobiles to have intimate conversations with a distant person, in front of groups of strangers
- Live another 'life' through an alter-ego in a virtual-reality world
- Participate in 'social networking' via the internet
- Publish our thoughts and images for the whole world to see in a blog
- Get filmed dozens of times a day on CCTV
- Have unprecedented continuous access to news, opinion and archived stories and data
- Shop, consume images and ideas, play games, search for a new partner – all in a solitary state without leaving our homes.

Many people can and do choose the extent to which they wish to engage with the activities and possibilities that technology offers, but these potentialities have a pervasive influence on culture, nonetheless. Frank Zingrone (2003) maintains that:

> *Mass media simplify experience and thus make reality more complex, and they speed up the rate of cultural change to the point of creating a pervasive panicky angst ... Information overload disintegrates reality. Inhibition holds things together. The inhibited individual, however, is not leading a full life. This is an antievolutionary condition, if consciousness is the result of an ever-increasing complexity in cerebral development. When we resist in engaging in ultracomplex human activity, we reverse the dynamic of expanding awareness.*

Zingrone (a co-worker with Marshall McLuhan) further asserts that the simplifying effect of media 'leaves us too often stumbling about the edge of meaning'. We might view the consultation, in this light, as exemplifying engagement with 'ultracomplex human activity' and providing a means whereby the person can navigate towards the centre of meaning.

So today, the self stands exposed by means and to a degree never before known. The person is multiplied, echoed, fragmented, super-sized, plasticized, uploaded/downloaded, wired, stored away, expressed, preserved, distorted, reconstituted. And in the midst of this ferment, we continue to carry on ancient acts and practices – such as going to see a healthcare practitioner for a consultation. The practitioner now meets a person who is in a process of 'change', who possesses 'options' and who can make 'choices'. Choosing to see a phytotherapist, for example, may be one among several purchases or creative acts relating to ongoing work on the self. The practitioner may assist, inhibit or adapt this work. The consultation can provide a sacred space in which rites relating to the review, modulation, collapse, repression or reinvention of the self may be enacted.

Perhaps worldly status and success have always been associated with one's ability to make connections and manipulate information and we are currently participating in only a more concretized and extended version of age-old activities. We might suggest that healthcare practitioners have always been in the business of making sense of information (about the world, the patient and healing options) in order to make connections between the patient and healing strategies. Today, the patient may view the practitioner more explicitly as an information filter and strategy connector. Overloaded and overwhelmed by information saturation and a wearying multiplicity of potential choices, the patient may ask the practitioner to perform the role of selector and adviser – which information is credible and which options are viable? The patient may arrive with a handful of print-outs and a head full of questions … The practitioner is no longer the font of wisdom of the paternalistic model, instead she is an adviser – one of many 'consultants' that the patient may employ in order to navigate through the information-strewn and data-heavy world.

Yet the practitioner need not be passive, she can be critical and radical – challenging and aiding the patient to develop a deeper and more vital sense of self. Commenting on his world-view Andy Warhol (1975) said: 'I always suspected that I was watching TV instead of living life. People sometimes say that the way things happen in the movies is unreal, but actually it's the way things happen to you in life that's unreal. The movies make emotions look so strong and real, whereas when things really do happen to you, it's like watching television – you don't feel anything'. Audiovisual technology has manipulated the human image and human emotions, amplified on the big screen, diminished on the small screen – abstracted in either case and possessing a force that drives alienation from nature. There is a thread to this however, that can be followed back into prehistory. To what extent do cave paintings, cup and ring carving and hieroglyphs represent forms of alienating technology? And what of the shock-wave from the CGI-like blast of perspective that accompanied the Renaissance? Well, one issue has to do with quality – that is the extent to which the products of visual innovation aid insight into, and appreciation of the world and the human condition, and whether they are beautiful or not. Terrence McKenna (1996) has observed that: 'low production values made acceptable through tolerance of TV (are) allowing people to accept material into their own story which should actually end up on the cutting room floor'. The practitioner is in a position to facilitate the patient in telling their story about their self and challenging them to question and scrutinize the sections that smack of cheap hack-work. McKenna's assertion was a phenomenological one, that: 'the truth is not in the public space, or the historical space, the truth is in the felt space of the body in the moment' – and this is perhaps the physician-healer's greatest offering, in the cyber-age as in the stone-age, to ground the patient in their body, in the moment – and in so doing to help them make sense of their lives and find meaning. This self-remedial power has not been removed by current technology; it is still possible to lift the multiple veils or masks of the composite contemporary self to reveal our primordial core-self. This self comes from nature and is still connected with nature, this self still belongs in the world and is part of the world. This self *is* nature. If a herbalist will not remind us of this fact then who will?

One problem with the notion of self is that it naturally suggests that there is something which must therefore be non-self. From the contrast of self with non-self, we generate essential duality and separate existence into parts rather than a whole. The definition of self, producing non-self as a consequence, is commensurate with the Christian idea of 'the fall'. As the self is formed, it is cast out of union with the non-self and is thereby capable of feeling loss, grief, loneliness, isolation. The human self becomes separated from other selves in nature – those of animals and the elements for example. A finer gradation however, continues to separate each individual human from all others. The concept of self then is the driver of alienation from nature and from our fellows and allows such a degree of distancing that it becomes possible for humans to harm their environment and each other. The sense of self is not then an attainment to be sought or desired, since it brings separation and pain. Not all peoples and cultures have developed or maintained a notion of the separate self and in those that have the aspiration to achieve union with others has persisted and even been institutionalized – as in marriage.

The interaction between the selves of practitioner and patient may in some circumstances achieve an at-oneing that can relieve alienation and loneliness and rouse hope. This may happen even when, or perhaps especially when, the practitioner is not able to cure but still communicates care: human warmth, empathy, love. These qualities and behaviours transgress the boundaries of the two selves present in the consultation and touch on a mystic human communion. Such a closeness is not always thought desirable in the consultation and various approaches to the healing arts take differing stances on how the person of the practitioner should be applied to the person of the patient. Rowan and Jacobs (2002) posit three types of self used by practitioners in psychological therapies which lead to particular ways of being in the consultation:

1. The *instrumental* position: The client is usually regarded as someone who has problems, which need to be put right … specific techniques have to be learned and put into practice … which nearly always include identification of a clear focus or problem … the key things is that there should be an aim … key words here are 'contract', 'assessment', 'treatment goals', 'empirically validated treatments', 'boundaries' and 'manualization'.
2. The *authentic* way of being: The therapist (is) much more closely identified with the client and more openly concerned to explore the therapeutic relationship. The idea of the wounded healer is often mentioned, as is the idea of personal growth … key words here are 'authenticity', personhood', 'healing through meeting', 'being in the world', 'intimacy', 'openness' and 'the real relationship'.
3. The *transpersonal* way of being: (here) boundaries between therapist and client may fall away. Both may occupy the same space at the same time, at the level of what is sometimes termed 'soul', sometimes 'heart' and sometimes 'essence': what they have in common is a willingness to let go of all aims and assumptions … key words here are 'interbeing', 'linking', 'transcendental empathy', 'resonance', 'dual unity', 'communion', 'the four-dimensional state' and 'ultimate reality'.

In order to operate as the *instrumental self* the practitioner must have received education and training in techniques but in order to occupy the other two modes the practitioner must have had additional experiences that have opened up new ways of being to the practitioner as a person. Rowan and Jacobs state that in order to be the *authentic self* the practitioner must have experienced 'authentic consciousness' and to be the *transpersonal self* must have experienced 'the "Subtle" level of psychospiritual development'. In other words – the practitioner's own experience and personal development, additional to basic education and training, determine both how the practitioner is *able* to work and how they *wish* to work.

The instrumental mode clearly corresponds to the biomedical self but this will also be the mode that is most typically applied in the training of herbal practitioners. For phytotherapists some awareness of the other two modes of being might usefully be encouraged in undergraduate courses but appreciation of them is only likely to substantially develop from a combination of personal experience, self-study and post-graduate training.

These three ways of being can be distinguished in terms of the proximity of the practitioners' and patients' selves to each other. In the *instrumental* mode the patient and practitioner are separate, the boundary between the two is clearly defined and clinical distance is maintained – a practitioner–patient relationship is established which may be paternalistic in nature and described as practitioner-centred. In the *authentic* mode, there is a greater closeness and openness between practitioner and patient and a person–person relationship is established that lends itself to the patient-centred model. The *transpersonal* mode might be identified with the partnership-centred model but this fit hardly seems tight enough to do the transpersonal dimension justice. In the transpersonal state of being, the boundaries between 'patient' and 'practitioner' dissolve; as does the separateness implicit in the term 'person–person' – rather there is the mystical union and at-oneing referred to above. Incidentally, Lawrence and Shapin (1998) remind us that while such talk will inevitably bring to mind the influence of late eighteenth- or early nineteenth-century notions of Romanticism, we would be mistaken to place too much emphasis there since Romanticism's 'use of notions of mystic union between knower and known have ancient and medieval antecedents'.

The skilled, experienced, advanced and personally-developed practitioner may be able to utilize all three of these selves, or ways of being, placing emphasis on this one or that one as appropriate and as the opportunity presents itself. In the practice of phytotherapy the use of the instrumental self will be most extensive in novice practitioners but will be applied by all practitioners to some degree since the practice of phytotherapy does fundamentally set out to identify the patient's condition and apply herbal medicines to remedy it. The practice of phytotherapy is involved with identifying 'a clear focus or problem' and setting therapeutic goals. Such work is not incompatible however with authentic and transpersonal activity. As the practitioner recognizes, and develops some facility in applying, *herself* as a healing agent, she will move the locus of her being in the consultation into the authentic or transpersonal modes. Being based in one or other of these modes she is still able to access and exert her instrumental self. Although the elision that obtains in the transpersonal mode may rarely be achieved it still represents a radical and deep potential that phytotherapists can remain open to.

The way that the consultation itself shapes the 'selving' (to use Fast's, 1998, term which denotes the dynamic and changing nature of the self) of patient and practitioner, should be remembered in conclusion. The self/selves that practitioner and patient bring to the consultation are not necessarily exactly the same as those that pertain outside of the consultation. The act of the consultation itself demarcates a territory where certain aspects of the self tend to be deployed or withheld. Where certain types of behaviour are allowed or disallowed. Rowan and Jacobs (2002) describe the origins of this selectivity regarding the use of the self in practitioner training:

> ... the self that the trainee therapist is invited to develop is nevertheless a type of act, a form of role-playing: to listen rather than interrupt as they otherwise might in an argument; to accept without passing judgement, where in another situation they might want to challenge a moral position; to select a response carefully, rather than spontaneously react.

These are the normative behaviours expected by both patients and practitioners in the consultation and they represent normal courtesy or etiquette in the consultation. As the advanced practitioner becomes more *herself* in the consultation then she may modulate or constructively transgress these 'rules'. This creative process needs to be conducted with care therefore, but, since it can move both practitioner and patient to an enhanced place of understanding and satisfaction, it is one of the great rewards of long-term practice.

## GENERALIZING ABOUT INDIVIDUALS

Illich (1976) has cautioned against making the mistake of 'equating statistical man with biologically unique men' – yet this error is made every time that the findings of quantitative medical research are uncritically applied to individual patients. We have previously (in Ch. 3) described the trinity that composes evidence-based medicine – namely, the union of: best available research evidence; clinical expertise; patient values – and noted that the first of these elements tends to be asserted to the neglect (commonly indeed to the *utter* neglect) of the other two. The researcher and the statistician then (facilitated by the health manager and the state legislator), rather than the clinician or the patient, become the arbiters of which care should (and which should not) be given and how it should be administered. Abstraction is placed above engagement and positivist scientific values are accorded greater credence than human experience and preferences. Researchers draw conclusions and make pronouncements about groups, which are then taken to be relevant to individuals. A grotesque mismatch arises in the relationship between the researcher and the clinician (or rather the non-relationship, since the two generally exist in separate worlds and rarely meet) given that the former only studies groups and the latter only treats individuals. The gulf between the two is compounded given that researchers prefer *really* big groups – the bigger the better, or rather, the bigger the more statistically significant. This predilection for super-sizing on the part of the researcher takes her ever further away from the realities of the individual practitioner and, moreover, the individual patient, while creating an illusion of greater-knowing.

Carl Jung (2002; first published 1958) was alive to this state of affairs when he wrote that:

> Judged scientifically, the individual is nothing but a unit which repeats itself ad infinitum and could just as well be designated with a letter of the alphabet. For understanding, on the other hand, it is just the unique individual human being who, when stripped of all those conformities and regularities so dear to the heart of the

> scientist, is the supreme and only real object of investigation. The doctor, above all, should be aware of this contradiction. On the one hand, he is equipped with the statistical truths of his scientific training, and on the other, he is faced with the task of treating a sick person who, especially in the case of psychic suffering, requires individual understanding ... This illustration in the case of medicine is only a special instance of the problem of education and training in general. Scientific education is based in the main on statistical truths and abstract knowledge and therefore imparts an unrealistic, rational picture of the world, in which the individual, as a merely marginal phenomenon, plays no role. The individual, however, as an irrational datum, is the true and authentic carrier of reality, the concrete man as opposed to the unreal ideal or normal man to whom scientific statements refer.

Positivist medical scientific research aims to detect the commonalities between patients sharing the same medical diagnosis and determine treatments that will benefit a substantial number of them *regardless* of their individual peculiarities. Such research generally overlooks the difficulties inherent in the notion of 'diagnosis' in the first place, as discussed earlier, and it is incapable of discerning the individual patient who will eventually consume the fruits of the research. Indeed the individual must be *effaced* in order for the research to be able to be conducted. The ideal is to return findings that can be applied to large groups of people sharing similar broad (let us rather say crude) characteristics so that the findings are said to be 'generalizable' to a particular section of the public or group of patients. A number of authorities have criticized the notion of generalizability, however including Fendler (2006) who has characterized generalizability as in actuality 'a local phenomenon ... not generalizable to other times and places' and Bonell et al. (2006) who noted that while an estimation of generalizability is usually deemed desirable when reporting randomized trials 'a framework for empirically assessing and reporting this is lacking'. If medical research is not generalizable then it is not only inherently worthless but also has the potential to mislead and, in so doing, to cause harm.

While medical research begins with the group and then conjectures about the individual, medical practice can trace this route in reverse – through accumulation of experience with individuals the practitioner forms views about the general characteristics pertaining to specific groups of patients. This latter process represents a form of pattern recognition which may consequently be formalized into a system that is then taught to students. The result of this circular process is that the student then learns how to classify patients into groups and subsets based on the perception that certain commonalities exist between particular 'types' of patients or conditions. This process is one factor determining the classification and diagnostic systems of traditional medicine such as Chinese, Ayurvedic and Greek humoral medicine – but only one factor, and not necessarily the most significant one. Unschuld (1985) describes how sociopolitical and philosophical influences have tended to shape the development of Chinese medical thought and practice:

> *The concepts of demonic medicine mirror human experiences during the period of the Warring States; the increasing amorality and continuing uncertainty of personal and collective existence were reflected in the way the age perceived the nature of*

*illness and its prevention and treatment ... the medicine of systematic correspondences reflects ideas and socio-political structures resulting from efforts to overcome the chaos of the Warring States and from the subsequent conditions accompanying the first unification of China.*

So observation of the patient is only one element contributing to the generation of medical theory and patient classification. There *is* a thread that begins with individual patients and extends to the categorization of groups of patients, leading from the particular to the general, but this is interwoven with many other threads, including those deriving from general observations about nature that lead to particular descriptions of patients. For example, nature provides macrocosmic information regarding dualistic phenomena such as heat and cold which can be applied to people at the microcosmic level. The sun/day/summer axis is hot while that of moon/night/winter is cold. Patient's conditions may be characterized by hot features (e.g. fever, restlessness, redness, aggression) or cold ones (e.g. chills, lying still, pallor, listlessness). Herbal medicines may be brought to bear on the patient's hot/cold picture since they have remedial properties based partly on the thermal qualities they can impart to the patient such as cooling (e.g. bitter herbs such as *Rehmannia glutinosa*; Sheng di Huang) or warming (e.g. pungent herbs such as *Zingiber officinale*; ginger). It can be seen in nature that cold and heat possess particular properties, such as the tendency of cold to slow movement (e.g. freezing water in streams in winter) whereas heat stimulates movement (e.g. boiling water over a fire in cooking). Numerous other related properties can be observed so that cooling herbs are seen to be contracting, calming and draining downwards in the body whereas heating herbs exert influences that are expansive, stimulating and moving upwards. A set of correspondences between nature, people and plants is so discerned and constructed that it can then act as a system of medicine. The patient may be the end point rather than the origin of this process however.

The urge to systematize appears to be both ancient and universal – in medicine it enables classification and management of the patient's condition. A degree of artificiality tends to be a feature of all classification systems however, with certain anomalies or challenges to the system being ignored or forced to fit the overall model. Unschuld (1985) identified a key characteristic of Chinese medical theorization and systemization as being its tendency to *syncretize* conflicting viewpoints or awkward interpretations. In other cultures, opposing systems have fought for prominence, with many falling by the wayside. Nutton (2004) has observed that: 'History is an art of forgetting as well as of remembrance. Many of the voices of the past, especially of the losers in any conflict, can be heard faintly at best ...'. While approaches related to the notion of Hippocratic medicine dominated western medicine until very recent times, Nutton has discussed other Greco-Roman medical approaches that have become obscure, such as the Methodists, Democriteans, Asclepiadeans, Pneumatists and Empiricists, and that of Leonides of Alexandria: 'whose soubriquet, the "Episynthetic", implied that he was bringing together all that was best in others' teaching'.

Medical classifications (of people, their conditions and remedial strategies) have always been strongly disputed. Let us remind ourselves of the Hippocratic author (in Lloyd, 1983) railing against those who would seek to ignore the complexities and subtleties involved in prescribing an appropriate medicinal diet for patients:

> I am utterly at a loss to know how those who prefer these hypothetical arguments and reduce the science to a simple matter of 'postulates' ever cure anyone on the basis of their assumptions. I do not think that they have ever discovered anything that is purely 'hot' or 'cold', 'dry' or 'wet', without it sharing some other qualities … It would be useless to bid a sick man to 'take something hot'. He would immediately ask 'What?' Whereupon the doctor must either talk some technical gibberish or take refuge in some known solid substance. But suppose 'something hot' is also astringent, another is hot and soothing as well, while a third produces rumbling in the belly. There are many varied hot substances with many and varied effects which may be contrary to one another.

Traditional schemata for classifying individuals have tended to incorporate both physical and psycho-emotional aspects. In the humoral tradition, for example, the person who has an excess of yellow bile is not only prone to hot and dry medical conditions but also exhibits the choleric temperament. Eysenck (1985) describes the choleric temperament as a personality type who is: touchy, restless, aggressive, excitable, changeable, impulsive, optimistic, active (Fig. 4.1). Eysenck's adaptation of the classical four temperaments to

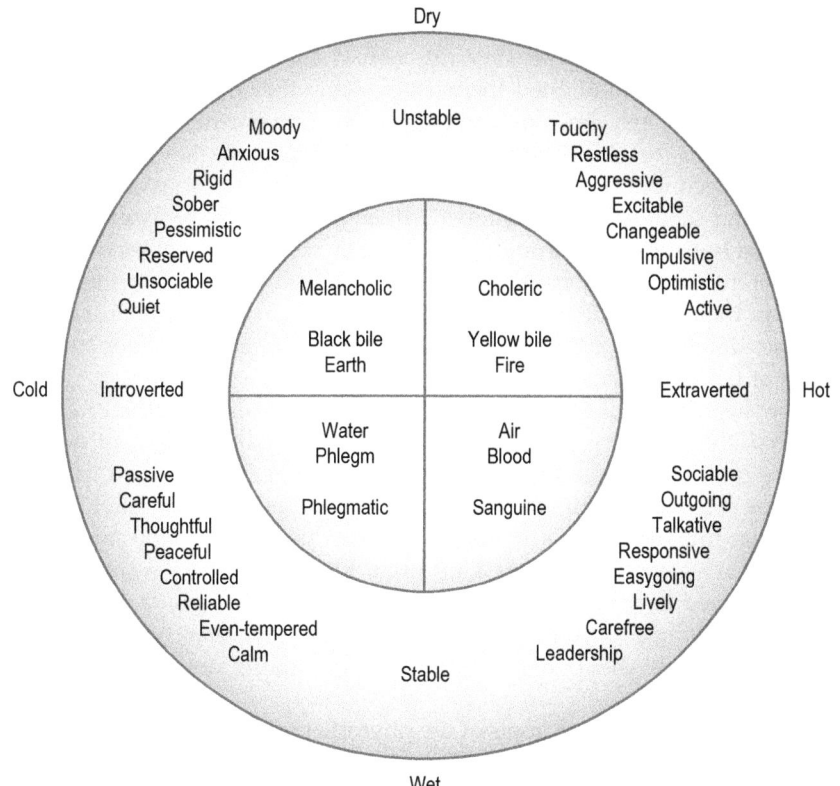

**Figure 4.1** Eysenck's Four Humours Model. *(Adapted from Eysenck (1985), with permission.)*

include the concept of introversion/extraversion, for example, his association of it with the autonomic nervous system, and his extrapolation of the model into personality profiling questionnaires, demonstrates both the persistence and the mutability of this ancient model.

The four humours model thus stands revealed as an early example of psychological profiling and continues amidst a plethora of profiling and classification 'tools' used in connection, not only with the patient but with the worker, the criminal, the consumer, the manager, and so forth. The person, then, can be categorized in numerous ways, as an 'early adopter' of new technology (Moore 1991) say or a 'maven' – someone who has expert knowledge about which products to buy and how to get a good deal on them (Gladwell 2000). Changes in culture are matched by new ways of defining people.

Tracy (1998) has discussed the revival of interest in constitutional approaches to the patient that occurred in America between 1920 and 1950 and has explored how: 'In their efforts to investigate the nature of the individual sick person, constitutionalists ambitiously constructed new human taxonomies based on body type, behaviour pattern, endocrine function and predisposition to disease'. Examples of their work included arranging people into categories based on body types such as asthenics, athletics and pyknics and William Sheldon's categorization based on the preponderance of structures derived from embryonic tissue layers: 'endomorphy (body roundness and softness); mesomorphy (body squareness and firm muscularity); and ectomorphy (body linearity and fragility)'. This latter system was known as somatotyping. Although the constitutionalists aimed for an integrated view of the individual and aligned themselves with other holistic movements of the time (such as 'psychosomatic medicine, the movement to integrate social services within the clinical arena, and social medicine') they were utilizing ideas and techniques such as heredity, laboratory investigations and the body-typing schemas just mentioned which allows Tracy to assert that they 'embraced holistic goals through reductionistic means'. This observation pins the inherent contradiction of approaches that attempt to assess individuals based on their categorization within group types. In the act of classification the practitioner is essentially limiting and diminishing the broader truth and reality of the patient and her unique predicament.

How then can we know patients? How can we be specific about individuals? First, the patient is always seen through the reducing lens of our own practice goals and formed in the image of our remedial tools and capacities – so these must be identified and questioned. Second, once we have clarified our goals and are aware of how our tools shape our expectations and behaviours, we can identify the kind of information that we want to gather. Third, we need to appraise and respond to the patient's agenda and expectations and take appropriate action to advise and/or refer when there is a poor fit between the patient's agenda/expectations and our achievable goals/capacities.

So what are the practice goals of the phytotherapist and how do our 'tools' (i.e. herbs and related strategies) shape our expectation of the consultation? We have discussed these issues in the previous chapter and returned to some of these themes earlier in this chapter. While phytotherapeutic goals are broad and the capacities afforded by plant medicines are similarly so, phytotherapists are still in the business (in the main) of using the instrumental self to assess the patient's condition, formulate aims around benefiting the patient's condition and implement a treatment plan to achieve these aims. So phytotherapists need to acquire a wide range of information about the patient, most substantially through questioning and discussion, including information that is part of the classical medical consultation. In addition, the phytotherapist desires to know who the patient is – what are her preoccupations, opinions, preferences and wishes. This 'getting to know' the patient is an ongoing process throughout a course of consultations or on re-engaging with the patient after an extended period of time during which they have not met. The practitioner must seek enough information of the type required to enable the goals of the consultation but must not close the book after doing so – there is always more to know and the practitioner must always stand ready to be surprised by her patients. More importantly still, the practitioner must remain open to the patient's change and development lest she act as a force of restriction inhibiting such change. At every meeting it is important to view the patient afresh – not starting from scratch but supplementing, reviewing and adjusting the existing base of knowledge that the practitioner holds about the patient.

The following questions are examples of ways of finding out more about the patient as a person, which are less familiar than those of the standard case history routine. There is no complete set of possible questions to be posed and practitioners should feel empowered to view question formulation as a spontaneous and creative art – improvising freely in the live consultation. The sample questions below seek to gather input about the patient's characteristics, preferences, views, opinions and 'taste'. They could be set alongside other questions as part of a questionnaire, yet so much additional information and so many opportunities for linked discussion will be lost by reducing them into this format. The consultation is a live dynamic non-linear process, whereas a questionnaire possesses all the opposite qualities. I would urge the phytotherapist to see herself as a performance artist rather than a data collector …

- Would you describe yourself as an 'early bird' or a 'night owl'?
- Do you like music, theatre, books, film? Tell me what kind of things you like and dislike.
- Which of the seasons (spring, summer, autumn, winter) do you feel most affinity for? Which do you like the most and least?
- Do you enjoy your own company?
- How are you in groups of people?
- What kind of places do you like to visit?
- Would you rather be outdoors or indoors?
- Tell me about your home. Is there anything you would like to change about it?
- What would an ideal holiday be like for you?
- How do you think those who know you well would describe you?
- What kinds of things or experiences make you feel alive/happy/joyful/sad/upset?

- If anything comes to you as a recurring worry, what would that be?
- If I could grant you one personal wish – what would it be?

## ON THE NATURE OF PATIENTS (AND PRACTITIONERS)

In the previous chapter, we mentioned Frank's (1995) description of three types of illness narratives:

- Restitution
- Quest
- Chaos.

These designations describe the types of stories that patients tell and the agendas they bring to the consultation and in doing this they tell us something of the nature of patients and provide a good matrix for us to add other ideas about the nature of patients and their practitioners to. In the discussion below I have added my own reflections to Frank's themes – some of which he might take issue with. I have also occasionally referred to the 'restitution/chaos/quest patient' for ease of discussion and as a useful generalization. Frank has not used this term and would, I suspect, disapprove of it – for the very good reasons given immediately below. I would suggest however that patients can, temporarily, be predominantly in one narrative mode or another. I do not mean to imply that the narrative variations represent permanently fixed types of patients. The categories described here should not be used as cages to confine the patient but merely as rough guides to understanding. Frank is keen to make clear that his:

> ... suggestion of three underlying narratives of illness does not deprecate the originality of the story any individual ill person tells, because no actual telling conforms exclusively to any of the three narratives. Actual tellings combine all three, each perpetually interrupting the other two.

The *restitution narrative* refers to an expectation that the patient will become fully well again, that they will become 'as good as new'. They will take their medicine, follow their course of treatment and be fully restored to their former non-ill self. Ideally, restitution will occur swiftly and with minimum disruption to the person's life and sense of self. This means that the restitution mode provides little opportunity for learning or change as a result of an illness episode. Despite this, restitution behaviour is prized and praised in western cultures, and may sometimes be envied. There is a political imperative to approve and encourage restitution behaviour, since this mode is the one that gets the patient back to work as quickly as possible. Restitution scenarios are played out as media stories such as the one about the politician who gets cancer but is back at her post conducting 'business as usual' the week after surgery; or the one about the Hollywood actress who 'gets her body back' and returns to filming within a few weeks of having a baby. Restitution patients may be relatively compliant and may accept, or even demand, a paternalistic style of practice – 'just tell me what I need to do to get better and I'll do it'. In fact the paternalistic model is only at ease with the restitution narrative and it requires that patients adopt this mode. The restitution patient therefore fits the classic sick-role – they seek treatment, comply with it and strive to get better. Restitution narratives and their associated agendas may be quickly expressed and patients may require little discussion about suggested treatment. As such the restitution narrative may fit within the short duration consultation that is characteristic of conventional medical practice. When the patient is in restitution mode they may be unwilling to respond to practitioner requests to explore the meaning and significance of their predicament more deeply and unwilling to hear practitioner explanations that describe their condition as complex, requiring long-term treatment or necessitating changes in thought or behaviour – 'look, can't you just fix me?' We can suggest that the restitution dominant patient is most likely to visit a conventional medical practitioner for help. When they do visit CAM practitioners, it may be because they have failed to achieve restitution from conventional medical care but still hope an alternative practitioner may be able (swiftly and without further disruption) to help them get 'back to normal'. In other words, they may bring the same agenda to the CAM practitioner that they brought to their doctor – the patient has not been altered by their experience so far and does not appear to be learning from it. CAM practitioners will generally be uncomfortable with such a state of intransigence and attempt to move the patient to reflect on their condition and shift their perspective. This may result in the patient taking on the quest perspective as a dominant mode of thinking, or, stuck in restitution mode, she may seek out other practitioners to find one who possesses the magic formula, in the meantime bemoaning that 'nobody seems to be able to sort me out'. In its extreme negative form, the restitution narrative describes a situation where the patient is in denial about the reality of her condition, unwilling to accept any responsibility for it, unwilling to adapt her thinking or behaviour to improve it and not prepared to accept that she may have to accept some long-term loss or limitation as a consequence of it. That something approximating this scenario might arise in patients for a period of time is unsurprising, especially when we consider that the patient-as-consumer may have had a lifetime of exposure to restitution marketing messages from pharmaceutical companies, nutritional supplement and herbal product companies, proponents of diets and exercise regimes, and practitioners both conventional and alternative that one only has to take this pill/food/class/practitioner and you will be restored to your former glory as if by magic.

Of course some conditions are susceptible to quick and relatively easy restitution – many conditions are self-limiting and therefore will tend to clear up regardless of whether the patient has taken any particular steps to address them. There is also nothing wrong with the desire to get better rapidly and to 'get on with one's life' with the minimum of interruption (although the implied suggestion that periods of illness do not constitute part of life but rather represent gaps or breaks in living is unsustainable and is part of the problem side of the restitution concept). The major issue with the restitution narrative has to do with its tendency to obstruct the patient in fully engaging with the dimensions and meaning of their predicament and thereby limiting learning and self-development.

Frank points out that a primary limitation of the restitution narrative is that: 'when it doesn't work any longer, there is no other story to fall back on'.

The restitution narrative understands itself as being simple, direct and definitive. Its core message to the patient plays something like this: when you have a health problem it's your duty to solve it – you do this by consulting an expert – you follow their advice and you get better – then you carry on where you left off. There is no plan B. If this sequence fails to run smoothly, the restitution narrative is revealed as inadequate and the patient needs to find another story to take its place. This is one of the key therapeutic opportunities that can present to the practitioner – the chance to help the patient find a new and more helpful story. Frequently this is a starting place for the phytotherapy consultation: a patient has been seeing another practitioner (or practitioners) but has failed to achieve restitution; she is now seeking an alternative approach. The phytotherapist may be able to respond by assisting the patient in moving to a new narrative perspective. Alternatively, she may just offer an alternative means of achieving restitution suggesting to the patient that where drug A, homeopathic remedy B and acupuncture points C–Y failed, herb Z will succeed! Care needs to be taken when swimming in these waters.

While patients may spend some time in restitution mode so may practitioners – some may linger there and attempt to make a career out of it. The implicit message that every practitioner, by the fact of *being* a practitioner, sends out into the world is: 'I am here to help you'. The nature of this help varies however and practitioners need to reflect on, and be clear about, what their own message is precisely. Some options are given below:

*'I am here to cure you'.*

*'I am here to restore you'.*

*'I am here to heal you'.*

*'I am here to empower you'.*

*'I am here to facilitate your personal development'.*

*'I am here to enlighten you'.*

*'I am here to convert you to my way of thinking'.*

*'I am actually here for me'.*

*'I am not here'.*

The practitioner may set out her stall as a 'restitution woman' – 'come to me and I will make you better'. We have previously discussed that one of the most potent healing qualities a practitioner can possess is confidence. Saying anything other than 'I will make you better' may appear to suggest that the practitioner is lacking in confidence regarding her abilities and capacity to heal. Yet there is a difference between confidence and arrogance, between knowing one's abilities and hubris. The reality of effective helping practice is a nuanced and subtle one. We return here to notions of the practitioner as actor and trickster, remembering that these roles need not be incompatible with practitioner genuineness. We have previously asserted that the most effective and content practitioners are those who are aware of the multiple roles and strategies that the practitioner can deploy and who are able to do skilfully and appropriately. With regard to this discussion, the practitioner needs to:

- Know which narrative mode the patient is in
- Recognize when that mode is unhelpful for the patient
- Be able to aid the patient in moving to a more helpful narrative mode.

There is no set hierarchy or linearity involved in moving between the restitution, quest and chaos narratives – indeed all three are usually present, to varying degrees, simultaneously. The issue has to do with which mode is dominant and where a shift in emphasis may be helpful.

Frank states that the *chaos narrative* represents: 'the opposite of restitution: its plot imagines life never getting better'. Chaos stories are hard to hear and hard to bear partly because their message is bleak and desperate and partly because they are told in a manner that is disordered – lacking in 'coherent sequence' they are actually non-narratives, or as Frank calls them 'anti-narratives'. As Frank explains: 'The teller of chaos stories is, pre-eminently, the wounded storyteller, but those who are truly *living* the chaos cannot tell in words. To turn the chaos into a verbal story is to have some reflective grasp on it' [original italics]. The chaos patient then does not tell a coherent story because they *cannot* do so, the teller tends to be stuck in 'an incessant present with no memorable past and no future worth anticipating' – the perspective provided by a clear sense of time is absent from these stories. Of course all patient stories tend to be told in a non-linear way, moving back and forth in time, but chaos stories seem to be hard to take in part due to their claustrophobic and overwhelming simultaneity – with no separating and sense-enabling time perspective provided. Chaos narratives may be read as lacking in variety and colour – 'they just keep going on about the same thing'. One implication for the consultation is that chaos narratives need a lot of time to be told, or rather, they do not have a beginning, middle and end so that it is hard to initiate chaos consultations ('the patient just jumps right in') or to draw them to a conclusion. Chaos consultations tend to run over time, since the patient is rarely aware of the practitioner's need to contain the narrative within a specific time period. Ellis (1996) has observed this phenomenon: 'I was working in chronological time against the surgery clock, but the patients seemed to have limitless time and to be detached from the reality of time passing'.

Chaos patients tend to feel a lack of control regarding their condition and their lives more generally. The practitioner may read such a patient as being a victim and respond by trying to rescue her by setting in place case-management strategies to enable the patient to attain greater control of her condition and situation. Such efforts will tend to be met with resistance, rejection, non-compliance and/or rebellion by the patient. Such patients are rarely seeking control and may see attempts to promote control as evidence of a lack of appreciation or even a denial of their predicament. They are actually seeking understanding and meaning. Ellis (1996) has diagnosed chaos-type narratives as evidence of 'chronic unhappiness' and reflected on his own journey in coming to appreciate how to help such patients, including what this exploration revealed about himself as a practitioner:

*Did these unhappy patients select a sympathetic doctor whose need was to be needed? I sensed that, for these patients, I was not only a medical expert but also a revealer of meanings and a healer. The patients were asking me to heal them of being human. My role was, therefore, to bear witness to their suffering and allow the unhappiness to exist or surface ...*

Yet Ellis felt personal resistance to working in this way:

*Because of my ingrained drive to cure and my massive armoury, I found it hard to accept that this was my role and often my only role.*

Phytotherapists too may find it frustrating or unsatisfactory to set aside our *materia medica* and focus on the human aspects of healing. As practitioners we tend, inevitably, to identify ourselves with our therapeutic modality so that as we work with patients who have more need of *us* as persons than our remedies we may feel inadequate to the task. This underlines the importance of the practitioner recognizing that she, in and of *herself*, is a medicine – sometimes distinct from, and sometimes entangled with, her therapeutic tools. In order to work comfortably and usefully with chaos narratives, the practitioner must be able to step into the foreground in her personhood and human healing presence, leaving all other therapeutic options in the background for the time being. Certainly the kinds of patient cases we are discussing here are likely to derive some benefit from such phytotherapeutic strategies as pertain to the use of, for example adaptogenic and nervous trophorestorative herbs, but the use of such strategies should not be allowed to stand in place of the human elements of caring. The practitioner should not use her materia medica as a screen to hide behind.

Ellis (1996) concludes that: 'The expectations and needs of chronically unhappy patients are neither met nor meetable in the current medical paradigm', and he recommends that:

*Different roles, apart from curative or therapeutic, should be taught to family practitioners for caring for patients suffering from a troubled existence. Practising patient-centred care, teaching and learning the art of healing and the relief of suffering, and just being there as a refuge and empathetic listener will help us to care for and comfort these patients.*

Not all practitioners come to such an appreciation of the chaos dynamic. Patients telling chaos stories may be considered to be 'difficult' and identified with the label of 'heartsink', a term whose coining with reference to medicine is commonly attributed to O'Dowd (1988) who explained it thus:

*There are patients in every practice who give the doctor and staff a feeling of 'heartsink' every time they consult. They evoke an overwhelming mixture of exasperation, defeat and sometimes plain dislike that causes the heart to sink when they consult.*

Booker (2006) has described her reflections on such a patient for whom 'Nothing pleased her, and whatever I did was wrong. Despite my best efforts, little changed as time passed ...'. Delany (2007) advises that practitioners should listen to what their heart is telling them about the patient:

*Our hearts sink for the best of reasons. Feelings are always true and always rational, that is, they are always appropriate and proportional to their original cause. They can therefore be trusted even when it may be impossible to link them to anything in the patient's present circumstances; and even though their original cause remains undiscovered during all our consultations together. Our difficulty in 'getting the picture' may indicate we are dealing with a patient's repressed experience, re-enacted in exact but obscure ways, using the listener/doctor as a ready-to-hand and convenient figure of transference.*

The suggestion is that practitioners react defensively against such patients in order to protect themselves from receiving the projected (transferred) pain, anxiety, fear and despair that chaos patients embody. Such practitioner reactions might then be offset to a large degree if they appreciated the concept of transference (this is mentioned again in Appendix 1).

Wilson (2005) contends that positive outcomes for the practitioner can result from working with 'difficult' patients:

... *'difficult' patients can be superb triggers for learning about important issues in modern medicine: awareness of self within the doctor–patient relationship, professional maintenance, models of healthcare.*

Mathers et al. (1995) questioned the role that factors related to the practitioner rather than the patient might play in determining what constituted a 'difficult' patient. They quoted previous studies that suggested: 'irritation with patients might arise from the doctor's own intolerance, impatience, fatigue, hunger or pressure of work'; that the greater the practitioner's experience the less frequently they experienced 'troubling patient encounters'; and that three prominent themes had previously been identified with the notion of the difficult patient:

- 'A lack of control grounded in the doctor's frustration ...
- The feeling that stalemate with the patient had been reached ...
- A fear of opening Pandora's box and being overwhelmed with problems ...'

Their own research revealed that: 'The greater a doctor's perceived workload and job dissatisfaction, the more heartsink patients he or she is likely to report ... Having a relevant postgraduate qualification was also associated with doctors reporting fewer heartsink patients'. Phytotherapists generally have less intensive workloads than doctors but this is not a given – all practitioners need to be clear when they are exceeding their capacity to care (see Appendix 2 on Self-care). When practitioners have training in areas such as communication skills, they cope better with challenges and are better equipped to help patients. Regular participation in relevant postgraduate skills' training can significantly improve practitioner competence in these areas.

Chaos narratives are *not* synonymous with notions of 'difficult' or 'heartsink' patients but chaos stories may often be told in cases so labelled. In working with chaos narratives, we need to learn, as Ellis did, to set aside (which does not mean to abandon) our 'ingrained drive to cure' and our therapeutic 'armoury' and to simply be there with the patients. Frank discusses the analysis of recordings of interviews with Holocaust survivors, which revealed how: 'Very subtly the interviewers direct witnesses toward another narrative that exhibits "the resiliency of the human spirit". The human spirit certainly is resilient, but ... *that is not what the witnesses are saying*' [original italics]. Similarly, practitioners tend to try to steer chaos narratives in the direction of a more positive perspective on their situation in the belief that this is a therapeutic strategy that will help the patient to 'move on' or to take a more optimistic and constructive view – this is a means of pushing the patient into a restitution scenario. The problem is that by attempting to move things on prematurely, or to do so without allowing a full hearing and exploration of the story and its issues, the practitioner may be read as showing a lack of appreciation of, and a disregard for the depth and dimensions of the patient's predicament. This amounts to a denial of the patient's experience and, as Frank says, this not only 'compounds the chaos' but also 'makes its horror worse'. Practitioners may be unwilling to linger in the chaos zone, fearful of encouraging the opening of Pandora's box as we previously stated, and keen to extinguish the feelings of anxiety that the chaos state is arousing in themselves. Frank contends that:

> *The challenge of encountering the chaos narrative is how not to steer the storyteller away from her feelings ... The challenge is to* hear. *Hearing is difficult not only because listeners have trouble facing what is being said as a possibility in their own lives. Hearing is also difficult because the chaos narrative is probably the most embodied form of story ... Ultimately, chaos is told in the silences that speech cannot penetrate or illuminate. The chaos narrative is always beyond speech, and thus it is always* lacking *in speech. Chaos is what can never be told; it is the hole in the telling.*

These are deep waters; spaces that some phytotherapists may feel should only be navigated by psychological therapists. Certainly practitioners should be trained in the appropriate concepts and skills to help them work with chaos pictures, as sources already quoted have recommended, and indeed some (perhaps most) chaos patients will benefit from specifically psychological therapies and should be referred for these as appropriate – but to vacate this territory entirely would severely limit the scope of phytotherapeutic or other types of 'non-psychological practice' (if any practice can be said to constitute such an entity). Moreover, such a dereliction would leave the notion and the actuality of the whole person *in pieces*.

Frank considers that:

> *The need to honour chaos stories is both moral and clinical. Until the chaos narrative can be honoured, the world in all its possibilities is being denied. To deny a chaos story is to deny the person telling this story, and people who are being denied cannot be cared for.*

In order to care for the chaos patient, the practitioner must hear their story and honour it. This cannot be achieved in a superficial manner. The wounded storyteller must be met by the wounded healer: the practitioner has to be aware of, and be able to safely enter, her own woundedness alongside that of the patient. From this point of deep human connection, the practitioner is able to listen and to bear witness. Such an act of loving acceptance may be accompanied by a degree of recognition on the part of the patient and perhaps a consequent shift allowing new story elements to emerge. In considering the implications for the practitioner in being able to work in this way, we might bear in mind Jung's injunction (Jacobi & Hull 1992) that: 'If the doctor wants to help a human being, he must be able to accept him as he is. And he can do this in reality only when he has already seen and accepted himself as he is'.

Frank introduces the *quest narrative* comparing it with the foregoing narratives:

> Restitution stories attempt to outdistance mortality by rendering illness transitory. Chaos stories are sucked into the undertow of illness and the disasters that attend it. Quest stories meet suffering head on; they accept illness and seek to use it. Illness is the occasion of a journey that becomes a quest. What is quested for may never be wholly clear, but the quest is defined by the ill person's belief that something is to be gained through the experience.

We might posit the following correlations:

- The restitution narrative is that of the typical conventional medicine patient, fitting the paternalistic model (and required by it)
- The quest narrative is that of the typical CAM patient, prepared to embark on a holistic journey of the self (and required to do so by the CAM practitioner)
- The chaos narrative is that of the typical psychotherapy patient, in need of psychological rehabilitation.

But these are stereotypes rather than archetypes: holism and paternalism are not limited to any one field or modality of practice and the patient is not limited to one narrative – recall that patients may move through the three types under discussion within one consultation. Yet the patient who is predominantly in quest mode is actively seeking alternative or additional ways of understanding and working with her predicament, so is fundamentally oriented in the direction of the holistic approach. The quest position allows for free movement and development because these goals are being actively sought. The patient in quest mode is self-empowered and, at least to a degree, self-directed. While the restitution story speaks of a delegated self (the dominant healing power lies with the practitioner or the medication) and the chaos story references an absent, lost, suppressed or deferred self; the quest self is present in the consultation as the primary active healing force. Quest patients are therefore a challenge to paternalistic practitioners – they have their own opinions and views and want to be treated as a partner, at the very least, in the consultation. Quest patients will sometimes seek opinions and advice from more than one practitioner in more than one modality, using them sometimes as consultants in the business sense – strategy advisers whose views are there to be weighed up, contrasted and considered rather than meekly followed.

The quest narrative can extend fluidly back and forth in time, providing the coherence that is lacking in the chaos picture. Part of the quest process involves the creative use of the self so that quest stories may contain significant interpretive elements formulated to improve the quality of the story in terms of generating greater meaning, sense and purpose. This cohering drive may then involve allowing for a degree of artistic licence. This is not to suggest that quest stories are 'untrue' but rather that the successful quest narrative is one that will make use of the best available links and connections but will remain open to replacing these if ones that fit better become available. The patient's quest narrative can reach such proportions of coherence and sense-making that the patient may construe it as a tale with universal application as a means of providing insight and perhaps instruction – Frank refers to this as 'automythology'. Not all quest narratives are so grandiose however.

Frank notes how the quest has become associated with the concept of 'New Age' thinking and practices. The quest has been linked with the New Age construct just as holism has been linked with the CAM construct, neither concept (i.e. 'quest' and 'holism') belong wholly or exclusively in these places and both constructs are re-castings that incorporate ancient elements with modern ones. Just as herbal medicine and acupuncture, for example, are simultaneously both ancient traditional medical systems seen from one perspective and new 'emerging professions' seen from another, so the quest is both common to ancient mythologies and a creation of New Age ideology. Frank notes the profundity of Joseph Campbell's influence on contemporary ideas about the quest, especially in his book *The Hero with a Thousand Faces* (Campbell 1949). Campbell's delineation of the steps involved in the quest process (broadly – departure, initiation and return) continue to be widely referenced in books aimed at teaching story construction to writers, including screen writers (such as Vogler 1998) to the extent that many novels and Hollywood movies (especially) have drawn heavily on Campbell's quest structure over the last few decades and so new spins on the quest notion have permeated popular culture. One thinks particularly of examples such as Peter Jackson's film version of *The Lord of the Rings* where Tolkien's original mythic take is adapted and layered by newer views of how the quest dynamic works.

The quest approach implies openness to experience and to learning – though this process is not necessarily free from episodes of resistance and self-doubt. While the notion of the quest implies a hero to undertake it Frank suggests, drawing on Campbell, that: 'heroism is evidenced not by force of arms but by *perseverance*' [original italics]. This thought returns us to the idea of life as a labyrinth, mentioned in the previous chapter: since the labyrinth is not a maze (i.e. it contains no blind alleys, although it may give that illusion as it twists and turns), the key to arriving at the centre, the place of meaning and renewal, is to simply keep moving, to keep putting one foot in front of another, to persevere. The ordinariness of the 'hero' has been emphasized in works of art and entertainment in popular culture, with increasing emphasis placed on the hero's flaws and idiosyncrasies, despite which he or she manages to succeed – through sticking to their goal and persevering. This is now the staple stuff of pulp print, television and film and is repeated endlessly, almost to the point of nausea. Because the quest narrative is a coherent, sense-making one, it can easily be reduced and trivialized to anodyne cliché where McKenna's 'poor production values' hold sway. Mass-media versions of the quest story influence our own perception of its meaning and process and may be so imprinted that it leads to pseudo-quest behaviour in the patient. Where restitution was once the approved narrative matching the cultural model of illness in paternalistic medical culture, now the quest narrative is becoming the norm in consumer medical culture where the patient is *supposed* to take responsibility for their own illness and select between healthcare options. This leads merely to pseudo-quest stories where the imperatives of restitution are dressed up in the clothing of the quest – when the assertion that the 'patient is being guided by the practitioner in making choices' really amounts to the same old restitution story 'the patient is being told what to do'. The practitioner needs to be on-guard both to detect pseudo-quest stories, and more importantly, to avoid colluding with the patient in generating them. I would suggest that a good number of CAM consultations result in the latter.

The keynote of the authentic quest narrative is that the patient speaks with her own voice. The core of the restitution narrative is really spoken by the practitioner, not the patient, since the patient defers to the practitioner's advice. The core of the chaos narrative is left unvoiced since the patient is unable to get close to articulating it – it exists in 'the silences'.

Several researchers have made use of Frank's narrative types in studying the illness experience of groups of people such as women who have had breast cancer (Thomas-McLean 2004), people with chronic fatigue syndrome (Whitehead 2006) and people living with HIV (Ezzy 2000). Thomas-McLean praises the fact that Frank's narrative types are (uncommonly): 'accessible to social and cultural theorists, as well as clinicians and those who have experienced illness'. One issue here however, demonstrated in the studies just cited (and in my own discussion in this section), is that the narrative types are loose enough to be open to individual readings that may be contentious between authorities – although it has ever been thus with stories …

Ezzy (2000) draws interesting comparisons between Frank's narratives and other classification models, including Davies' (1997) three forms of temporal orientation. Davies' model derived from work looking at the perspectives of people living with HIV and AIDS. Since people in this group have been diagnosed with a condition that has a high potentiality to be life-shortening but where the timescale for the experience of morbidity and mortality is unclear then a disruption in the relationship with time becomes 'one of the main existential problems faced by people living with an HIV positive diagnosis' (Davies 1997) as they come to terms with living a 'provisional existence'. Davies' three forms of temporal orientation are:

- *Living in the future* (where people) refuse to relinquish their routine future orientation, thus refusing to entertain the possibility of the imminence of their death
- *Living in the empty present* (where people) tend to believe that they will die soon, refusing to commit themselves to any project because of the fear of failure. They retain a desire for a long future, but mourn its loss and as a consequence of this lost future resign themselves to an empty present
- *Living with a philosophy of the present* (where) the provisional existence of the HIV positive person is embraced as an opportunity to discover new meaning and values oriented to enjoying the present.

(This list is compiled from Ezzy 2000 and contains partly Ezzy's words and partly those of Davies 1997 – I have omitted distinguishing each voice to aid ease of reading).

Ezzy suggests that 'living in the future' parallels the restitution narrative; that 'living in the empty present' parallels the chaos narrative; but that 'living with a philosophy of the present' has both overlap and differences with the quest narrative. This latter pair share an emphasis on self-development but while the quest narrative projects into the future (since there is an expectation of living into the future), the people living with HIV (at least at the time of Davies' study) did not have such an expectation and so focussed on the present. Yet this may have a positive effect since: 'Davies suggests that living with a philosophy of the present involves a liberation from a need to fight towards the future' (Ezzy 2000). A similar assessment may be made of other patients facing terminal illness and is suggestive of the ways in which time orientation may adapt Frank's narratives.

Ezzy also draws a distinction between what he describes as polyphonic and linear narratives. Polyphonic ('many voiced') narratives:

> ... are characterised by overlaid, interwoven and often contradictory goals, values, temporal assumptions and attitudes ... (they are) associated with the embracement of uncertainty about the future, a more communally oriented morality and politics and an acceptance of the reality of death at some stage in the future. In contrast, linear narratives tended to be secular, self-centred and attempt to colonise the future, believing the future to be almost completely controllable through human action and open-ended, with death a distant and relatively unimportant concern.

We might rename polyphonic and linear narratives as complex and simple narratives – with the polyphonic/complex narratives (despite, or because of, their contradictory elements) providing a better and more comfortable fit with reality than linear/simple narratives; as we would expect from the greater robustness and adaptability of a complex system. The linear narratives seem to be striving for 'too much order' and too much control – seeking to grasp life and force it to fit the person's desires rather than 'going with the flow'. We could suggest then that when dealing with linear/simple narratives the practitioner might seek to introduce new perspectives to the patient in order to sow the possibility of new narratives emerging that might amplify polyphony, increase complexity and therefore enhance robustness and resilience. Ezzy also considers that polyphonic narratives 'involve a reenchantment of everyday life and a communally oriented ethics' and allow 'the narrator to embrace uncertainty and contradiction as integral to the human condition'.

Let us conclude this section by mentioning a few helpful associated considerations regarding the nature of patients. In this section, and the preceding one, we have attempted to discuss some of the ways in which we might appreciate patients, while emphasizing the need to take an integrated and individual view of each unique person. The distinction between focussing on a precise delineation of each separate trait that a patient might show as opposed to combining such traits into broader systems of interpretation is highlighted in Cronbach's (1956) categorization of psychologists as *splitters* (interested in specific knowledge) and *lumpers* (concerned with broad knowledge). Splitters are associated with the reductionist-specialist axis, whereas lumpers are connected with the holistic-generalist axis. Judge et al. (2002) have pointed out that, while the specific approach has generated thousands of personality traits 'these labors have produced independent literatures that evolved from related traits with little consideration of their possible common core'. When research and hypothesizing fails to take account of, and make comparisons with, previous research and existing models it risks replicating (or more likely approximating) already known concepts under another name. When commonalities between concepts go unobserved, unnecessary confusion can arise and the opportunity for a greater understanding arising from the synthesis of near-concepts can be missed. In an attempt to test the extent to which factors in personality psychology might overlap or coincide, Judge and colleagues (2002) compared several of the key traits described in this field, including:

- Self-esteem
- Locus of control (internal and external)
- Neuroticism (also known as emotional stability or emotional adjustment).

In summary, they found that: 'Although these traits are usually investigated in isolation, in many cases they seem to operate similarly in theory'. For example:

- Self-esteem and neuroticism are 'conceptually related in that the positivity of self-description has been used to operationalize both'
- Self-esteem and locus of control are related; low self-esteem correlates in some ways to an external locus of control and the correlate scenario applies – high self-esteem is related to an internal locus of control
- Locus of control and neuroticism overlap and 'the relationship between locus of control and stress is strong, in some cases nearly as strong as the relationship between neuroticism and stress'. I take this to mean that the pairing of internal locus of control with emotional stability results in better adaptation to stress than the partnership of external locus of control with emotional instability.

It seems odd that, as Judge and colleagues observe: 'Despite the prominence of these traits and some rather obvious connections between them, relatively few investigations have explicitly considered their interrelationships'. Here we see the tendency of reductionist science to work in isolated and ever more introspective ways, failing to reap the benefits that may accrue from joining-up research and risking the dangers that may accompany this failure. The various benefits and risks associated with the presence or lack of comparison of concepts and findings have been well summarized by Judge and colleagues and their observations are listed below (with acknowledgement of their sources):

- This diffusion in the literature is not a problem if measures of these traits are orthogonal
- However, if there is substantial communal or redundant variance shared by the measures, the problem is well summarized by Block

(1995): 'To the extent a variable correlates with other variables ... it is said to be "explainable" by these other variables and conveys no unique information'. In such a case, at best, there is redundancy in that more measures are used than are necessary to account for psychological phenomena
- At worst, the Tower of Babel problem noted by Block (1995) exists, whereby results with respect to one trait are ignored in research investigating the same phenomenon but using a different trait
- The resulting jangle fallacy (Kelley 1927) wastes scientific time and serves to 'prevent the recognition of correspondences that could help build cumulative knowledge' (Block 1995).

As with research, so with the patient and with the consultation ... this returns us to Ezzy's notion of polyphonic narratives – where advantage is associated with the ability to hear and combine several voices. The utilization of an approach that incorporates the comparison and synthesis of multiple perspectives with the allowance of seemingly contradictory elements is vital in independent work on the self; in the consultation; and in conducting and interpreting research. In the consultation, if we fail to gather a broad range of information about the patient (her expectations, agenda, characteristics, self-perception, etc.) we operate under the 'jangle fallacy' failing to 'build cumulative knowledge' about the patient and consequently wasting her time at best and, at worst, giving her inadequate, unnecessary or harmful treatment and advice based on lack of knowledge and poor appreciation of her situation. The term 'jangle fallacy' is apt, since jangle implies a discordant note and fallacy can be read as 'unsound' – when we fail to appreciate the concordance between differing voices on the same theme, we *mishear*.

The urge to distinguish between voices in positivist science derives from the conviction that there exists one definitive, authoritative voice (the linear narrative) that is truer or more reliable than others and so should be discerned to the exclusion of those others. This conviction originates from a world-sense that hears complexity as cacophony – the world is discordant and messy, it stands in need of ordering, clearing up, sifting and refining. The aim is to tune in to the lead soloist while blotting out the rest of the orchestra. Monophony is the voice of reason that describes truth, whereas polyphony represents the multiple voices of confusion and illusion. While pursuing this metaphor let us also note how unwanted or inexplicable research data is referred to as 'noise'. By contrast, the use of polyphony is appropriate since it suggests a way of listening that hears the world as symphonic, complex yet harmonious. This is the way that the holist perceives the world – oriented to discern (or construct) concord rather than discord.

It is interesting to observe here the connection between positivistic science and monotheistic religion, which the former eschews. The one God and the one Method are versions of the monophonic way of hearing and pronouncing the world. Holistic science is then closer to archaic pantheistic approaches to the sacred – polyphonic ways of hearing the world – and possibly to some instances of pre-Counter-Reformation Catholicism where 'the "polyphonic" nature of tradition (had) historically allowed for a plurality of voices in biblical interpretation' (Feldhay 2005). The Counter-Reformation brought a more authoritarian Catholic stance where such plurality was inhibited. Staines and Clark (2005) have described how, in the period of the Reformation in England: 'Church musicians found themselves at the centre of the storm ... Up to the 1540s, the country's choral traditions had been tied to the ancient practices of worship at the monasteries and chantries, in which florid polyphony was the dominant style' but this changed significantly with the introduction of the *Book of Common Prayer* in 1549 which 'replaced at a stroke long-established Catholic services' and led to a change where 'religious music, as the reformist Thomas Cranmer put it, should not be "full of notes", but instead communicate the meaning of the words, ideally in a strictly syllabic arrangement ...' The sixteenth century period of the Reformation and the Counter-Reformation overlaps the birth of what is known as the 'Scientific Revolution', conventionally given a precise birth date with the publication of Copernicus's *De revolutionibus orbium coelestium* (On the Revolutions of the Heavenly Spheres) and Vesalius's *De humani corporis fabrica* (On the Fabric of the Human Body), both in 1543. (Incidentally, let us note that 1543 is also the year in which Henry VIII enacts the 'Herbalist's Charter', which 'enshrines the right of all the King's subjects having knowledge of herbal medicine to practise it'). Here we have a confluence of would-be definitive voices:

- The Protestant and Counter-Reformation Catholic (the Council of Trent begins in 1545) Churches attempt to assert the dominant voice on doctrine and to precisely define the body of faith
- Copernicus speaks of the true nature of the body of the universe
- Vesalius opens and defines the body of man.

We can discern in these enterprises a complementarity having to do with their shared efforts to pronounce an authorial voice on a distinct body of knowledge. Polyphony is abandoned and as a consequence, it becomes increasingly difficult to hear multiple voices. It is a large leap from this point, but let us make it in any case, to say that when we listen to the patient it isn't just about what we hear it's also about *how* we hear. Our mode of listening, the style in which we conduct it and the concepts that we are able to register, has a history.

Returning to Judge et al.'s (2002) finding of correspondences between three of the core concepts in personal psychology, is it *too* obvious then to suggest that the following assertion holds true: Internal locus of control, high self-esteem and emotional stability are related and people possessing this trinity of attributes will cope better with stress and be happier than people who have the contrasting trio of traits, namely external locus of control, low self-esteem and emotional instability? The relationships between locus of control, self-esteem and emotional adjustment could be pondered at length but for the purposes of our discussion we will focus on locus of control for a moment.

Development of the theory of locus of control is generally attributed to Rotter (1966) who suggests that people's explanatory models for what happens to them in life derive from their early learning experiences. Those who were rewarded for good behaviour and punished for bad behaviour supposedly develop a sense of internal control – achievements in life are based on one's own efforts. People who were rewarded and punished indiscriminately in early life tend to feel a lack of personal control of events so that the locus of control lies elsewhere (in 'luck' or 'fate' for instance). Wallston et al. (1978) revised Rotter's concept and adapted it into an assessment tool called the multidimensional health locus of control (MHLC), which Wallston (1992) later described as 'no longer adequate'. Stainton Rogers (1992) has criticized locus of control as a concept but especially as a psychometric test in the form developed by Wallston: 'Its problem is that it is grounded within a modernistic, scientific, methodological approach – psychometrics – in which a limited number of predetermined categories are all that are available for response. Psychometric method thus imposes the researchers' view of 'how the world works' upon participants' responses, and then interprets their responses only within that framework'. This reminds us of Judge and colleague's critique of using psychological models separately rather than in combined form. Yet, there remains something interesting in the notion of locus of control as an open concept for reflection, divested of much of its historical baggage. My personal reading of it is below.

The person with an *internal locus of control* is 'comfortable in their own skin' and has a positive engagement in the world since they feel their inner selves and the outer world are connected, that 'the universe' is ultimately good and that it is exciting to have novel experiences – even if these are occasionally unpleasant, one can learn from them. They are self-empowered and more likely to make their own health choices, creating their own programme of care when such is needed. The quest narrative is their dominant mode and they push the therapeutic relationship in the direction of the partnership-model. In the consultation, the power associated with control lies predominantly with the patient.

The person with an *external locus of control* is lacking in self-confidence and has a largely negative relationship with the world, since it is seen as existing at a distance from them. The nature of 'the universe' is uncertain or clearly known but fraught with danger – novel experiences are risky, since one may be exposed or damaged by them. They are likely to act on the authority of others, following prescribed treatment courses but doubting their efficacy. The restitution narrative is their dominant mode and they tend to push towards a paternalistic relationship. In the consultation the power associated with control lies predominantly with the practitioner.

We might also suggest a third category of 'absent locus of control' or 'displaced locus of control' to match the chaos narrative. In the consultation in this case, the power of control is missing – it does not lie with the patient or the practitioner but is lodged inaccessibly within the trauma that has led to the chaos state.

So, if the separate split pieces covered in this section really are indicators of a unified higher order construct, then how might we lump these together to suggest such a construct? At the risk of fallaciously mangling the constituent parts, I will suggest a tabulation which can form the basis of an endless parlour game wherein the various elements can be debated, moved around and added to. Let us put Frank's narrative types at the head, since we started with these:

*Restitution narrative* – linear narrative – living in the future – external locus of control – low self-esteem – emotionally unstable

*Quest narrative* – polyphonic narrative – living in the present – internal locus of control – high self-esteem – emotionally stable

*Chaos narrative* – non-narrative – living in the empty present – displaced locus of control – the self is absent – emotionally devastated.

There are thousands of additional types of classification schemes that can be drawn into this game of contrast and combine and added to the collage – from other psychological models to the five phases/elements of Chinese medicine and other traditional medical models. From familiar pairings such as introversion/extraversion and optimist/pessimist to less familiar ones such as infophilic/infophobic and naturephilic/naturephobic. There is huge room for discussion around these groupings and they are certainly not offered as fixed diagnostic pictures – far from it, possible patient scenarios are infinitely variable but in order to begin to work with them it is helpful to have indicative models that can be modified or discarded as appropriate. Nonetheless, this type of exercise may act as a stimulant to reflection on the nature of patients and to the exercise of creativity in determining how we might best be able to appreciate and assist them.

## ON THE NATURE OF CONDITIONS

This section will consider two controversial hypothetical models that offer radical perspectives for reassessing the nature of conditions, after which we will revisit Stacey's 'certainty–agreement' model then move on to provide a brief assessment of the nature of acute conditions and a longer reflection on chronic pictures, since the latter form the bulk of practice in phytotherapy.

Hyland (2003) proposes that the combination of two theories: Extended Network Theory and the Theory of Generalized Quantum Entanglement, will help explain the processes by which CAM therapies work. He calls the result of the conflation of these two theories Extended Network Generalized Entanglement Theory. We are not concerned here with whether this is a helpful model for appreciating CAM therapies in general, especially since it would appear to be applicable, to a degree, to any system of medicine. Rather, we are concerned to identify what this model has to offer in appreciating conditions seen from the perspective of phytotherapy, and to this extent, we will focus on the Extended Network Theory.

In describing Extended Network Theory Hyland (2003) states that:

*The underlying assumption of the theory is that the body has a superordinate system, the extended network, that sets the parameters ... of the body's control systems ... This superordinate system is assumed to be a network-based intelligent system that has the ability to co-ordinate conflicting requirements of a system that requires temporal specialization of function ...*

This description fits with concepts in psychoneuroimmunology (PNI), where Hyland's nebulous 'superordinate system' would be more specifically described as being constituted as a complex interaction between psychoemotional information and the nervous, endocrine and immune systems. Hyland considers the superordinate system (which we can posit as a PNI construct) to be a parallel processing network system that possesses the properties common to such systems including pattern recognition and adaptive self-organization. Hyland sees the superordinate system as a higher-level control system which 'using genetically conferred rules ... self-organizes so as to create more effective self-regulation at the lower-level control systems'. Hyland considers lower-level systems to include 'immune activity, bowel motility, glucose levels ...', factors which, from the perspective of PNI, would tend to be described as integral effects and modulators of PNI activity as opposed to representing a separate tier or level of function. Hyland posits that if the 'rules that create' self-organization at the level of the superordinate system change adversely then this will result in 'less effective self-regulation (which) creates the distal cause for chronic disregulatory disease'. There seems to be some confusion in the use of the terms 'proximal' and 'distal' in the paper under analysis but I take Hyland to mean the following, which I will call the first and second realms:

- First realm: The proximal (i.e. 'more central') locus of disease causation is at the extended network/superordinate system level which has to do particularly with self-organization
- Second realm: The distal (i.e. 'more peripheral') locus of disease causation lies with the lower-level control systems which are involved specifically in self-regulation.

Hyland contends that conventional therapy, which he calls 'robust therapy' exerts influences primarily in the second realm and is therefore, as I read it, more associated with symptom alleviation, whereas 'subtle therapy' (which he associates with some types of CAM) acts principally in the first realm and is associated with disease prevention. Hyland divides the CAM therapies that act as subtle therapy into 'push therapies and pull therapies'. Push therapies 'provide the extended network with information that the network is in a more disregulated state than it actually is' in response to which influence the 'network compensates by self-organizing in the direction of greater regulation'. Hyland suggests that this fits with the idea that conditions may have to get worse (in response to the remedial activity) before they get better (as a result of enhanced regulation). Hyland cites this example in relation to homoeopathy but we might argue that the push concept also applies to some phytotherapy strategies such as counter-irritation: if one whips an osteo-arthritic joint with stinging nettles (*Urtica dioica*) this will exacerbate the local joint inflammation ('warming a cold and stagnant picture' would be an alternative but equivalent explanation) leading to an increase in endogenous anti-inflammatory activity that may subsequently provide pain relief for several weeks. It would be hard to convince most patients that this constituted 'subtle' therapy though. A second example would be the use of diaphoretics, where herbs with this action will tend to exacerbate the sensation of heat and increase sweating in mild to moderate fevers causing the fever to peak and then reduce.

'Pull therapies' by contrast are ones that, using the language associated with chaos theory, act as health attractors that compete with disease attractors and, if successful, act as a kind of 'network guide that shows the network the route it needs to take in order to achieve a more healthy, regulatory state'. Numerous strategies in herbal medicine could be explained in this way, such as the use of adaptogens, nervous trophorestoratives and immunomodulators (note that these herbal actions influence the key integrated control systems of PNI: the endocrine, nervous and immune system). Hyland considers self-organizational change to be slow in nature (while suggesting that there are advantages associated with such a pace) so that subtle therapy is 'the catalyst for a slow self-healing process'. Robust therapy, on the other hand, may achieve more rapid symptomatic or cosmetic results. I would suggest that the slowness of self-organizational change/self-healing is necessary to enable deep processing and modulation of function with the result that change can be either *held* more effectively (conferring substantial long-term control of the original condition) or become embodied to the degree that profound and persisting change occurs (definitive healing or 'cure'). Subtle therapies acting slowly to promote self-healing at the extended network level may be described as 'nudging' the body into an improved pattern of behaviour. 'Nudging' (subtle) is better than 'shoving' (robust) in the long run, since nudged messages meet less resistance and so are more likely to be heard and incorporated. There is an opportunity to develop a 'nudge theory' for herbal medicine. I first heard the idea mentioned in lectures given by the phytotherapist Simon Mills; recently the economist Richard Thaler has extended his political-economical 'nudge theory' to include giving advice on 'health and happiness' as well as 'wealth' (Thaler & Sunstein 2008).

We can argue then that phytotherapy has the ability to act as a subtle therapy, both in terms of push and pull mechanisms, *but also* can act as a robust therapy since herbs possessing actions similar to conventional medicines, such as herbal anti-inflammatories and anodynes, influence lower-level control symptoms providing symptom relief in the manner of robust conventional drugs. Phytotherapy then has a huge range of potential influence, across the spectrum of causal levels in disease. Using Hyland's Extended Network theory may be helpful in helping phytotherapists determine the 'level' or locus of the problem in order to better focus treatment.

It should also be noted that Hyland suggests that conditions may optimally reside at the superordinate system level with little formal extension into the lower-level systems (Fig. 4.2). For example chronic fatigue syndrome, irritable bowel syndrome, fibromyalgia (and many pictures currently lacking even pseudo-diagnostic labels) are located as disruptions at the extended network/superordinate level but, while they have symptoms associated with them, they do not demonstrate consistent pathophysiological changes, i.e. they are considered functional rather than organic.

Golbin and Umantsev (2006) studied, and reflected on, the nature of medical conditions and considered that some represented a picture of 'low dimensional dynamical chaos' and that, when applying the framework of the control system theory to the body 'chaotic regime in one subsystem may be compensating for the loss of chaos in another subsystem for the sake of stability of the whole system'. It should be remembered that 'chaos', as used in this context does not mean 'complete disorder and confusion', rather, from the perspective of mathematical chaos and chaos theory it refers to the dynamic, fluid functioning of healthy natural systems. In terms of the body, chaos is assumed to be the default state in healthy resiliently adaptive individuals, 'too much order' on the other hand results in a lack of dynamic flexibility and

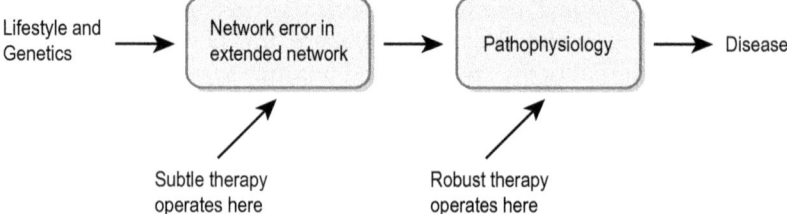

**Figure 4.2** Hyland says that: 'Particular combinations of lifestyle and genetics create self-organizational change in the extended network, which is then responsible for the emergence of pathophysiology. Disease for which there is no consistent pathophysiology (e.g. irritable bowel syndrome, chronic fatigue syndrome) are limited to extended network error'. *(Reproduced from Hyland (2003), with permission.)*

impairs vital functions leading to pathological change. What Golbin and Umantsev are suggesting is that where chaos is 'lost' (or conversely where 'too much order' is gained) in one subsystem of the body (say the cardiovascular system), another subsystem may become, let us call it 'more chaotic' (or possessing 'too much chaos') in order to attempt to compensate and maintain the overall resiliently chaotic state of the body as a 'whole system'. The key, and important, suggestion that Golbin and Umantsev make after following this line of logic is that the 'chaotic behaviour of different organ sets in a human body as an *alternative* to serious diseases or even death' such that 'adaptive disorders with chaotic symptoms *should not* be aggressively treated; if (they) are overtreated, the whole organism may be thrown into a more regular state, which eventually will lead to a chronic disease or even death' [my italics]. Such a hypothesis requires, and easily generates, a number of responses around its implications – here are a few:

- There has always been a popular awareness that some types of disorder may in fact be both necessary and beneficial. They may be described as 'your pressure valve', or people may say 'your weakness is actually your strength', or yet again 'its better to come out like that than to stay inside and fester'. Seen in the light of the foregoing discussion, these statements can be read, when appropriately applied, as examples of profound popular wisdom.
- Imposing control of symptoms is not invariably desirable and the appearance of order that may arise with the control and supposed resolution of symptoms may in fact herald a shift in the disorder to a more dangerous level of activity. Seen in this way, the suggestion that the suppression of symptoms may 'drive the problem deeper' should be taken seriously.
- 'Adaptive disorders with chaotic symptoms' should be treated gently and aggressive treatment should be actively avoided. Subtle therapies working in the 'pull' mode and acting at the extended network/PNI/superordinate system level should be utilized.
- It is imperative to be able to discern, as far as possible, which conditions represent 'adaptive disorders with chaotic symptoms'. One suggestion is that these may be the conditions which are located at the extended

network/superordinate system level and which do not develop pathophysiological changes in the lower-level control systems, i.e. functional as opposed to organic disorders.
- The lack of response to treatment, or difficulty in resolving, these adaptive disorders with chaotic symptoms (e.g. chronic fatigue system, etc.) may be a sign of their robustness and an assertion of their *value*. These conditions cannot be easily resolved because, for the sake of the organism as a whole, they *should not* be easily treatable.

So where does this leave the phytotherapist? 'Very well placed to help' would be one response. Having access to both subtle and robust remedies and being able to work at the core PNI/extended network level and/or with the lower-level control systems the phytotherapist has *only* to work out in which circumstances to deploy which strategy! I oversimplify of course, but to aid us in navigating the assessment/diagnostic territory that has been (hopefully) cast in a new light by the above reflections, we might usefully return to the 'certainty–agreement' model mentioned earlier.

The 'certainty–agreement' model was described by Stacey (2001, 2002) and is a decision-making concept that helps to guide thinking across three regions: simple, complex and chaotic. These regions are defined with regard to the degree of certainty that exists around the nature of the issue or problem at hand and the degree of agreement between the parties, or authorities, involved on how to proceed. Where both certainty and agreement are very strong (or their levels of accord are 'high') the issue is said to be simple. Where both are very weak (or 'low') it is said to be chaotic. In the interzone, where varying shades of agreement–certainty reside, the issue is said to be complex (Fig. 4.3).

Let us speculate on applying this model to medicine. Simple conditions might be those where the assessment or diagnosis is clear, where a number of colleagues could easily and independently come to the same conclusion, and where the patient finds the practitioner's assessment makes sense and fits well with her own views of the condition. Simple conditions are rarely to

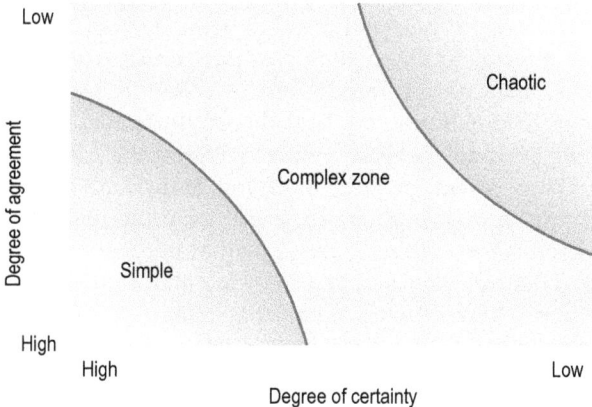

**Figure 4.3** Certainty–Agreement model. *(Adapted from Stacey (2002), with permission.)*

be found but may include some of the organic diseases. Note that 'simple' does not equate, necessarily, with 'non-serious' or 'easy to treat'. If a simple condition can be discovered and if it can be treated relatively easily, then a restitution story may be told about the experience. The chaotic region is the place of chaos narratives – nobody knows what's going on or what to do. The complex region is a zone of uncertainty yet possibilities suggest themselves and may be attempted, and quest stories may be generated.

With regard to steering through the implications of Golbin and Umantsev's hypothesis, we may suggest that the further one drifts from the simple zone, the more cautious one should be in intervening aggressively. The less sure one is about what is going on and how to proceed the more subtle and gentle should be the approach. In the zones of complexity and chaos nudges should be attempted in the direction/s thought best and then re-nudged in the light of the response. The practitioner working in these regions needs to become comfortable with uncertainty and learn to tolerate, and assist the patient in appreciating and tolerating, a degree of ongoing 'illness' if need be – since a low level of 'illness' may be seen as promoting a relative degree of 'wellness'. Herbal medicine is well suited to the slow game of adaptation that should be the default position in complex and chaotic conditions, using herbal strategies such as those related to the adaptogens, nervines, immunomodulators, hepatics, lymphatics, digestive tonics and so forth as subtle attractors. Monitoring and recalibrating treatment alongside providing ongoing support, care, reflection and exploration of the patient's self and their predicament's meaning – these are the core processes that define herbal practice. In the simple region robust herbs may be deployed and, in suitable cases, may yield rapid and powerful results. The herbal forte however, is in the regions where the complexity and chaos of the plants themselves as multi-chemical pharmacological entities, part revealed to science, part mysterious, have particular affinity and applicability to complex and chaotic patient states.

In moving on to consider acute and chronic illness we may begin where we are leaving off. Acute conditions may call for initial aggressive palliative treatment with robust herbs (at higher dosages and given more frequently), whereas chronic conditions tend to require more subtle therapy (at lower doses given less frequently).

Additionally an assessment will need to be made in acute severe pictures as to whether referral to emergency medical services is required. Certain herbal strategies may be contraindicated in acute disease as the following example drawn from Chinese medical theory illustrates. In Chinese medicine, acute infections are generally classed within the category of 'exterior syndromes' where 'sweet, cloying tonifying herbs and sour or astringent herbs should not be used because they will keep the pathogenic factors in the body and reduce the strength of herbs that expel the exogenous pathogenic factors. This mistake is called "closing the door and keeping your enemy in"' (Yang 2002). Rather herbs that release the exterior should be used, assisting the free expression, movement and hence the resolution of the acute phenomenon.

We can suggest here, thinking of Golbin and Umantsev's theory, that acute conditions represent a temporary situation of what we might term 'high dimensional dynamical chaos' as opposed to the more chronic 'low dimensional dynamical chaos' that their suggestions are based upon. As such it may generally be more appropriate to provide short-term aggressive treatment of acute symptoms. Of course in some acute cases (severe haemorrhaging; overwhelming infection, etc.), aggressive intervention is essential to provide the patient with ease and to save their life but treatment is not always necessary beyond appropriate nursing and basic care in some other acute pictures, for example in self-limiting infections.

Acute conditions arise quickly and have strong, pronounced symptoms. The consultation around acute cases should reflect these qualities, which is to say that the consultation will need to respond rapidly to the nature of the condition because of the urgency in needing to assess the severity and significance of the situation and take decisive action with regard to treatment, management and referral. 'Acute consultations' are therefore different in nature from 'chronic consultations' – there is less space for nuance and subtlety, less time and opportunity (and often less necessity) for reflecting on the broader personal meaning of the condition, greater need to focus on diagnosis and usually a greater emphasis on examination and investigation. In the face of extreme symptoms and pronounced patient distress questions of certainty and agreement become more pressing, it is essential that the consultation zones in on short-term questions regarding how to make the patient more comfortable and whether referral or additional help and perspectives are required. In future consultations, once the acute phase has settled, a broader perspective should be sought including the consideration of whether adaptive and/or preventive ideas and strategies need to be considered/implemented. Acute pictures may be seen as episodes of frank communication on the part of the body which need to be heard and appreciated fully, directly and immediately – these are occasions for the practitioner to speak plainly and clearly. Some acute episodes may be seen as healthy expressions of release or self-development – outbursts or performances that, although spectacular, are 'all to the good'. An example here would be the view that many acute infections serve a useful purpose in exercising and maturing the immune system.

Acute phenomena may arise *ex novo* (suddenly appearing, seemingly 'out of the blue'); with reference to a discernible lead-in period (following a period of, e.g. stress, lack of self-care or alcohol abuse); or within the context of a chronic condition where the acute episode represents an exacerbation, flare or relapse (e.g. in inflammatory bowel disease or systemic lupus erythematosus). In all cases, triggering or precipitating factors should be sought.

Let us turn to consider chronic conditions, the bulk of current herbal practice in the UK and other developed nations. These frequently represent manifestations of 'low dimensional dynamical chaos' so our earlier discussion on this matter should be borne in mind as we proceed. First let us list some general basic considerations regarding chronic conditions and phytotherapy:

- Some chronic conditions are unlikely to be curable
- In this case long-term management is required – perhaps over many years

- Chronic disorders significantly affect the patient's sense of self and issues to do with self and meaning are key ongoing aspects of supporting patients with chronic pictures
- Specific herbal treatment aims should be realistic
- Achievement and then maintenance of maximum improvements is the key therapeutic aim
- Dosages of herbal medicines used over the long term should be at the minimum effective dose
- Specific herbs may need to be changed for others with similar actions from time to time to maintain a good impact
- Regular review should take place, perhaps a maximum of every 6 months for long-term stable treatment
- When a patient is seen over a period of years for a chronic condition, it is important to keep a fresh approach, remaining open to new developments in the patient
- Worsening of chronic disorders should be noted and appropriate referral made if required
- The patient should in any case be referred for supplementary treatment where appropriate to aid recovery and improve symptom management
- Patients with chronic disorders can receive enormous benefit from regular check-ups with herbal practitioners, where careful assessment and support can be given
- In chronic disorders, ongoing emotional support is important – chronic illness can be demoralizing and is a factor in depression, enhancing mood is also associated with improving immune function
- If a patient is taking conventional medication it is particularly important that herb-drug interactions (HDIs) are borne in mind, especially since pharmaceutical treatments may accumulate over time leading to highly complex and unpredictable patterns of influence on the patient (the best orientation on the issue of HDIs can be found in Mills and Bone 2005)
- In serious cases, consultations should be frequent enough so that important changes can be noted and responded to quickly
- In serious chronic disorders especially, it is essential to have a deep understanding of the condition, its management and an appreciation of the latest research in the area (including the conventional treatment)
- The herbal practitioner should communicate with the patient's other healthcare professionals when appropriate
- It can be argued that herbal medicines are uniquely suited to use in chronic conditions given: their chemical complexity and relative safety when used for extended periods (including their lack of cumulative side-effects), and their ability to address many of the physiological and psychoemotional needs of the long-term ill
- Nervine herbs can help manage mood disorders connected with long-term illness, including the psychophysiological impacts of lowered self-esteem
- Adaptogenic herbs are of great importance in improving mental and physical performance, endurance and stamina and in protecting from psychoemotional, physical and environmental stress

- Immunomodulators enhance long-term disease resistance and may mediate neurotransmitter and hormonal activity (in the psychoneuroimmunology model)
- Organ/system specific tonic/trophorestorative herbs will support the general function of long-term affected body parts/systems.

Nettleton (2006) has described some of the factors that constitute the complexity of chronic conditions:

> ... chronic illness can impact upon sufferers' daily living, their social relationships, their identity (the views that others hold of them) and their sense of self (their private views of themselves) ... responses to illness are not simply determined by either the nature of biophysical symptoms or individual motivations, but rather are shaped and imbued by the social, cultural and ideological context of a person's biography. Thus illness is at once both *a very personal* and *a very public phenomenon*.

A crucial role of the practitioner in chronic situations is that of a mediator between the patient's personal experience and three types of public phenomena:

1. The *public influence* on how the patient's condition is understood and perceived
2. The *public reception* of the patient's state
3. The *public expression* of her condition by the patient; how she talks about and expresses herself with regard to her condition.

## Public influence

This category includes social conditions, cultural norms, public opinion, media messages and so forth. The patient is impacted by such influences and they will play a part in shaping her own view of her predicament and those of her circle. The practitioner can act as an interpreter with regard to these factors – translating, critiquing, explaining and re-contextualizing. The practitioner may reinforce, call into question, strongly criticize or offer an alternative perspective. It is especially important that the practitioner inhabits this role and uses it effectively where the patient's sense of self, or their practical support, is compromised by unhelpful, unfair or ill-informed public influences. Such difficulties may arise, e.g. where the patient has a disputed diagnosis such as chronic fatigue syndrome (CFS).

## Public reception

The practitioner's role here may be very closely connected with public influence since the doctor's opinion, particularly, can shape public opinion. This category has been kept separate however, since it refers to the practitioner's own part in the public construction of the patient's situation as opposed to that of other players. Doctors have power to confer legitimacy to patient pictures of illness, and thus hold power over how the patient's predicament is publicly received, in large part through the making of the diagnosis and the provision of treatment – or the lack of these. If the patient remains undiagnosed and unmedicated then the public contract that is described by Parson's 'sick role' cannot be established; which is to say that in the absence of medical legitimacy the patient may not be publicly seen to be entitled to sympathy; to exemption from normative roles and behaviour and to statutory benefits such as sick leave and disability pensions. Woodward et al. (1995) are one of the teams who have highlighted the tensions around this area. They studied doctors' and patients' perspectives on CFS, finding the pairing of doctors' reluctance to ascribe a diagnosis of CFS (due to feeling constrained by the 'scientific uncertainty regarding its aetiology and by a concern that diagnosis might become a self-fulfilling prophecy') with CFS patients' emphasis on the 'negative effects of having no explanation for their problems' and the 'enabling aspects of singular coherent diagnosis'. In providing a diagnosis the doctor is actually contributing to the formation of two holons of coherency – that concerning the patient's self and that concerning the patient's harmonization with their social circle and wider culture. Yet the practitioner may decide to withhold her cohering power if she feels its application cannot be justified since it may summon into being a fictitious creature that nonetheless may be capable of causing harm. (We will leave to one side discussion of the dangers regarding the self-fulfilling nature of scientifically 'certain' diagnoses.)

Since phytotherapists are not members of the dominant medical hierarchy, our ability to confer a legitimizing diagnosis that significantly alters public perception of the patient is weak since we do not have the status that confers the authority to make uncontested diagnoses. The very act of visiting a CAM practitioner will have an influence, however. This act will usually meet a mixed public reception depending on the particular take on CAM that the member of the public has. While figures can be provided to show that a huge percentage of people in the UK use some form of CAM therapy each year (Conway 2005), this mostly represents self-medication with over-the-counter remedies (herbal, nutritional, homoeopathic) rather than consultations with practitioners. The experience with, and acceptance of, CAM generated diagnoses is still a publicly disputed area, especially since many CAM practitioners offer diagnoses from within a non-biomedical framework, the concepts and language of which may not be widely shared in the public sphere.

**Public expression**

The phytotherapist's work will likely have a more profound effect on patient's self-perception and sense of self-coherence than on factors directly adapting a positive public reception of the patient's predicament. By aiding the patient in determining meaning and by offering support, care and encouragement however, the phytotherapist is able to influence the patient's public expression of their condition. This will include how the patient carries herself in public contexts – how she refers to her condition and what she projects about it. If a patient is sufficiently supported in this way, her own sense of greater coherence is likely to positively affect perceptions in her immediate social circle, if not those in the wider public context. Clarke and James (2003), again studying CFS, found that: 'As people with CFS, lacking an uncontested medical diagnosis, search for meaningful self-identities, they resist previously available discourses to take up an alternative discourse, one that we call radicalized selves'. Herbal practitioners can provide elements of alternative explanatory models that help to support the radicalization of patients but in order to act effectively in such a way practitioners need to be clear about, and confident in, the radical nature of their own work.

The practitioner needs to be aware of the public and personal issues affecting the patient in chronic disease; of the connection between the two; and of the work that may be required to adapt both of these – on the part of both practitioner and patient. Nettleton (2006) describes more specifically the background lack of resources that may affect the chronically ill and references a model for the types of work that chronic conditions involve:

*The experience of chronic illness can very often mean a severe reduction in resources in terms of energy, skill, strength, time, money, friends and so on. Consequently, sufferers adopt strategies to overcome these restrictions. These have been conceptualized as forms of work. Corbin and Strauss (1985) understand chronic illness in terms of three types of work:* illness work, *which consists of regimen work, crisis prevention and management, symptom management and diagnostic-related work;* everyday life-work *which refers to the daily round of tasks that keep a household going, such as housekeeping, occupational work, child rearing, sentimental work and activities such as eating; and* biographical work, *which involves the reconstruction of the ill person's biography.*

The type of work that most closely and most often mirrors the focus of practitioners is illness work. Yet practitioners also need to appreciate patient's everyday life-work and utilize the opportunity they have to fundamentally support biographical work. The phytotherapy consultation is well suited to provide a place where this latter type of work can be undertaken. With reference particularly to patients with rheumatoid arthritis Bury (1982) discussed chronic illness as a 'major kind of disruptive experience' that affects the patient's biography, which is to say their understanding of and their account of their own life, its course and its meaning:

*My contention is that illness, and especially chronic illness, is precisely that kind of experience where the structures of everyday life and the forms of knowledge which underpin them are disrupted. Chronic illness involves a recognition of the worlds of pain and suffering, possibly even of death, which are normally only seen as distant possibilities or the plight of others. In addition, it brings individuals, their families, and wider social networks face to face with the character of their relationships in stark form, disrupting normal rules of reciprocity and support. The growing dependency involved in chronic illness is a major issue here. Further, the expectations and plans that individuals hold for the future have to be re-examined. Thus, I want to maintain that the development of a chronic illness like rheumatoid arthritis is most usefully regarded as a 'critical situation', a form of biographical disruption ...*

Bury initially identifies and links 'three aspects of disruption to the unfolding of a chronic illness'. These are summarized below:

- First, there is the disruption of taken-for-granted assumptions and behaviours: the breaching of common-sense boundaries ... This 'what is

going on here' stage involves attention to bodily states not usually brought into consciousness and decisions about seeking help.
- Second, there are more profound disruptions in explanatory systems normally used by people, such that a fundamental re-thinking of the person's biography and self-concept is involved.
- Third, there is the response to disruption involving the mobilization of resources, in facing an altered situation'.

The practitioner can offer significant support, care, advice and perspective at each of these junctures.

Williams (2000) has noted that biographical disruption is not limited to illness but accompanies other major life events or 'normal crises' and that both illness and such life events are conceptualized and dealt with differently by different groups of people. Williams draws on Cornwell's (1984) work which:

> ... highlights the cheerful stoicism and pragmatism with which much illness is greeted by many (London) East-Enders, including notions of 'normal illnesses' and 'health problems which are not illnesses' ... illness, like hard work itself, is only to be expected ... These East-Enders, in direct parallel to their attitudes towards work and life more generally: (quoting Cornwell) ... take seriously the idea that having the 'right attitude' is the passport, if not to good health, at least to a life that is tolerable. The moral prescription for a healthy life is in fact a kind of cheerful stoicism, evident in the refusal to worry, or to complain, or to be morbid. [original emphasis]

Williams goes on to conclude that:

> Health, from this viewpoint, may indeed be an important moral category which few if any of us wish to relinquish, but the biographically disruptive nature of illness is perhaps most keenly felt amongst the privileged rather than disadvantaged segments of society. Biographical disruption, in other words, carries particular class- and age-related connotations, as well as gender and ethnic dimensions, which remain, at present, under-played and under-researched.

Again we are reminded that explanatory models must always be applied flexibly and adapted or abandoned as necessary so that there is space for the individual to be discerned in her or his own uniqueness. Williams' constructive critique of biographical disruption (only one part of which is mentioned here) in the above regard calls into question the more general matter of practitioners' expectations of patients. We may expect patients to experience illness in certain ways and according to certain models which, because we consider them to be enlightened and holistic models, we mistake as having universal applicability. We might suggest that practitioners should understand their models profoundly, but wear them lightly and be wiling to combine/defer/reject/modulate them gladly. The further reminder that we have from Williams' observations is the extent to which patient's *experiences of illness* are shaped by their *expectations of life*.

Wagner et al. (2001) note that although the number of people experiencing chronic illness is significantly increasing, their medical care is often inadequate to meeting their clinical, psychological and informational needs. They hypothesize that: 'The primary reason for this may be the mismatch between their needs and care delivery systems largely designed for acute illness'. The assertion we will make here is that current biomedical systems and biomedical thinking arose from and are still crystallized around the demands of acute medicine. Conventional medical services are not only based on but also biased towards acute care; yet the methods of the hospital do not belong in the clinic. The classic brief consultation in general practice is modelled on acute hospital practice and is both inappropriate and inadequate to the task of *comprehending* the dimensionality of chronicity. The origin of 'acute' lies in Latin *acus* meaning 'needle', which lends itself only too easily to the following excruciating pun in that the acute consultation is about 'getting to the point'. In acute severe cases, the practitioner must be especially sharp, precise, pointed, incisive and single-minded in focussing on making a diagnosis and prescribing appropriate treatment to relieve pronounced suffering. Even then it may not be possible to discern a diagnosis or effective intervention – but the attempt must be rigorously made. The origin of 'chronic' lies in Greek *khronos* 'time' and describes both the nature of the situation and of the type of care required – persisting for a long period of time. The acute consultation needs to be diagnostically oriented, conducted and concluded quickly in order to move on to delivering treatment as rapidly as possible, and there may not be a need for medium- to long-term follow-up. The chronic consultation needs to adapt to and reflect the characteristics of chronic illness – being complex; only initially concerned with diagnosis then over time more with understanding and meaning; focussed on care, support and adaptation as well as, and commonly more than, treatment.

Conventional medicine has not coped well with the shift in emphasis from acute to chronic conditions – as acute dramatic pictures increasingly vacate centre stage (at least in the developed world), the mass of chronicity in the background stands revealed. As twentieth-century medicine developed more effective tools for dealing with acute conditions, then such conditions came to be associated with the ideal of medical practice: clear, readily-diagnosable, florid pictures that respond quickly to aggressively effective medical treatment delivered by the doctor as hero. Chronic conditions then represent the ill-fitting and unacknowledged failures of such a system. In coming to terms with chronicity biomedicine must address its failures and its shame – which may act as more powerful catalysts to philosophical reflection and practical change than any other imaginable.

Herbal medicine has always treated both acute and chronic disorders and has always existed as a (and usually *the*) major therapeutic strand in mainstream medicine in all cultures through all time. As expectations of medical treatment changed and in light of the dramatic effects of, especially, antibiotics and steroids in treating acute severe infections and inflammatory disorders herbal medicines came to appear relatively ineffective. Throughout the mid to latter part of the twentieth century, the use of herbs to treat acute disorders declined but it has not disappeared. Rather there is a resurgence of popular use of herbal medicines such as echinacea (*Echinacea* spp.) to treat acute viral infections particularly, albeit that the vast majority of over-the-counter echinacea (and other herbal) products are of poor therapeutic quality, conventional medicine has little to offer in competition and the conditions treated are usually self-limiting. As conventional medicine has dominated acute medicine, herbal medicine has been increasingly applied to chronic disorders – the complexity of herbs, their relatively gentle nature, suitability for long-term use and vast scope makes them particularly suited to utilization in chronic pictures.

Biomedicine is particularly fixated on acute medicine to the point that it tends to treat all disease in an acute manner – that is to say with brief consultations focussed on diagnostic and treatment questions where the patient is essentially passive. CAM therapies are mostly focussed on working with chronic pictures but problems could arise if CAM practitioners attempted to treat acute conditions in a manner suited to chronicity.

In closing, we can posit that acute and chronic illness represent two types of *emergency* with reference to the origin of that term as 'to arise; to bring to light'.

Acute situations represent a *medical emergency*, where the nature of the condition and the appropriate mode of treatment need to be urgently brought to light. Such goals are facilitated by the 'acute consultation'.

Chronic situations represent the opportunity for *emergency of properties*, to slightly adapt the notion of 'emergent properties' as used in connection with complexity and chaos theories. The nature of the person needs to arise and a mode of living needs to be brought to light. These goals are enabled by the 'chronic consultation'.

## MOVING WITH THE PATIENT

To summarize, let us assert that the task of attempting to understand the patient and her predicament is a complex, fascinating but hugely rewarding one that involves work on the practitioner's self as well as the patient's. Awareness of a wide range of models that can be used to help contextualize, assess and appreciate the patient is useful but the practitioner should be able to overlap and move between them as appropriate. Diagnosis is not always the key component of the consultation, and phytotherapists should guard against making the error of treating chronic pictures as if they were acute.

It is important to move with the patient, appreciating their trajectories and selecting and applying what seem to be the best and most relevant strategies but always remaining open to being surprised by patients and to learning from them. These are among the greatest joys and rewards of practice.

In the following chapter, we will extend our discussion regarding how we might come to appreciate patients by focussing on the case history. It includes several subjects that would have been equally at home in this chapter, such as evaluating the four aspects of being, remembering the six non-naturals and using intuition ... but it's time to move on; let's set 'the history' in context first.

# REFERENCES

Barry CA, Bradley P, Britten N, et al: Patients' unvoiced agendas in general practice consultations: qualitative study, *British Medical Journal* 320:1246–1250, 2000.

Block JA: Contrarian view of the five-factor approach to personality description, *Psychological Bulletin* 117:187–215, 1995.

Bonell C, Oakley J, Hargreaves J, et al: Assessment of generalisability in trials of health interventions: suggested framework and systematic review, *British Medical Journal* 333:346–349, 2006.

Booker R: Heartbroken, not heartsink, *British Medical Journal* 332:894, 2006.

Bury M: Chronic illness as biographical disruption, *Sociology of Health and Illness* 4(2):167–182, 1982.

Butler CC, Evans M, Greaves D, et al: Medically unexplained symptoms: the biopsychosocial model found wanting, *Journal of the Royal Society of Medicine* 97:219–222, 2004.

Campbell J: *The hero with a thousand faces*, 1949, Princeton University Press.

Clarke JN, James S: The radicalized self: the impact on the self of the contested nature of the diagnosis of chronic fatigue syndrome, *Social Science and Medicine* 57(8):1387–1395, 2003.

Collins S, Britten N, Ruusuvuori J, et al, editors: Understanding the process of patient participation. *Patient participation in healthcare consultations*, Milton Keynes, 2007, McGraw-Hill/Open University Press.

Conway P, O'Sullivan C, editor: *Reshaping herbal medicine: knowledge, education and professional development*, London, 2005, Elsevier.

Corbin J, Strauss A: Managing chronic illness at home: three lines of work, *Qualitative Sociology* 1985:1(3); 224–247.

Cornwell J: *Hard-earned lives: accounts of health and illness from East-End London*, London, 1984, Tavistock.

Cronbach LJ: Assessment of individual differences, *Annual Review of Psychology* 7:173–196, 1956.

Daghio MM, Ciardullo AV, Cadioli T, et al: GPs' satisfaction with the doctor-patient encounter: findings from a community-based survey, *Family Practice* 20(3): 283–288, 2003.

Davies ML: Shattered assumptions: time and the experience of long-term HIV positivity, *Social Science & Medicine* 44(5):561–571, 1997.

Delany GA: Farewell to heartsink? *British Journal of General Practice* 57(540):584–585, 2007.

Ellis CG: Chronic unhappiness: investigating the phenomenon in family practice, *Canadian Family Physician* 42:645–651, 1996.

Epstein RM, Shields CG, Meldrum SC, et al: Physicians' responses to patients' medically unexplained symptoms, *Psychosomatic Medicine* 68:269–276, 2006.

Eysenck HJ: *Personality and Individual Differences: a natural science approach*, New York, 1985, Kluwer Academic/Plenum.

Ezzy D: Illness narratives: time, hope and HIV, *Social Science & Medicine* 50:605–617, 2000.

Fairhurst K, May C: What general practitioners find satisfying in their work: implications for healthcare system reform, *Annals of Family Medicine* 4(6):500–505, 2006.

Fast I: *Selving: a rational theory of self-organization*, London, 1998, Routledge.

Feldhay R: Recent narratives on Galileo and the Church: or the three dogmas of the Counter-Reformation, *Science in Context* 219–237, 2005.

Fendler L: Why generalisability is not generalisable, *Journal of Philosophy of Education* 40(4):437–449, 2006.

Foucault M: *The Birth of the Clinic (first published 1963)*, London, 2007, Routledge.

Frank A: *The wounded storyteller: body, illness and ethics*, 1995, University of Chicago Press.

Golbin A, Umantsev A: Adaptive chaos: mild disorder may help contain major disease, *Medical Hypotheses* 66:182–187, 2006.

Gladwell M: *The tipping point: how little things can make a big difference*, New York, 2000, Little, Brown and Company.

Gordon JS: Holistic medicine: advances and shortcomings, *Western Journal of Medicine* 136:546–551, 1982.

Greaves D: *Mystery in Western Medicine*, Aldershot, 1996, Avebury.

Hadler N: *The last well person: how to stay well despite the health-care system*,

Montreal, 2004, McGill-Queen's University Press.

Hyland ME: Extended network generalized entanglement theory: therapeutic mechanisms, empirical predictions, and investigations, *Journal of Alternative and Complementary Medicine* 9(6):919–936, 2003.

Illich: *Limits to medicine*, London, 1976, Boyars.

Iwasaki K, Takahashi M, Nakata A: Health problems due to long working hours in Japan: working hours, workers compensation (*Karoshi*), and preventive measures, *Industrial Health* 44:537–540, 2006.

Jacobi J, Hull RFC (eds): *C.G. Jung: Psychological reflections: a new anthology of his writings, 1905-1961*, 1992, Princeton University Press.

Judge TA, Erez A, Bono JE, Thoresen CJ: Are measures of self-esteem, neuroticism, locus of control and generalized self-efficacy indicators of a common core construct? *Journal of Personality and Social Psychology* 83(3):693–710, 2002.

Jung CG: *The undiscovered self*, London, 2002, Routledge.

Katz J: *The silent world of doctor and patient*, Glencoe IL, 1986, The Free Press.

Kelley EL: *Interpretation of educational measurements*, New York, 1927, World.

Lawrence C, Shapin S: *Science incarnate: historical embodiments of natural knowledge*, 1998, University of Chicago Press.

Leder D: Clinical interpretation: the hermeneutics of medicine, *Theoretical Medicine* 11(1):9–24, 1990.

Levenstein JH, McCracken EC, McWhinney IR et al: The patient-centred clinical method. 1. A model for the doctor-patient in family medicine, *Family Practice* 3:24–30, 1986.

Little CV: Simply because it works better: exploring motives for the use of medical herbalism in contemporary UK health care, *Complementary Therapies in Medicine* 17:300-308, 2009.

Lloyd GE, editor: *Hippocratic writings*, London, 1983, Penguin Classics.

Malterud K: The art and science of clinical knowledge: evidence beyond measures and numbers, *The Lancet* 358:397–400, 2001.

Maslow AH: *Toward a Psychology of Being*, New York, 1968, Van Nostrand Reinhold.

Mathers N, Jones N, Hannay D: Heartsink patients: a study of their general practitioners, *British Journal of General Practice* 45:293–296, 1995.

McKenna: *A few conclusions about life*. Psychedelic Salon podcast No. 136, 1996. Released 14 April 2008.

McWhinney IR, Epstein RM, Freeman TR: Lingua medica: rethinking somatization, *Annals of Internal Medicine* 126(9):747–750, 1997.

Middleton JF, McKinley RF, Gillies GL: Effect of patient completed agenda forms and doctors' education about the agenda on the outcome of consultations: randomised controlled trial, *British Medical Journal* 332:1238–1242, 2006.

Mills S, Bone K: *The essential guide to herbal safety*, London, 2005, Elsevier/Churchill Livingstone.

Moore GA: *Crossing the chasm: marketing and selling technology products to mainstream consumers*, New York, 1991, Harper Collins.

Nettleton S: *The sociology of health and illness*, Cambridge, 2006, Polity.

Nishiyama K, Johnson JV: Karoshi – death from overwork: occupational health consequences of Japanese production management, *International Journal of Health Services: Planning, Administration, Evaluation* 27(4):625–641, 1997.

Nutton V: *Ancient medicine*, London, 2004, Routledge.

O'Dowd: Five years of heartsink patients in general practice, *British Medical Journal* 297:528–530, 1988.

Parsons T: *The Social System*, Glencoe IL, 1951, The Free Press.

Peck BM, Ubel PA, Roter DL, et al: Do unmet expectations for specific tests, referrals, and new medications reduce patients' satisfaction? *Journal of General Internal Medicine* 19:1080–1087, 2004.

Rotter JB: Generalised expectancies for internal versus external control enforcement, *Psychological Monographs* 80(1):1–28, 1966.

Rowan J, Jacobs M: *The therapist's use of self*, Milton Keynes, 2002, Open University Press.

Schilling C: *The body and social theory*, London, 1993, Sage.

Shapin S: The great neurotic art, *London Review of Books*, 5 August, 2004.

Sorabji R: *Self: ancient and modern insights about individuality, life and death*, 2006, Oxford University Press.

Stacey RD: *Complex responsive processes in organizations: learning and knowledge creation*, London, 2001, Routledge.

Stacey RD: *Strategic management and organisational dynamics: the challenge of complexity*, Harlow, 2002, Prentice Hall.

Staines J, Clark D: *The rough guide to classical music*, London, 2005, Penguin.

Stainton Rogers W: From psychometric scales to cultural perspectives. In Beattie A, Gott M, Jones L, Sidell M, editors: *Health and wellbeing: a reader*, Milton Keynes, 1992, Macmillan/Open University.

Summerton N: Making a diagnosis in primary care: symptoms and context, *British Journal of General Practice* August: 570–571, 2004.

Thaler RH, Sunstein CR: *Nudge: improving decisions about health, wealth and happiness*, 2008, Yale University Press.

Thomas-McLean R: Understanding breast cancer stories via Frank's narrative types, *Social Science & Medicine* 58(9):1647–1657, 2004.

Times Higher Education: Editorial. A suitable subject for teaching. *Times Higher Education* 30 October, 23, 2008.

Tracy SW: An evolving science of man: the transformation and demise of American constitutional medicine, 1920–1950. In Lawrence C, Weisz G, editors: *Greater than the parts: holism in biomedicine 1920–1950*, 1998, Oxford University Press.

Unschuld PU: *Medicine in China: a history of ideas*, 1985, University of California Press.

Usherwood T: *Understanding the consultation*, Milton Keynes, 1999, Open University Press.

Vogler C: *The writer's journey: mythic structure for writers*, Studio City, 1998, Michael Wiese.

Wagner EH, Austin BT, Davis C, et al: Improving chronic illness care: translating evidence into action, *Health Affairs* 20(6):64–78, 2001.

Wallston KA, Wallston BS, DeVellis R: Development of the multidimensional health locus of control (MHLC) scales, *Health Education Monographs* 6:161–170, 1978.

Wallston KA: Hocus-pocus, the focus isn't strictly on the locus: Rotter's social learning theory modified for health, *Cognitive Therapy and Research* 16(2): 183–199, 1992.

Warhol A: *From A to B and back again: the philosophy of Andy Warhol*, London, 1975, Michael Dempsey/Cassell.

Whitehead LC: Quest, chaos and restitution: living with chronic fatigue syndrome/ myalgic encephalomyelitis, *Social Science & Medicine* 62:2236–2245, 2006.

Williams SJ: Chronic illness as biological disruption or biographical disruption as chronic illness? Reflections on a core concept, *Sociology of Health and Illness* 22(1):40–67, 2000.

Wilson H: Reflecting on the 'difficult' patient, *Journal of the New Zealand Medical Association* 118(1212), 2005.

Woodward RV, Broom DH, Legge DG: Diagnosis in chronic illness: disabling or enabling – the case of chronic fatigue syndrome, *Journal of the Royal Society of Medicine* 88:325–329, 1995.

Yang Y: *Chinese Herbal Medicines: comparisons and characteristics*, Edinburgh, 2002, Elsevier/Churchill Livingstone.

Zingrone F: Multimedia overload produces 'symplexity', *Psychiatric Services* 54(3):311–316, 2003.

# Case history-taking
## Hearing the patient's story

**5**

## CHAPTER CONTENTS

**General considerations 207**
   Taking the history 207
   Summary of the aims of history-taking 209
   The history of the case history 209
   The 'conversation' 212
   The nature of history 214
   Clinical hermeneutics 217
   Narrative-based medicine 218
   On hearing, speaking, moving and recording 224
   Posing questions and listening to replies 227
      *Ask for more information* 229
      *Seek clarification* 230
      *Use echoing (repetition)* 230
      *Share thoughts* 230
      *Summarize* 230
      *Interrupt* 232
      *Use silence* 233
      *Use humour and play* 234
      *Questioning style* 235
      *Keep questions separate* 236
      *Keep questions simple and clear* 236
      *Proceed from open to closed questioning* 236
      *Avoid leading questions* 239
      *Non-verbal questions* 240
   The consultation environment 240
   Children 242
   The older patient 248
   Using intuition 251
   Assessing the four aspects of being 253
   The six non-naturals and the prioritization of the individual 256

**History formats 261**
   Opening questions 261
   Opening answers 263

**Follow-up consultations 264**
   Preparation 265

Enactment 266
'By the way …' 268
Four territories 268
Change and recollection 268
**The initial consultation 269**
 The blank sheet 270
 To be continued … 271
 Questioning prior conceptions 271
 Recognizing limitations 272
 Complexity, non-linearity and flexibility 273
**Welcoming 273**
 Personal details 275
  Patient's name 275
  Address 275
  Preferred contact telephone number 276
  Date of birth 276
  Gender 277
  Occupation 277
  Relationship status 278
  Children 279
  Who lives at home? 280
  GP details 281
  'How did you hear about me?' 281
 Personal details leading into the history 282
 Phytotherapy orientation 282
 The presenting complaint 283
 History of the presenting complaint 283
 Expectations 1 284
 Previous medical and life history: sensitivity to initial conditions 284
 Allergies, intolerances or sensitivities 286
 Family history 287
 Drug and treatment history 288
 Social history 289
  Smoking 290
  Alcohol 291
  Illicit substances 294
  Exercise and relaxation 295
  Interests and pastimes 297
  Home or/and working life 297
 Vitality 298
 Energetic assessment 301
 Temperament, personality, mood and outlook 304
 Personal style 306
 Diet 306
  Dietary intake and pattern of eating 307
  General dietary factors 308
  Food history 310
  Financial limitations 310
 Systems enquiry 311

Digestive system   311
   Urinary system   312
   Integumentary system (skin, hair and nails)   312
   Musculoskeletal system   313
   Cardiovascular system   314
   Respiratory system   314
   Immune system   314
   Nervous system   315
   Reproductive system   315
 Comprehensive versus comprehension   317
**Expectations 2 and transiting to the physical examination   317**

## GENERAL CONSIDERATIONS

### TAKING THE HISTORY

Case history-taking, as we discussed in the previous chapter, is the key means of getting to know the patient. The majority of diagnoses in phytotherapy, conventional medicine and many other modalities are based principally on the case history. For example, Peterson et al. (1992), studying medical doctors, found that in 76% of cases: 'the leading diagnosis after taking the history agreed with the diagnosis accepted at the time the record was reviewed two months after the initial visit'. Yet, despite its central importance, in conventional medical practice, it has been suggested that 'skilled history-taking is in danger of becoming a lost art' (Schechter et al. 1996). We can propose that this is likely to be primarily due to biomedicine's emphasis on acute medicine (where history-taking tends to be pointed and abbreviated) and over-emphasis (leading to over-reliance) on investigative technology. Herbal practice remains a place where the case history is accorded central importance and where adequate space is made available for its exploration. This is in part because herbal practice has been less occupied with acute medicine and more focussed on chronicity (especially since around the mid-twentieth century) and the attendant need of the chronically ill patient for more profound personal exploration of their predicament; and since herbal practice has been excluded from mainstream medicine it has not had direct access to, and therefore has not become excessively entangled with, technological methods of patient exploration.

Regardless of the orientation of one's therapeutic discipline towards it, however, history-taking remains a tricky art. Students are generally exhorted to 'maintain objectivity' and 'keep a clinical distance', while engaging with the patient's story but such directions represent forlorn hopes raised to protect against the fact that case taking is a subjective phenomena and therefore a suspect area of activity viewed from the perspective of positivistic medical science (and this is another reason why history-taking is a threatened species in biomedicine). So we need to ask whether a history can ever be 'taken' as if it existed as a solid object that can be 'extracted' (*Note*: it is common for clinical texts to purport to instruct students on how to 'extract the history') from the patient and then held up to the light for analysis. To 'take' or 'extract' a history is to de-contextualize it and risks rendering it an insipid and flimsy simulacrum – great care needs to be taken when basing clinical decisions on such an untrue-to-life creature. Rather the practitioner needs to be aware of the fact that she cannot help but be actively involved in building, constructing and creating the 'case history'. The case history, as written, is an artefact, and one that usually requires interpretation when being exhibited to others – even colleagues trained in the same style of questioning and documenting. One practitioner's precise clinical record is another's incomprehensible screed.

The practitioner is involved in the construction and presentation of the patient's history *of necessity* and this fact should be negotiated rather than resisted. The practitioner cannot help but set the patient's story within her own frame of reference, which is based on her theoretical and clinical training, personal history (early education, parental influence, etc.), political bias, social status, cultural milieu and so forth. In other words, since the practitioner cannot be other than who she *is*, then the limits to her capacity to comprehend patient's stories are set by the expansiveness and subtlety of her worldview. The greater the practitioner's own fund of experiences and stories, and the greater her degree of subtlety of thought, the broader will be her capacity to appreciate the experiences and stories of her patients. The practitioner's formative influences and inner and outer journeys determine her ability to *leave* the history in the context of the whole patient as opposed to *taking* it from them. This is analogous to the herbal practitioner's insistence on leaving active phytochemicals within the context of the whole plant (amidst a mass of material that is indeterminate or only partially appreciated) rather than extracting isolated active constituents (in order to only deal with factors that are precisely and concretely known).

As the practitioner is 'taking the history', she is selecting, editing, omitting, mishearing, 'overhearing', interpreting and developing the patient's picture – by all these means, she constructs a version of events and builds a thesis regarding their significance and meaning. While direction of the patient in this process can be minimized (e.g. by posing 'open' questions and avoiding 'leading' ones; see below), it cannot be eradicated. Even with the greatest awareness of the various issues involved the practitioner cannot be aware of every factor in the clinical encounter that adapts the way that the patient tells her story, nor, even with identification of the issues, can she change (or predict the impact of) some of these, e.g. the practitioner's gender, skin colour, accent, age, etc.

Histories are not consistent entities, they change in the telling and retelling and depending on the audience. Patients may discover new insights as they tell their story (a desirable and often therapeutic outcome that should be one of the key goals of history-taking) but alternatively, they may mechanically repeat an oft-told and negatively reinforced self-tale (a scenario to be detected and challenged), or creatively 'play' with adding new elements to the storyline to see if they fit or to 'play tricks' on the practitioner (strategies that may confuse or mislead the practitioner if they are not picked up on).

So then, the case history is a fascinating, if slippery, place to visit; let us go and take a look around …

## SUMMARY OF THE AIMS OF HISTORY-TAKING

Since we have discussed many of the concepts and issues related to the aims of history-taking in the phytotherapy consultation in previous chapters, we need only briefly state them at this stage:

- Enabling patients to reflect on their predicament and to:
  - Identify key themes and issues
  - Gain insight into their situation
  - Explore the meaning of their situation
  - Develop a more coherent sense of self
- Allow the practitioner to provide assistance in:
  - Bearing witness
  - Conveying human warmth and care
  - Facilitate self-discovery and self-development
- Access information to help form a diagnosis (less important in follow-up consultations)
- Determine areas that stand in need of:
  - Support
  - Care
  - Learning
  - Treatment
- Elucidate areas where referral is indicated.

## THE HISTORY OF THE CASE HISTORY

Epstein et al. (1997) maintain that: 'For generations, there has been little change in the method of recording information from the history', but is such an argument sustainable? Certainly the 'method of recording' has changed dramatically, at least in biomedicine, in that patient records are now computerized, although we will save discussing the intrusion of the computer as the 'third person in the consulting room' for later. I take Epstein to mean, however, that the *process of taking the history* is little changed, but again this is hard to credit. As doctors have moved from the bedside to being desk-bound, there has also been a shift of location of emphasis from the context of patient (represented by 'bed': resting, sleeping, dreaming, copulating) to that of doctor ('desk': acting, writing, filing, working). Factors such as the means by which information is recorded and the setting in which information is obtained affect the conduct and content of the consultation itself, including history-taking.

We should not assume, despite the emphasis placed on the importance of the history at the beginning of this chapter, that the 'case history' – meaning a verbal dialogue between patient and practitioner – has always been the dominant means of knowing the patient or that 'case history' has always equated to 'verbal dialogue'. Kuriyama (1999) provides an alternative perspective:

> In the second century B.C.E., in the earliest case histories of China, the sick summon Chunyu Yi not with vague pleas for succor, but with the specific wish that he come and feel their pulse. And that is just what the great doctor does. In each case, he

*arrives, straightaway grasps the pulse, then prescribes a remedy, explaining, 'The way I knew the ailment is that when I felt the pulse ...' As if it were all a ritual, and his role was that of pulse interpreter.*

Primary focus on the pulse was not limited to China but, based on the pronouncements of Galen, dominated diagnosis in the west until recent centuries. Kuriyama names the four ways of assessing patients used in ancient Chinese medicine as: 'gazing (*wang*); listening and smelling (*wen*); questioning (*wen*); and touching (*qie*)', but asserts that 'in practice ... attentions concentrated mainly on *qiemo*, palpating the *mo*'. *Mo* can be translated as (but without being limited to) *blood vessels* or *pulse*. This focus on the pulse contrasts with the diagnostic hierarchy outlined in various classic Chinese medicine texts described by Kuriyama. For example in the *Nanjing*:

*... to gaze and know the illness is 'divine' (*shen*), to know by listening or smelling is 'sagely' (*sheng*), to question and know was 'crafty' (*gong*), to touch and know only 'skillful' (*qiao*).*

Whereas the *Shanghanlun* 'was blunt: the physician who knew by gazing belonged to the top class (*shanggong*); the physician who questioned and knew was average (*zhonggong*); the physician who touched and knew was inferior (*xiagong*)'.

Kuriyama concludes that: 'Mastery of medicine was defined first by an exceptional eye', and proceeds to discuss the subtleties of what was represented by the concept of the diagnostic 'eye' and the 'gaze'. We might consider the progression of this emphasis on visual knowing to extend through X-ray machines to MRI scanners though the notion of the doctor's ability to 'see inside' the patient is an ancient one.

Commenting on the case reports collected in the Hippocratic *Epidemics*, Nutton (2004) observes that the authors 'are already selective in their presentation of signs and symptoms, focussing in particular on things that would, in future, enable the writer (and later his audience) to estimate the severity of a similar condition, forecast its outcome and, where possible, intervene successfully'. Nutton lists the relationships and features associated with disease described in the case histories in *Epidemics 1*:

*... the common nature of all things and the particular nature of the individual; the disease and the patient; the regimen prescribed and the prescriber; the constitution of the heavens and the region, in general and in particular; the custom, way of life, practices and age; talk, manner, silence, thoughts, sleeping or not; dreams, plucking, scratching, tearing; exacerbations, stools, urines, sputa, vomit; the stages of a disease, and its potential for crisis and death; sweat, rigor, chill, cough, sneezes, hiccoughs, flatulence, haemorrhoids and haemorrhages. Behind all this lies shrewd, careful and accurate observation, using all the senses.*

Yet these are reports dealing with acute cases and we hear fewer stories regarding chronicity from ancient medical texts, partly because, as Nutton explains: 'given the age structure of the population, the degenerative diseases characteristic of the twentieth century will have been fewer in number', and partly due to a different conceptualization of disease, in that 'ancient doctors saw the gradual physical and mental deterioration of old age as part of an inevitable process' so that consequently, 'it is not the infirm we hear of, but the exceptions, the hale and hearty, like the Elder Pliny's centenarian friend Antonius Castor, still pottering around his herb garden'. Nutton points out the importance of prognostic ability in early Greek doctors, as a means of establishing trust in their capacities. Prognostic skill was a means by which the doctor 'could establish his credentials and, at the same time, protect himself against accusations of malpractice. By being able to predict the likely outcome of a disease ... he could gain obvious credit for a cure ... [but] should the patient die, he had a strong defence if he had already announced that this was a likely outcome'. An emphasis on prognosis then served as a 'tactical' strategy regarding 'both advertising and insurance' but was not limited to these goals since it was also 'essential to the understanding and treatment of the individual patient, ensuring that whatever is prescribed will be appropriate for that patient'. Furthermore, 'the doctor who professes the art of prognosis declares that his particular technique deals with the past, present and future of his patient, a bold claim incorporating what today would be termed obtaining the case history, diagnosis and prognosis'. This attempt to stand in the present and yet be able to look backwards and forwards in time continues to be one of the hallmarks of the clinician but also constitutes one of the key characteristics of the shaman. 'Shaman' can be translated as 'one who knows' (or 'clever fella' as McKenna reports) and figures occupying the shamanic role typically act simultaneously as repositories of the history of the tribal group; authorities on the present; and seers who are able to predict future events. Healthcare practitioners, then, partake in a shamanic tradition at least in being accorded the status of possessing an uncommon temporal facility. The origin of case history-taking in the consultation then might be extended back to shamanism in archaic cultures.

The case history represents a gathering together of information about the past and the present in order to be able to see into, and to make predictions about, the future. The current emphasis in conventional medicine on diagnosis, prognosis and acute cases therefore does not represent a particularly recent trend. However, the reliance on technology and the extent to which the individual personal characteristics of the patient are excluded from consideration do signify breaks with a long medical tradition and are major current influences preventing mainstream medicine from adapting to meet the requirements necessitated by the shift in burden from acute to chronic disease. Current mainstream medical methods of assessing past impacts, present influences and future likelihoods, including imaging technology and genetic testing could be considered as a concretization of archaic visionary capacities or as phenomena emerging within an ancient project. The major concern surrounding the point now reached has to do with the extent to which this continuum has shot beyond the human dimension to a place where the patient is viewed differently – de-personalized and disembodied.

The relationship between herbal medicine and shamanism is profound but complex. In ancient indigenous cultures, the possession of substantial personal knowledge of the healing properties of a wide range of plants is commonplace and tends to be seen as ordinary or basic knowledge that is therefore considered unremarkable, although some people have greater knowledge than others and are accorded 'practitioner' status. Lenaerts (2006) studied the

Asheninka people who live on the Peru–Brazil border and found a distinction in that: 'Shamans are deemed to have a superior knowledge, since they are able to heal illnesses that ordinary people or herbalists cannot' although herbalism and shamanism do not represent 'two specialized, separate fields of healing, (rather) they form two distinct *expressions* of the same issues' [original emphasis]. The shaman's advantage does not rest in his superior knowledge of plants (in fact Lenaerts suggests that, in some cultures at least, the shaman may know *less* about healing plants than other types of healers) but rather in his status as a 'specialist in relationships with other beings'. The Asheninka shaman is able, with the assistance of ingested 'entheogenic' plants (*entheogen* means 'God generated within', and is an alternative way of viewing and describing so-called 'hallucinogenic' plants) to meet other beings such as plants, animals and stones *as people*. Discourse with these beings can lead (among other things) to diagnostic insights and the subsequent implementation of therapeutic strategies.

Such encounters also give rise to creation stories, human–environment relationship schemas and rationales for the interpretation of experiences. They are the source of philosophies, religions and medical systems and they unify and hold together the distinct cultures that the agglomeration of these elements give rise to. We are engaged here with the construction and interpretation of worlds, plunged into the matrix of myth, story, saga, fairy-story, morality-play and 'case history' that spin out of this generative centre. Although it may seem at this point that we have travelled a long way in this chapter, and very quickly, the suggestion remains that if we follow the thread of what the case history actually *is* (i.e. an attempt to temporally comprehend one person, to understand their predicament and to discern ways of assisting them), back far enough it will lead us to the root of art, science, philosophy and medicine that resides in the person of the shaman and in the presence of the entheogen.

It is difficult to perceive the sacred worldview from the perspective attending that of the profane but the shaman and the physician share a common origin. Both are 'ones who know' and what they know has to do with *nature* – they know the *nature of nature*. In origin and essence both encompass the roles of artist, scientist, philosopher and healer. Although the scope of the physician (whether phytotherapist, doctor or other) has diminished to the generic mediocrity of 'healthcare practitioner', the territory and the possibility of the shaman remain available and are accessible through means of 'taking the history', since the case history is the place where all our stories come together and where time travel is the mandatory mode of transport.

**THE 'CONVERSATION'**

Referring to the 'case history' may seem somewhat inadequate to the task of describing a way of looking that includes assessment of the present and speculation about the future, since 'history' is commonly perceived as referring to the study of what is past. *Collins English Dictionary* (2000) describes 'history' as deriving from 'Latin *historia*, from Greek: enquiry, from *historein* to narrate, from *histor* judge' and gives one definition of history as a: 'Narrative relating the events of a character's life'. Enquiry, narrative, events, judgement – these are all features of the consultation that can easily be identified with the case history. *Churchill's Medical Dictionary* (1989) defines the case history blandly as: 'A recording of information relating to a particular case …'. This view, emphasizing the production of a historical record by a neutral observer, lacks any sense of the assessment and dynamic interplay that occurs during the process of history-taking – of what the practitioner gives to the encounter alongside what she takes away from it. So perhaps there is a better term to describe the question and answer session that transpires during the consultation, and which, in contemporary phytotherapy at least, forms its most significant part?

It was the convention in medical textbooks on clinical examination until recent times to describe it as 'the interrogation' (e.g. Hunter & Bomford 1956; Macleod 1967). This term refers to formal and detailed questioning but it also suggests aggression and its use in medicine is now hard to countenance since the word 'interrogation' is inextricably linked with a visual image of a bright light being shone into one's face. The negative associations we have with the concept of interrogation are disturbing, since we now connect the word with torture. Many authors have described and considered the history of, and continuing involvement between, medicine and torture (e.g. Maio 2001; Lifton 2004; Klein 2007). A recent questionnaire-based study (Bean et al. 2008) exploring the attitudes of one population of American medical students (336 students at the University of Illinois College of Medicine) to the 'permissibility and ethics of the use of torture' found that '35 percent of students agreed that torture could be "condoned" under some circumstances. Moreover, 24 percent … disagreed that torture should "be prohibited" as a matter of state policy and a similar 24 percent disagreed that torture was "intrinsically wrong"'. This is a hugely complex as well as troubling area but we may suggest that an excessive, indeed a pathological, emphasis on objectivity and clinical distance is one amongst a number of underlying factors that enable medical torture. If objectivity extends to the objectification of bodies, and if clinical distance ranges to the point where human connection and feeling is lost, then some of the conditions in which unforced torture can be conducted are set. Clinicians are still encouraged to 'put the spotlight on the patient' and 'keep yourself out of the picture' but we should remain aware of the double reading that is possible when this type of language is used.

More recent textbooks on clinical examination have tended to refer to history-taking as 'the interview'. This can be read as an attempt to retain the formality and the objectivity/neutrality of the practitioner implicit in the use of 'interrogation' while losing the negative correlations that word now gives rise to. The move from 'interrogation' to 'interview' also represents a shift from the practitioner as 'policeman' to the practitioner as 'manager'. To be interviewed is to be cast in the role of applicant or news item. The practitioner-as-interviewer has a power role where she can:

- Act as a manager in approving the patient's application ('following a successful interview') to be a sick person by conferring a diagnosis and a course of treatment to be followed
- Act as a journalist in taking the patient's information and spinning it into a (more or less reliable) story. In this role we can see the short

conventional medicine consultation as a form of rushed TV interviewing where only pre-formulated sound-bites can register and a nuanced discussion of the complexity and multidimensionality of a given issue is impossible.

Some clinicians have suggested the use of 'conversation' (e.g. Kaplan 2001), which is certainly informal and devoid of unpleasant connotations but seems a little, well, aimless and insipid. We know that a lot of conversations 'don't go anywhere', that people tend to make 'polite conversation' and do things 'just for the sake of' conversation. Perhaps it would help if we medicalized it by calling it the 'clinical conversation'? Or therapized it by calling it the 'therapeutic conversation'? Or how about we try something else – the 'discussion' anybody?

Perhaps, after all, 'the history' still works best since it suggests a comprehensive view and implies an attempt to take in and make sense of the big picture. In which case, it may be helpful to explore the notion of 'history' as applied to the consultation in a little more detail.

## THE NATURE OF HISTORY

The way that history is practised varies but the archetypal model reflects the dominant scientific values of contemporary western culture. This type of history is based on objectivity, chronology and classification. Complex, sinuous themes and elliptical notions are forced into ill-fitting (and sometimes delusional) categories such as that of 'the baroque period' or 'the scientific revolution'. Other forms of historical method focus more on contextualization and interpretation but even here the preference is to begin deconstructive work on what purport to be finished objects. The patient represents history-in-process and only becomes a finished project when the heart stops beating – a study option that is not consistent with the aims of the clinician!

Gadamer (1989) addresses the issue of historical analysis and its temporal separation from its topic of study, commenting with reference to works of art. He recognizes that in historical studies, it is generally believed that: 'objective knowledge can be achieved only if there has been a certain historical distance' from the creation of the object, and maintains that 'it is true that what a thing has to say, its intrinsic content, first appears only after it is divorced from the fleeting circumstances that first gave rise to it'. A person is not a 'thing' and does not materially endure for long, although the same could be said of 'the baroque period' or 'the enlightenment' and yet, these continue to be topics of historical study. We can consider previous events in the patient's life (or their 'previous medical history') to represent 'things', however – at the time of the consultation the patient may have achieved enough distance from the event for it to be open to analysis and be capable of yielding its 'intrinsic content'. Yet the practitioner is frequently trying to make sense of events as they happen, to make sense of 'fleeting circumstances' especially in acute medicine. At these times it is necessary to make the best judgement one can and then to keep that assessment continually open to revision.

Gadamer (1989) further describes the dominant historical perspective:

*The positive conditions of historical understanding include the relative closure of a historical event, which allows us to view it as a whole, and its distance from contemporary opinions concerning its import. The implicit presumption of historical method, then, is that the permanent significance of something can first be known objectively only when it belongs to a closed context – in other words, when it is dead enough to have only historical interest.*

In terms of living patients, 'relative closure' is the only type of closure available and it will rarely be possible to gain much distance from 'contemporary opinions'; such an achievement is only attainable when we view events-as-things in older patients where sufficient sociocultural and medical change may have occurred within one lifetime for that event to be viewed differently (as has happened with, e.g. HIV/AIDS). Even then we can never be certain that this 'different view' represents the definitive, ultimate, true or *truest* view – it can only appear to be relatively such. Let us return once more to Gadamer as he criticizes the historical method previously outlined, saying that it represents a paradox since:

*... the discovery of the true meaning of a text or a work of art is never finished; it is in fact an infinite process. Not only are fresh sources of error constantly excluded, so that all kinds of things are filtered out that obscure the true meaning; but new sources of understanding are continually emerging that reveal unsuspected elements of meaning. The temporal distance that performs the filtering process is not fixed, but is itself undergoing constant movement and extension.*

The same argument holds for people and it well describes the potentiality of practice – to increasingly discover the self and discern enhanced meaning. It also holds for texts about those no longer living. Consider the ways that successive biographies written about people (e.g. Joan of Arc, Napoleon, Bernard Shaw, Sylvia Pankhurst, Orson Welles) follow the process described by Gadamer. Each successive work (if it is any good/worth reading) filters what was previously known, finds new information and arrives at new meanings and each new biography reflects the time it was written in. There is no closure, then, on a remembered life long after it has been lived just as the same is true of life as it is *being lived*. There is no closure, only a state of natural chaos fluxing with the eternal emergence of new phenomena. The search for absolute objectivity in the human case history constitutes the pursuit of an unrealizable goal that should therefore be abandoned. Rather the practitioner ought to relish the challenges and breakthroughs that result from engaging dynamically with the contingent, latent and emergent worlds of patients, learning to work with relative wholes and testing theories and refining approaches in the light of feedback.

In the introduction to their exceptional book looking at emotions and their connections with the 'histories of art, music and medicine' Gouk and Hills (2005) describe an approach to the practice of history that fits with, and contains insights for, that pertaining to the taking of the case history:

*The essays collected here do not, and of course could not, constitute a chronological or geographical survey of the representation of emotions in Western Europe since the*

*Greeks. More significantly, we have not privileged those historical conjunctions conventionally identified as crucial for changing patterns in emotional articulation (for instance, the Ancient World, the medieval era and the eighteenth century), nor singled out those thinkers most usually credited with formulating new approaches (e.g. Plato, Aristotle, Augustine, Descartes, Le Brun, Spinoza, Rousseau, Voltaire). Instead, our principal aim has been to focus the investigative spotlight on specific moments when one formulation of emotions conflicts or converges with another, or when gaps or ellipses in one discourse on emotion are illuminated by another. In adopting this dual approach, we draw attention both to the necessarily non-disciplinary ways in which emotions have been conceived and to the complex processes by which some ideas eventually achieve authoritative status while others wither, neglected.*

With a little work, the above could be adapted to form a manifesto for the holistic case history, one especially suited to chronic pictures, bearing in mind the points made in the previous chapter and given that:

- Chronological and geographical considerations are similarly difficult in the consultation – recall the non-chronological chaos narrative and the difficulty of anatomically locating conditions such as chronic fatigue syndrome.
- It is important to avoid privileging one particular model or authority in conducting the consultation lest one's ability to work synthetically and see creatively is impeded.
- We could use identical language to describe one of the primary aims of the case history as being to: 'focus the investigative spotlight on specific moments when one formulation of emotions conflicts or converges with another, or when gaps or ellipses in one discourse on emotion are illuminated by another'. This statement of intent has even wider utility if, in place of 'emotions' we broaden the remit to 'emotions/symptoms/stories'.
- This approach is better suited to detecting which features, aspects and themes in the patient's picture are of greatest significance and which are less deserving of attention.

Foucault (1963) has distinguished between the 'historical' and 'philosophical' perception of disease. Here, 'history' has to do with such matters as the symptoms and course of the disease whereas the philosophical approach calls 'into question the origin, the principle, the causes of disease'. In practice these are not separate but rather interweaving lines of thought – as soon as we have some sense of the historical features of the patient's condition we philosophize as to their meaning. The ebb and flow of this process is strongest in the early part of the consultation where multiple philosophical analyses may be made rapidly and, indeed, intuitively, in response to historical information until the field of options becomes clearer (note that this does not necessarily mean narrower). The practitioner cast as historian, then, needs to be a historian–philosopher; but what use would a historian lacking in philosophy be in any case?

## CLINICAL HERMENEUTICS

Leder (1990) argues that: 'clinical medicine can best be understood not as a purified science but as a hermeneutical enterprise: that is, as involved with the interpretation of texts' and he identifies four textual forms that relate to the consultation:

- The 'experiential text' of illness as lived out by the patient
- The 'narrative text' constituted during history-taking
- The 'physical text' of the patient's body as objectively examined
- The 'instrumental text' constructed by diagnostic technologies.

Of these, the central two constitute the texts available in the consultation, the last is a subtext that may inform the consultation and the first refers to the patient's life outside of the consultation. This latter text is the most important to the personal experience of the patient but the least accessible in the consultation – although all three of the other texts can combine to attempt some degree of approximation of it. The narrative text of the case history most particularly represents the practitioner's effort to appreciate the experiential text of the patient's lived experience. The history represents the practitioner's best chance of understanding the patient's life and its attendant phenomena.

How far can/should we take the concept of textual analysis? Leder suggests we should follow the hermeneutical thread a long way down because, at root: 'certain flaws in modern medicine arise from its refusal of a hermeneutical self-understanding (such that) in seeking to escape all interpretive subjectivity, medicine has threatened to expunge its primary subject – the living, experiencing patient'. The case seems an urgent and crucial one then, except this analysis fails to factor in the substantive rebellion that takes place daily at grassroots level on the part of both patients and practitioners who reject being treated/treating people like automata rather than persons. Churchill (1990), however, argues that Leder does not go far enough and that it is insufficient to limit the hermeneutical argument to medicine, it should be extended to recognize that science itself is, at its core, a hermeneutic enterprise. Baron (1990) meanwhile queries the notion of the textual metaphor since it 'runs the risk of conceptualizing patients as more static than they are' and because it does not fit the characteristics of the consultation in that 'the qualities of mutuality and determinacy are not those one usually associates with texts'. Baron ends by calling for a different metaphor that captures the uncertainty resident in practitioner's comprehensions of patients. OK, Baron says, you've told us to look at the patient's texts – but it just doesn't work like that; that doesn't fit the reality of the clinical encounter – even if one is well disposed to the hermeneutical way.

Churchill (1990) argues that it is necessary to question the foundations of medicine and science and discover that they rest on a base that has to do with hermeneutics. Upshur (2002) questions the notion of a 'base' for the practice of medicine with regard to a discussion of evidence-based medicine (EBM) and suggests that, if we are to talk of bases and foundations, they must be pluralistic in nature. Upshur sees no reason why there should be any 'sharp conflict between facts and values' and references medical and scientific theorists who are attempting to overcome this duality. He perceives a growing appreciation of the 'complex values, perceptions and beliefs that frame how medicine is practised' and notes that the 'focus on interpretation, subjectivity, natural language and qualitative methods highlights dimensions of practice that escape the methods of EBM'. Such a focus on combining interpretive approaches 'is likely to lead a move from the metaphor of a uniform base for medicine as the consideration of the qualitative domain acknowledges multiplicity of perspectives and meanings'. Furthermore, Upshur asserts: 'medicine and health care are not in need of a single solid foundation, but can operate well in a dynamic emergent framework' that is woven from these multiple ways of perceiving. This brings us back to the fund of stories that represent the roots of knowing and how we might make sense of these 'texts' as they form within and around the individual patient and returns us to Baron's query about how we can work with patient's texts in a way that reflects the inter-relational plasticity of the clinical encounter and which takes account of the underlying uncertainties in this dynamic. We can best deal with this by moving on to the next section considering one key interpretive method that can be applied to case history-taking.

## NARRATIVE-BASED MEDICINE

> *narrative* ... **1** *an account, report, or story, as of events, experiences, etc.* **2** *... the part of a literary work that relates events ...* **4** *telling a story ...*
> Collins English Dictionary (2000)

Much has been written about which techniques and behaviours constitute 'communication skills' and how they can be developed and we will draw on some of this work later in this chapter. We will also discuss the structure of the consultation format and the steps in its enactment in the 'History formats' section of this chapter. However, regardless of our knowledge and ability in applying such skills, and despite our structural awareness, what we hear in the case history and what we learn from it will be shaped by what we are listening out for (what we are tuned to hear). This tuning is adjusted by what we think are the aims of the consultation and what we think is *going on* in the case taking. The narrative approach considers that what is essentially occurring in the consultation is a process of storytelling, although this, in itself, tells us little – no more than the blank assertion that patients can be perceived as a collection of texts. What is key to unlocking both of these concepts (history-as-story and history-as-text) lies in the *interpretation* of these phenomena. Narrative-based medicine represents a contrasting approach to positivistic, deterministic, reductionist medicine in that it is interpretivistic, relativistic, holistic. But stating the case in this way is to suggest a polarity of thought and action that, while it is easy to set on the page (in the 'text') does not accurately reflect the reality of practice. Practitioners may, when they think about it (or more commonly when they are asked to think about it) come down on one side or other of an ideological divide between positivism and interpretivism but in the act of practising we tend to be pragmatic. I have already suggested, for instance, that different approaches come into play in dealing with acute and chronic cases. Practitioners in action do not pause to think 'hmm, shall I take a positivistic or an interpretivistic approach here?', rather, having an awareness of differing approaches and knowledge of a variety of models and techniques provides options and informs practice.

Narrative-based medicine (NBM) is not an alternative to evidence-based medicine (EBM). Patient narratives are a *form* of evidence just as research represents a type of narrative. If we recall Sackett et al.'s (2000) definition of EBM as 'the integration of best research evidence with clinical expertise and patient values', then we can easily see NBM as providing us with an appreciation of the patient's part in this triad but we can also view each element of EBM as a narrative type since each is a text and each is a story: 'research evidence', 'clinical expertise', 'patient values' – all stories. Research evidence is a collection of texts, accounts of (or 'stories about') studies conducted with an attempt at objectivity (quantitative research) or subjectivity (qualitative research) with each type being open to (and standing in need of) interpretation. Clinical expertise represents accumulated knowledge and skills *in action* but which can be assessed and described in the form of texts (supervision and peer-review reports; patient feedback forms; practitioner self-reflection documents and so forth) which tell stories that can be interpreted. Patient values (which I take to mean patient opinions, expectations, preferences, morals, etc.) can be assessed in the case history, written down as text and interpreted. Seen from this perspective, any notion of setting up NBM/EBM as opposing models breaks down and becomes unsustainable – they are in actuality merely different takes on the same *stuff*.

NBM has the potential to be used to scrutinize scientific research evidence and practitioner activity in addition to its usual area of application – the patient's story. We will shortly move on to focus on this latter domain but need first to point to the practitioner's involvement with the generation of the patient's narrative. The way in which stories are told (or performed) in the consultation space, and their content, to varying degrees, is potentially influenced by a number of factors, difficult to exhaustively enumerate and even more difficult to estimate in terms of the extent to which they may have shaped the story. Such factors, on the part of the patient, include:

- Topics that the patient does not wish to reveal to the practitioner
- Notions about what is allowable and what is not allowed to be said in the consultation
- Notions concerning what practitioners want to hear and what they do not want to know about
- Opinion on the manner in which information should be expressed in a consultation
- Thoughts of the possible implications of revealing or concealing information
- Feelings of security and comfort
- The extent to which the practitioner is sensed to be actually listening and genuinely interested in the patient and her story
- Time: whether the patient feels there is enough time available to express themselves (and whether they have enough time to give to the

consultation, e.g. they may be in a rush to get home or to another engagement)
- The level of trust the patient feels she can place in the practitioner
- The level of ability to communicate: influenced by emotion, inhibition, educational level
- External influences: the opinions of others such as family, friends, colleagues and other healthcare practitioners
- The patient's narrative style and bias
- 'Other things' that are on the patient's mind, displacing focus on the consultation
- The patient's mood and outlook at the particular time
- The extent to which the patient feels well enough and has sufficient energy to fully engage with the consultation.

The practitioner has some influence over some of these factors and, through active awareness of them, may be able to modulate them. A simple preamble to the consultation will go a long way, for example:

*'Before we begin let me just say that this is a safe place to talk, we have plenty of time available and I am very interested to know what you really think and feel about your situation'.*

Of course, one can only convey such signals if they are true (i.e. you really do have enough time) and if you mean them – you *really* do want to know the patient's story and are not secretly afraid of 'opening Pandora's box' (or at least not so afraid that it stops you trying). A simple strategy like this will only wield its power if the patient believes you and this will only happen if the statement is genuine. Patient's know when they are being sold a line and trust is diminished when they feel that this is occurring.

The practitioner normally initiates the patient's storytelling by saying something like:

*'So tell me what you would like help with'.*

Or:

*'So how have you been since the last visit?'*

These simple sentences act as catalysts for the construction of a narrative but they also set an orientation for the way the narrative should begin. This capacity can be utilized by the practitioner to direct the patient specifically or minimally. Consider, for example, an opening line in a follow-up visit where the patient had previously consulted regarding headaches:

1. *'So how has your headache been since I last saw you?'*
2. *'So how have you been since I last saw you?'*

These are virtually identical but radically different, since the first directs the patient straight to a targeted narrative and the second leaves an open space for the patient to bring in whatever is most significant for them. Line 1 invites the patient into a restitution narrative, whereas line 2 opens the possibility of a quest narrative. The patient *may* respond similarly to either question but there is a risk of missing valuable new information in scenario 1 since this line may be read by the patient as meaning that you only want to know about the headache and are not interested in any additional symptoms that may have arisen between this visit and the last. In scenario 2, you will get on to asking specifically about the headache if the patient has not already mentioned it but you give an opportunity for additional stories to be told first. It can easily be seen from this example that the practitioner partakes in the construction of the patient's narrative – somewhere along a spectrum from *extensively so* to *minimally so*. The practitioner is not, therefore, merely a witness to an improvised performance on the theme of the patient's autobiography (practitioner-as-audience) rather, she is an active participant in the creation of the story (practitioner-as-ghost-writer).

The practitioner must be aware of her role, power and opportunities in influencing the formation of the patient's narrative on the one hand but equally aware of her interpretation of it on the other. These two strands: narrative formation and narrative interpretation are the key strands of narrative-based medicine.

The practitioner interprets the patient's narrative with regard to a complex and fluctuating combination of her own reference points and influences, including her:

- Personal fund of story models (which include experiences, education, clinical models, etc.)
- Perception of the aims of the consultation and ethical and bureaucratic parameters/constraints
- Personal predicament (energy level, mood, degree of thirst/hunger/satiety, environment, other concerns on her mind, etc.)

So how and when should the interpretive exercise around the patient's narrative be done? Elwyn and Gwyn (1999) commend the use of discourse analysis which they describe as: 'the study of language in context … [which] has its roots in linguistics, sociology and psychology but … is really no more than the examination of the processes of naturally occurring talk'. This is a method of textual analysis which works with detailed transcripts of 'talk' that are written using notation to indicate pauses, breaths taken, intonations, coughs, etc. Some study is required in order to be able to write and read such transcripts, particularly with regard to learning the language of the symbols used for notation. Discourse analysis can reveal the signals that patient and practitioner give to each other, not only in the words spoken but by pausing, coughing, etc. Practitioner and patient can send signals that indicate their:

- Confusion or insight
- Wish to change the subject or go into more depth
- Desire to emphasize or underplay a point
- Wish to clarify or explain
- Attempt to register that they have been misunderstood
- Wish to make a request.

We tend to think that we notice these things automatically but discourse analysis reveals how much we miss – especially at the subtler end of the spectrum. Working with discourse analysis then can be hugely valuable in enhancing appreciation of what is actually being said in the consultation, what is wanting to be said and what is not being said. This method takes place in connection with written texts and therefore happens after the fact of the consultation. Nevertheless, it can help develop skills that can then be applied during the consultation. This is vital since practitioners do not deal with written texts, they work with living people and the discourse analysis cannot wait until after the consultation if it is to be helpful to specific patients – it must occur while the consultation is happening. We therefore need to practise a form of discourse analysis in action so that, as the concept of reflective practice maintains, the practitioner can conduct reflection *in* practice (during the consultation) as well as reflection *on* practice (after the event). The practitioner's task during the case history, then, is multilevelled and complex since it combines a number of overlapping or simultaneous foci that must be accounted for, comprising considerations given to:

- Analysis of the discourse to do with the patient's and the practitioner's messages and meanings
- Generation and consideration of differential diagnoses
- Reflection on potential treatment options or modulations
- The need for referral or additional strategies.

Although it might be suggested that these four steps be taken sequentially, that only tends to happen at the student or novice practitioner level since one of the hallmarks and necessities of highly skilled practice is the ability to continuously access maps, models and options and to generate and test hypotheses. This is what happens during the case history – this is the heart of it. The key to successful practice in narrative-based medicine lies with the ability to retain primary focus on the patient and what is *actually* being said *while* (and not instead of) reflecting and hypothesizing. Having said this it should also be appreciated that there are crucial moments where the practitioner should give total attention to the patient, consciously suspending all other considerations (as far as that is ever possible).

We tend to think of narratives as linear entities; after all, is it not so that all 'good' stories have a beginning, middle and an end? Patient narratives are not like this, as we observed in the previous chapter – patients generate multiple stories which overlap, intertwine, repeat, dissolve, mutate, conflict with each other, fizzle out, 'go nowhere' and are subject to continual revision. The method of construction of patient narratives is more reminiscent of William Burrough's cut-up technique than that prevailing in the eighteenth century novel. The practitioner working with narrative needs to pick up on cues, make connections, check for meaning and scry for potentials but should be on guard against, and resist the urge, to form the patient's narrative into a neatly comprehensible linear tale, let alone try to match and locate it within any single grand historical narrative. In reading about NBM, one gets the feeling that some authors see it as a new medical utopia. Let us guard against this impulse too. NBM, again, represents just one model that is there to be integrated with a multiplicity of others enabling an increased synergistic dynamic.

Gray (2007) has warned of the dangers of constructing grand unifying narratives in a searing critique of current utopianism and millenarianism:

*The dominant western myths have been historical narratives, and it has become fashionable to view narrative as a basic human need. Humans are tellers of tales, we have come to think, who cannot be happy unless they can see the world as a story ...*

Unhappiness, in persons and peoples, is associated with the lack of a coherent overarching narrative since: 'nothing is more threatening than the idea that (history) is a meandering flux without purpose or direction'. Life does meander and it is constantly in a process of flux – that is the nature of life, of people, of history. The recognition that life is chaotic (meander and flux) does not preclude the search for purpose, direction and meaning, however. The practitioner needs to work with this apparent paradox in the consultation – the navigation of patient's personal chaos is not incompatible with assisting them in their search for personal meaning. The synthesis of chaos and meaning is an old project as Gray recognizes:

*Seeing one's life as an episode in a universal narrative is a fantasy, and while it is supported by powerful western traditions it has not always been regarded as a good thing. Many of the world's mystics have aimed to achieve a state of contemplation in which the succession of happenings from which we construct the story of our lives is absent ... Taoists taught that freedom lies in freeing oneself from personal narratives by identifying with cosmic processes of death and renewal.*

It is difficult to talk in this way because the Taoist concept of transcending the illusion of the separateness of the self by fusing with the immanence of all things gathered together in the one is still an account of how things are, it is still a story, a narrative – albeit one offering a radically different perspective to dominant western views on the nature of existence. Which leads us to question the juxtaposition and relationship between the patient's and the practitioner's stories of 'how things are'. Patient-centred medicine has tended to imply a high degree of passivity on the part of the practitioner, and deference towards the patient (a polar swing from the patriarchal model it reacts against), which would suggest that the practitioner should subdue her own story in order to allow for the patient's to arise. At some point, however, the practitioner's story must come out too – in the form, at the least, of advice on treatment and other remedial strategies and care. Surely, the narrative approach allows for more than this though? If the practitioner is able to gather deep insights into the patient's predicament via appreciation of her stories there must be a correlate duty to sensitively challenge stories that appear counterproductive or harmful and to proffer means towards alternative modes of thought (such as those described in the previous chapter) that are more healthful? It is unacceptable that a clinician merely *hear* stories, there is also a moral requirement to question them and to enable and support change. In doing so the practitioner will be best equipped working dynamically from Upshur's 'domain [that] acknowledges (a) multiplicity of perspectives and meanings' guided by Gendlin's advice to be in our bodies 'in the felt presence of the moment'. A place, in other words, not of grand narratives but one alive with therapeutic possibilities.

## ON HEARING, SPEAKING, MOVING AND RECORDING

The key figures involved in the performance of the consultation are the history-giver (patient) and the history-taker (practitioner). The practitioner is an active co-creator of the case history but she is also an audience for the patient to play to. Practitioner formality and unresponsiveness will constrain the patient's performance, whereas an informal and appreciative manner will encourage the patient to give more of herself. The effect of the practitioner, both as actor and as audience, is partly set by the staging of the clinical environment (set design) and by the practitioner's clothes (costume), grooming and so on, but the key factors, which in a skilled practitioner can transcend any setting, have to do with the way in which she listens, speaks and moves.

The practitioner can help the patient to provide a fluent account of her predicament or contribute towards its lack of fluency or disfluency. As the history takes place, both practitioner and patient are constantly monitoring each other for cues regarding the conduct of their exchange – signals to go ahead, to pause, to clarify, to rephrase, and so on. A key behaviour here has to do with the direction of the practitioner's gaze, which Ruusuvuori (2001) maintains is 'of utmost importance ... as gazing at the speaker constitutes a display of attention by the recipient'. When the practitioner shifts her gaze away from the patient to her notepad, computer or other location, this will tend to trigger disfluency in the patient, since it signals inattention and it is hard to speak coherently to another person when they are perceived to be not listening. In this case the patient's mode of speech falls somewhere in-between the type of speech we use when we talk to another person and the type of 'speech' we use when we formulate thoughts silently within ourselves. In this in-between place, language falls apart due to the lack of a cohering locus – since the speech is not being received by the other person and is not being formed for the self. This is a meaningless place, a void where sense disintegrates and the patient's disfluent vocalizations are calls for re-engaged attention. Patient's halting, broken, disrupted and disconnected speech at these times is both a result of the difficulty of making sense in a non-cohesive void and an attempt to cause the correction of the situation by gaining the practitioner's attention since discordant speech may jar the practitioner into re-hearing.

It becomes immediately important then to consider how note-taking should be performed. The practitioner is caught between two imperatives – hearing the patient's account and recording it accurately; these two modes represent 'the patient embodied' and 'the patient inscribed'. Undue emphasis on either of these drivers will work to the detriment of the other. The situation is particularly marked with regard to the most crucial, significant and important moments in the history since these are the points at which the patient's need to be heard and the practitioner's urge to record are simultaneously at their strongest. At these times, especially, the practitioner needs to listen very closely, ideally suspending all note-taking until the crucial moment has concluded, at which juncture it may be both necessary and appropriate to prioritize note-taking and to make space for this by saying, e.g.:

> *'I just want to pause for a few seconds here to make some notes on what we've just discussed, if that's alright?'*

Throughout the history-taking, the balance of attention should lie heavily in the patient's favour, with maximal focus on the patient and minimal focus on recording. The practitioner who can hear the patient most effectively will be the one who has developed subtle skills and strategies in recording the exchanges of the history. Simple and brief notes should be taken discreetly, with the least possible time spent looking away from the patient. With practice, it is possible to write or type brief notes with only the briefest of glances towards the writing medium. Such brief glances away from the patient are useful, since training a continuous gaze on the patient amounts to staring and is unnerving. When more than a brief moment away from the patient is needed to set down the practitioner's observations, thoughts, self-reminders or queries, then a form of words can be used to suspend the history to accommodate a pause. Something like:

*'We've covered a lot of ground and I'd just like to take a few seconds now to jot some notes down before we carry on if that's OK?'*

This strategy, while breaking the continuous flow of the history, may be helpful in allowing the patient time to reflect and gather thoughts together before proceeding. If the practitioner thinks this is desirable she may speak to direct the patient towards this activity:

*'While I'm making a few notes perhaps you would like to just think for a moment about what we've just discussed.'*

The recording medium will generally be either some form of notepad, computer, printed form or combination of these. My preference is to use blank A4 paper to record the history (the same at first appointments and follow-ups), since this represents the most minimal and therefore least invasive intrusion into the patient–practitioner relationship and is the least diverting for the practitioner's gaze. Printed forms with boxes to fill in can suggest to the patient, even if they may only glimpse them, that their narrative is going to be split and contained and amounts to a form of subliminal suggestion. Computers go further in that they can give information as well as record it – this means that the computer can be a source of influence upon the consultation and may amount to being perceived as a 'third person in the room'. This sense is increased, particularly if the practitioner spends a lot of time looking at the computer, and is exacerbated by use of the computer to extract clinical information, work out risk-ratios, print off prescriptions and treatment plans and the like. More subtle messages are also conveyed by factors such as the patient hearing their story being tapped into electronic existence by a noisy keyboard.

If computers occupy a central place in the consultation (i.e. lots of time spent looking at it and typing on it; retrieval of evidence; calculation of risk; searching for data; printing off treatment plans, etc.) as they have come to in mainstream medicine then they can become not only the repository of information but the source of authority. In extremis then, the practitioner becomes a mere intermediary between patient and the computer-recorder-healer. If computers have to be used, then they will have the least detrimental impact on patient–practitioner communication if they are:

- Used minimally
- Glanced at rather than pored over
- Slight in size – a slim laptop is better than a hulking desktop
- Quiet
- Aesthetically pleasing (beautiful machines are less jarring and anxiety-inducing than ugly ones).

In other words, the use of computers should be as unobtrusive as possible. In phytotherapy practice, it is still possible to avoid the use of computers in taking the history, although some practitioners may want to use them to search databases and find information with or in front of patients, in which case I would recommend locating the computer in a different part of the consulting room if possible and 'going over to the computer' to consult it so that it maintains a peripheral rather than a central place in the consultation.

Direction of gaze is perhaps the most important non-verbal cue at play in history-taking but practitioners need to be aware of others that accompany the gaze. The practitioner who recognizes the potential she has to use her body to aid communication and who is able to use it accordingly will be mores successful in establishing positive relationships with patients. Posture, facial expression, movement and gesture, collectively considered as body language, are all significant. Stillness and motion, movements of hands and arms, composure of lips and eyebrows – all these convey information to the patient, most crucially around whether the practitioner is attending closely and is interested in what the patient has to say. For example, if the gaze is directed to the patient but the body is turned away (either only the head is turned towards the patient, or the head and upper body) this communicates that the practitioner's focus on the patient is only temporary and partial – their primary focus lies elsewhere, somewhere in the line described by the direction of the body. Body position can be looked at in terms relating to the position of three segments (Ruusuvuori 2001):

- Lower body (waist down)
- Upper body (waist to neck)
- Head and neck.

Positioning of the lower body denotes the 'home position', meaning that the direction of the lower body indicates the primary focus of the practitioner's attention, so it should be towards the patient whereas it is often towards the note-taking medium on the desk. Ideally, all body segments should face in the direction of the patient for most of the history – but not rigidly so. Some degree of movement, turning to reach a glass of water for instance, is useful to modulate the intensity of the direction of focus, just as shifting the gaze avoids turning into staring at the patient. Twisting of the body from the home position is said to generate 'body-torque' which is a state of physical tension arising from conflicts in attention (e.g. the practitioner's lower body points to the desk and their upper body and head point to the patient, showing movement in two separate directions of attention) which, if maintained more than briefly, communicate both the practitioner's physical state of tension and mental state of inattention to the patient. Ruusuvuori found that if the practitioner's home position was directed at the patient, then movements of gaze away from the patient resulted in less disfluency on the part of the patient than when both home position and gaze were directed away.

The practitioner's body is not used in the same way, and listening and speaking are not done in the same way, as happens outside of the consultation. A greater level of attention and intensity is applied to awareness and use of these capacities within the consultation. The patient is attended to more closely and more care is taken to avoid misunderstanding the patient than occurs in everyday discourse. Yet the practitioner, in acting out her role, must retain qualities of naturalness and genuineness. Although the practitioner's performance is contrived it must feel *real*, to both patient *and* practitioner; this occurs easily where the practitioner is truly interested in hearing the patient's story and where time and conditions permit this.

Ruusuvuori (2001) concludes her paper by noting the importance of being able to engage with the patient and warning of the dangers that may accompany inappropriate signals of disengagement made by practitioners, since these could:

> *... be seen as signalling disinterest to the patient's narrative, or even disregard for it ... withdrawal of gaze at moments proposed by the patient as relevant for recipiency, could result in the patient leaving out a particularly important part of his/her symptom description.*

## POSING QUESTIONS AND LISTENING TO REPLIES

> *Listening goes straight to the heart and helps to create empathy. Empathy opens our eyes to let us see what the CT scan has missed. The ear is as important as the eye in medical practice.*
>
> Spiro (1993)

Asking questions of patients infers receiving answers from them, so that talking and listening are dominant mutual occupations during the case history-taking. While it is easy to conceive of formulating questions, it is difficult to imagine formulating listening. Posing questions seems to be a concrete act of work, whereas hearing the response feels less tangible – doesn't it 'just happen?' It is important to appreciate talking and listening as two forms of action, since both are active processes. Listening is not the same as hearing – hearing implies the reception of sound, whereas listening has to do with making sense of the sound, making connections with it and interpreting it. Rogers and Farson (1988) discussed the notion of 'active listening' to make clear that listening is not a passive process. While listening, attention needs to be paid to:

- The words being spoken
- Their superficial and deep meanings
- What is being implied as opposed to what is being said
- How what is said links with what the speaker has said previously
- The speaker's tone, pace of delivery, inflexions, emphases, etc.
- The speaker's body language – posture, movement, gestures.

While all this is going on, the practitioner-as-listener is also *listening for* specific medically and therapy-related information, such as: diagnostic clues, differential possibilities, treatment indicators, evidence of progression or deterioration, etc. Additionally, work will be taking place on formulating the practitioner's response to what the patient is saying and/or generating the next question to be asked.

This is complex and demanding work. One of the greatest challenges to students is to reach the point where they can start to feel some ease in conducting this job of network processing. Until that point is reached, a key task for clinical supervisors is to constantly remind students of what they missed from the patient's response while their 'mind was elsewhere' as the patient was replying to their question. In the early stages of case history-taking, students tend to pose a question, then spend a lot of consciousness on formulating the next one, while trying to hear enough of the patient's first reply to keep up-to-speed. In fact, a type of dichotomous listening is occurring – the student is trying to listen to two voices at the same time, the voice of the patient and their own inner reasoning voice. This results in superficial listening – getting the gist of the patient's reply at best. Later on, with practice, it starts to become possible to 'read between the lines' of what is being said – a sign of the transition to 'deep listening', a notion described by Haskell (2001) as: 'training the ear to hear hidden and unconscious meanings'.

Active, deep, professional listening is demanding and tiring on the listener. There is a limit to how long any of us can sustain operating at this level of intensity. If we work long days and have large case-loads it will be difficult and depleting to continuously maintain the degree of focus that is being described here. Tiredness and deep listening are not compatible. It is important to have time when we are not listening so intently, when we use our other senses more actively or spend time in silence.

In considering the posing of questions, we must first of all be aware of the limitations of answers. Kuriyama (1999) describes these well:

*The truth about people is hard to know. There is much that they will not say, and much of what they say is only partly true. There is also much that people simply cannot say, because they themselves don't know, because many realities defy introspection.*

Questions that go unanswered or that are declined or that are incompletely answered can still yield valuable information however, clarifying which subject areas are sensitive, inaccessible or in need of further exploration. The formulation of questions does not have to be limited by decisions about whether they can be answered, as this can only be discovered by testing them out; by asking them. Routine questions may gather surprising replies, whereas questions that the practitioner thinks might engender profound reflection can be brushed off with a mundane comment. In some cases, the exact formulation of questions matters less than that a warm human regard for the patient is shown and that their plight is heard, witnessed, cared for. At these times, listening and simply being, may be of greater value than speech – listening to, and in, the silence that may accompany, e.g. severe illness or bereavement. Cassell (2004) articulates the mystical potential that exists in the shared humanity this type of listening enables.

*It cannot be said too often that in learning to communicate effectively with the very sick, listening, really listening, is as important as talking. Part of listening is learning to be completely open in the presence of the patient. As though there were a door to the inside of you – to your heart or soul, call it what you will – and you consciously opened it so the patient would flow into you.*

As Cassell says, this type of listening has been called 'sympathetic listening, empathic communication, or empathic attentiveness' – but is it adequate to call this 'listening'? Is this not also 'being', 'loving', 'healing'? Listening has the power to fuse with these capacities in ways that speech cannot. In listening at this level of scope and intensity, what is heard in the environment merges with the inner voices of the practitioner and the patient in ways that speech cannot describe. While there is something transcendental happening in these circumstances, the patient more commonly perceives that the practitioner is listening by noting practitioner behaviour that accompanies, and provides evidence of, listening such as head-nodding; meeting the patient's gaze; moving the eyebrows and other facial expressions such as smiling; posture (e.g. directing the body towards and leaning forward towards the patient); making affirmative sounds like 'mm hmm', 'uh-huh', 'yes'. These all demonstrate attention on the part of the practitioner but also give encouragement to the patient since they convey multiple messages such as: 'I'm really interested in what you have to say'; 'keep going'; 'tell me more'. Such signs of listening tend to arise spontaneously when someone *really* is listening and do not have to be simulated – if the practitioner pays much attention to these behaviours they can appear forced and therefore unconvincing. The best policy is to focus on the listening itself rather than giving the appearance of listening. Absence of these behaviours (e.g. expressionless face, lack of head movement, lack of affirmative sounds), or the presence of opposite behaviour (e.g. turning the body and head away from the patient) is taken as evidence of inattention but may further be interpreted as lack of interest or dismissal.

The ability to listen well will be enhanced by practice at listening in general terms, for example by careful, conscious listening to complex music and to subtle sounds in nature. Regular meditation can help to focus attention and quiet distracting background 'chatter' in the mind. Wide reading of literature including fiction, histories and biographies, including more experimental forms, will help to train narrative fluency and sharpen narrative insight (avoiding exposure to storytelling based on 'cheap production values' will help to prevent dulling it).

Forms of speech such as directions and requests, and other strategies, can be used to facilitate the patient in telling her story, help gain extra detail and to enhance the practitioner's listening. For example the practitioner can:

### Ask for more information

The simplicity of this strategy should not be allowed to obscure its essential importance. The simple act of asking the patient to 'tell more' is one of the most profound and deeply useful questioning techniques.

*'Can you tell me more about your headache?'*

*'Is there anything you would like to add?'*

### Seek clarification

*'Can you tell me what you mean by 'indigestion' – what are you experiencing?'*

### Use echoing (repetition)

The last word, or few words, spoken by the patient are repeated by the practitioner. This method tends to suggest itself when patients end a statement by introducing a new theme that they leave unexplored or when they finish without providing detailed information about a theme. Appropriate use of this technique can subtly encourage the patient to continue their story and provide more detail.

Echoing can be a simple restatement of what the patient has said:

Patient: 'It used to be okay but now I go more frequently'.

Practitioner: 'More frequently'.

Patient: 'That's the biggest problem, I could cope going to the loo five or six times a day but now its, you know, it can be twenty to twenty-five'!

Or, a restatement formed into a question:

Patient: ' ... and then things started to fall apart!'

Practitioner: 'Fall apart?'

Patient: 'Yes, that's when my life started to sound like a blues song – I lost my job and my marriage started to get rocky and then, around that time was when I first had the panic attacks'.

### Share thoughts

Here the practitioner explains why she is asking a particular question, or following a line of questioning, to test how the aim or hypotheses behind it seems to the patient and to elicit further information. This strategy may be particularly helpful if a patient seems to be uncertain in participating in a line of questioning.

*'The reason I'm asking questions about your mood and about stress is that sometimes these things can be associated with psoriasis. How does that idea sound to you?'*

### Summarize

Here the practitioner sums up the situation as she sees it and then checks to see whether the patient agrees that this is a correct version or interpretation of events. This is one of the most useful techniques, since it provides substantial evidence that the practitioner has been listening carefully and is also a potent means of clarifying the patient's situation. It is a way of checking with the patient that the practitioner has understood things accurately and as such may lead to a simple response such as: 'Yes, that's right'. Very often, summaries are considered, by the patient, to be only partially correct or to have left something out, leading to: 'Yes, that's mostly right, but …' – in which case the patient now offers clarification. Occasionally a summary may be met with: 'That's not really it at all, it's more like this …' – in which case new and important information may be offered.

Summaries may begin with phrases such as:

*'So let me see if I've got this right'.*

*'So let me check whether I've understood'.*

And/or end with phrases such as:

*'Is that right?'*

*'Would that describe things accurately?'*

Summaries can be used at any appropriate time during the consultation and with regard to numerous phenomena such as checking for sequencing of events; they can be used strategically in order to bring a patient to reflect on their predicament, simply collecting what the patient has said and offering it back to them for consideration. An example would be a case where a patient is caring too much for other people and not adequately prioritizing themselves. In such an instance the practitioner can use a summary instead of sharing thoughts, such as: 'So I'm thinking that you might be doing too much for other people and not enough to care for yourself. I wonder what you think about that idea?' This is perfectly acceptable and may work very well. In some cases, a summary which implies the same thing to the patient may work more powerfully, such as:

> Practitioner: 'So Julia, let me see if I have this right. You're 72 now and you're feeling very tired at the moment. You are looking after two small grandchildren five days a week; helping your son decorate his flat at the weekends; taking care of a large house and garden without help and you've recently become a school governor. Do I have that right?'
>
> Patient: 'Hmm, well when you put it like that perhaps I'm doing too much'.

The choice of summary points by the practitioner here makes it clear that this is not a neutral overview of the situation – a story line is embedded in the summary which leads to a subtle but potent accusation that the patient feels and responds to. Some skill is obviously needed to strike the right note so that patients know that the deep meaning read between the lines of what the practitioner is saying speaks of the practitioner's love and concern for the patient. The 'right note' here, as in other contexts, depends on a number of factors affecting the delivery of the performance of speech, such as:

- *Intonation, pitch and pace:* the way the voice rises and falls; high and low sounds; softness and harshness; soothing and shrill; slowness and fastness – the huge variety of combinations and gradations in these factors gives rise to the overall 'tone' of the practitioner's voice. Tone is not only about the way the voice sounds but also about what the speaker really means. Words can say one thing while tone implies another. Have you ever said to somebody: 'don't you take that tone with me'?

- *Phrasing:* the types of words and combinations of words that you tend to use
- *Emphasis:* which words are selected to be stressed and which are softened
- *Facility with language:* being able to 'put things into words'
- *Accompanying body language:* gazing at the patient, leaning the body towards them, use of facial expressions, etc.

All these factors can be skilfully combined to transmit a positive message that, beyond the actual words spoken, conveys: love, caring, concern, playfulness, gentle provocation, support, and so on. Alternatively, the message that gets through may be: shock, disapproval, disgust, indifference, disinterest, etc. One can certainly practise different intonations and so on and it helps to be aware of these issues but, again, too much focus on these details can end up with a performance that sounds artificial and unconvincing – or even bizarre! It comes down to this: while a certain amount of facility in modulating behaviour can be attained, the meaning behind words cannot be faked. Genuineness is all – if you really love and care for your patient then your behind-speech messages will tend to reveal this, without you having to focus on this area at all. Similarly, your indifference will be hard to mask.

The summary allows scope for the practitioner to work as a caring trickster, even by offering what are clearly false or parodic summaries in order to point to a situation and to gently and positively provoke a reflective reaction in patients. Trickster methods are rarely discussed in the literature on case history-taking, probably because they are considered to stray into shaky ethical territory, yet practitioners commonly use techniques that could be put into this category. Practitioners may feign a response in order to get a particular effect from a patient: mock surprise ('Oh, *really*?'), play dumb ('I don't know what that is, can you tell me about it?'), act as if they haven't heard ('Sorry, what was that, can you say that again?') – these are all forms of clowning that are regularly used to positive ends, i.e. they are attempts to gain information and clarification.

### Interrupt

Books on communication skills tend to emphasize the importance of letting the patient's story flow and not interrupting it. This is generally very sound advice, yet there are times when interruption is necessary, for example when patients have strayed too far from the point or presented an overwhelming amount of information such that the practitioner needs to pause to take stock. It is important to be confident in making appropriate interruptions in a way that does not upset the patient or upset the flow of the consultation. Body language is used to signal that an interruption is coming, e.g. by leaning further forward, raising a hand with a pause request gesture, opening the mouth as if to speak. Examples of forms of words to explain the interruption include:

- When patients have strayed too far from the point:

    *'Can we just pause there for a moment because I'd like to bring us back to focussing on ...'*

    *'Thank you very much for that but I also wanted to know about ...'*

    *'I'm sorry to break in but I'd really like to turn now to asking you about ...'*

    *'I apologize for interrupting but would it be okay if we shifted to look at ...'.*

- When an overwhelming amount of information is being presented:

    *'I wonder if we can pause for a moment because I just want to check that I've understood things so far ...'.*

## Use silence

Spoken directions, requests and questions may be followed by a period of silence before the patient speaks in return. I say *may* because sometimes, indeed more frequently than we tend to realize, speech overlaps. One party has begun talking as the other is finishing, or even as they are mid-flow. Where there is a silence, it may be brief or long. Long pauses may be useful as they allow time for reflection and formulation, especially where responses are complicated, difficult or profound. Practitioners need to be able to *allow* a silence to extend when appropriate, while reading the patient's body language, e.g. seeing internal struggle represented by facial expressions, body posture, utterances, perhaps tears. If the patient is clearly emotionally perturbed by a question but still seems to be in the act of considering it as opposed to rejecting it, the practitioner should resist the urge to rescue the patient, as sometimes these episodes can represent important breakthrough moments. At these junctures, the practitioner needs to hold the silence with integrity and care reflected in body language and, again, transcendental capacities to do with simply *being there*. Additionally, it may be both appropriate and helpful to say things such as:

*'This is a safe place to feel like this; it's safe to feel your emotions here; take your time; only speak when you are ready; this is important, it's safe to feel this way'.*

These are times of vulnerability and transition and assuring the patient that they are safe can be important to enable them to relax, release and connect with the feelings and thoughts that are coming through. If the patient appears to be on the verge of tears but is holding back this can be seen as teetering on the edge of going with the feelings/thoughts or drawing back from them. A very simple act tends to enable the patient to move into tears (and therefore into release and discovery), this just involves pushing a box of tissues towards the patient and saying: 'there's a tissue here if you need one'.

Once the patient is ready to talk, the practitioner should simply and deeply listen and be aware of the importance and potential that lies in breakthrough moments, being careful not to rush or press the patient. Once such an episode is coming to a close within the consultation, it is often helpful for the practitioner to acknowledge the patient's work and the importance of what has taken place before moving on in order to pay respect to the patient, to set the gains that have been made and to avoid striking a jarring note in making the transition of other topics. Something along the lines of:

> *'Thank you for what's just happened. That felt very important. Are you ready for us to move to discuss other things?'*

Such experiences are common in the practice of phytotherapy since the scope and depth of the phytotherapy approach and the time allowed for its enactment naturally provides opportunities for deep reflection and self-discovery. There is space in the typical phytotherapy consultation for enough silence to conceive deep exploration.

## Use humour and play

Humour and medicine go back a long way. The Latin origin of the word, *humor* refers to 'moisture' (the connection retained today in 'humidity') and was applied to the concept of the four humours (literally, bodily fluids: yellow and black bile, blood and phlegm) in Hippocratic medicine. Since the humours were associated with temperaments (the choleric, melancholic, sanguine and phlegmatic), they described people's personalities, emotions and moods. We still talk of someone being in a good or bad humour, as a remnant of this association. Medicine has long explored the gamut of human emotion and behaviour and all human emotions may arise or be referenced within the consultation. The consulting room represents a theatre of the emotions, just as the surgical theatre is a forum of the physical.

Humorous moments ('funny moments') will spontaneously arise in the consultation and patients and practitioners signal their willingness to use play and humour by 'smiling, twinkling eyes, and exaggerated hand motions or voice inflection' (Greenberg 2003). Laughter is a bit of a give away too … Humour and play will come to the fore more frequently when either patient or practitioner is predisposed to take a humorous view of life, but especially when both are. It is obviously important that humour, when ventured by the practitioner, is appropriate and that its use does not detract from other necessary areas of focus in the consultation – but this is equally true of every activity and behaviour in the consultation. Many of those who comment on humour and medicine, however, especially stress the need to control humour – this is partly because humour has an anarchic capacity that mocks and subverts notions of control. This is one of its most useful potentials – as a liberating and transformative force similar to that of sorrow. It is not uncommon for consultations to contain both laughter and tears; the masks of tragedy and comedy belong on the consulting room wall as much as above the theatre stage.

Humour can cheer, lighten the mood, ease loneliness and suffering, help us cope, keep us going; it can also offend and upset and be used as a means of avoidance. Humour may be used by patients and practitioners to diffuse tension, open up the consultation, enhance therapeutic connections and, sometimes, it may facilitate and accompany a breakthrough moment. Humour can also be used by both parties to signal uneasiness, to draw an exploration to a close, to minimize, reduce and diminish the significance of an issue, to distract and mislead, and to self-deprecate. Penson et al. (2005) consider humour to be a 'high-risk strategy' because of its potential to have adverse effects as well as positive benefits and they caution that 'clinicians should be careful not to initiate humour without a clear lead from the patient, as some patients will view it as hurtful'.

It may sound trivializing to describe the consultation as a place for play, since play is considered as something done for recreation and pleasure – as opposed to a serious and practical occupation. We distinguish between work and play, so it may sound odd to conflate the two. The sense of play that I am suggesting here is two-fold. The first has to do with the fact that there are periods of playfulness in the consultation – where amusing games are played between patient and practitioner, which may also be creative and instructive. These may arise spontaneously or be initiated by the practitioner. An example of the latter may be started as follows:

> Practitioner: 'If I could prescribe anything in the world for you – a holiday, a partner, a house – anything at all, what would it be?'

The idea of this game is to provide a play space where the patient can fantasize about their wishes, hopes and desires. In doing so, something might be learnt about these aspects of the patient and about their priorities.

The second sense of play begins with an appreciation of the origin of the word 'play' from Anglo-Saxon *plega* meaning 'singing or dancing gestures, clapping, quick movements' and Indo-European *plegan* meaning 'to risk, chance, expose oneself to hazard' (Ackerman 1999). This sense of play matches well with the performance of the consultation and of the history-taking especially – a dance with the patient where one is exposed to risk and hazard; this fits well with more serious, challenging or complex cases particularly. Which leads us to an end described by Ackerman (1999) as 'deep play' which:

> ... arises in such moments of intense enjoyment, focus, control, creativity, timelessness, confidence, volition, lack of self-awareness (hence transcendence), while doing things intrinsically worthwhile, rewarding for their own sake, following certain rules ... on a limited playing field.

## Questioning style

Medicine is seen as a vocation rather than a 'job'; it is something more than work and it can extend to include play. People who love their occupations sometimes say 'my work *is* my play' and this is how it can be for phytotherapists and other healthcare practitioners. There are dangers in this – the ability to find a self or a life outside of one's work can be lost and this situation has to be guarded against (see Appendix 2, on Self care) – but it is also a privilege.

The practitioner has a great degree of control over the way the consultation will play out depending on the way she poses questions. The aim in phytotherapy is to facilitate the patient in expressing herself regarding her predicament to the fullest extent possible. This necessitates a questioning style that is expansive and enabling. Key factors to consider in working in this way are covered below.

### Keep questions separate

Only ask one question at a time. The following represents a poorly focussed question in that it runs several separate questions together. How many separate questions could you make from this one 'question'?

> Practitioner: 'So I'm wondering how all this started. Things like what was going on in your life at the time, what you felt at first, what you thought was the problem and what treatments you tried. Okay?'

This question is actually a statement followed by a very brief question. Its literal meaning is something like: 'This is what I'm thinking. Is it okay with you if I think these things?' It is not actually an invitation for the patient to respond to any of the elements contained within the statement. Patients will, nonetheless, try and help the practitioner out and answer what they think the practitioner really meant rather than what was actually said. The potential for confusion and the undermining of confidence in the practitioner is large.

### Keep questions simple and clear

Frame questions so that they are simply (but not inelegantly) and clearly (but not patronizingly so) stated. This does not mean that they should necessarily be short – some questions will need to be longer than others – but economy should be aimed for.

### Proceed from open to closed questioning

Open questions provide a broad opportunity for the patient to select the information that she thinks is important and to talk about it in her own words. They also allow space for the provision of information that is surprising or unexpected by the practitioner. An example is:

> 'Tell me about your periods'.

A less open, more specific question would be:

> 'How often do you have your period?'

A highly specific, closed question would be:

> 'Does your period come every 28 days?'

The first question allows for a wide range of possible answers. The second narrows things to the timing of the period but still allows for a number of responses on this particular topic. The final, closed, question only permits a 'yes or no' answer. The journey from open to closed questions is one of diminishing possibilities. Each type of question has its place but open questions should be posed first, thereby enabling the patient to decide what is significant or important in the response (i.e. self-directed) rather than being led by the practitioner. If one starts with closed questions this narrows the patient's options and limits the scope of reply so that they are telling a story structured by the practitioner rather than one that is self-created (or rather as self-created as possible since even open questions point in a direction that is set by the practitioner).

Patients will tend to supply specific information in response to open questions but in a manner, order and language of their own. If the patient does not provide all the specifics that the practitioner wants, then a less open question can be posed followed by a closed one if necessary. For example:

Practitioner: 'Can you tell me about your periods?'

Patient: 'They're pretty straightforward really. Normal. Pain on the first day. A bit bloated. First couple of days are heavy, then it trails off. They've never really been a problem'.

Practitioner: 'So how often do you have your period?'

Patient: 'Normal I think. About every month. I don't really count'.

Practitioner: 'Every 28 days or so?'

Patient: 'I'd say 28 to 30'.

In this example, the patient provides a lot of information and the practitioner then focuses on a particular element that she wants to know more about. Note here however that the final closed question still allows some room for adaptation, which the patient takes by modulating 28 days to 30 days.

The process of moving from open to closed questions is known as a *funnel sequence* (Fig. 5.1) or an *open-to-closed-cone,* since it begins with a broad range

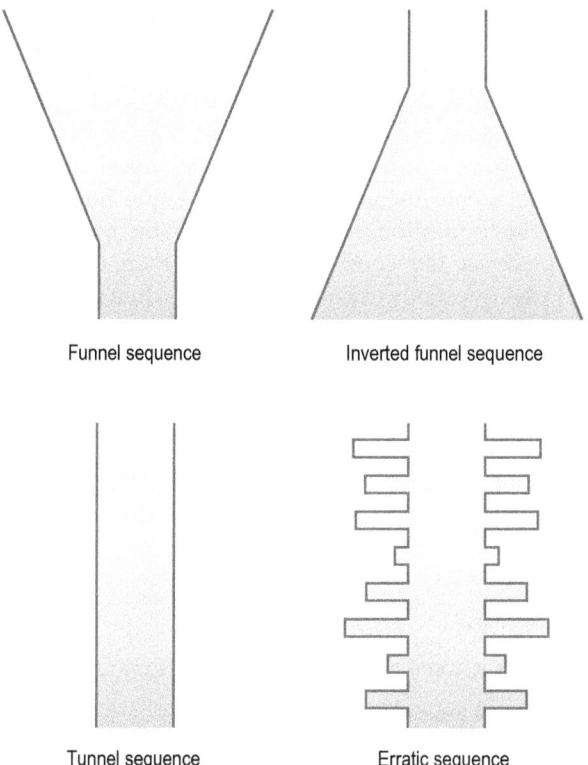

**Figure 5.1** Types of questioning sequence. *(Reproduced from Hargie et al. 1994, with permission.)*

of possible answers (represented by the wide end of a funnel/cone) and ends with a greatly restricted number of possibilities (the narrow end of the funnel/cone).

The opposite line of questioning is called an *inverted funnel sequence,* where one begins with a closed question and then proceeds to more open ones. This structure may occur in the consultation when the patient has presented a specific piece of information that the practitioner then seeks to contextualize and appreciate from a broader perspective. So here we start with a 'closed statement', as it were, from the patient, which leads to increasingly open questions from the practitioner. An example would be:

Patient: 'Another problem is my cycle. It comes every 36 days'.

Practitioner: 'How long has it been like that?'

Patient: 'For the last year or so'.

Practitioner: 'And how was it before then?'

Patient: 'Fine, no problems'.

Practitioner: 'So what do you think has caused this change?'

Patient: 'I'm really not sure. It just seemed to change'.

Practitioner: 'Okay. So tell me more about your periods'.

Another type of questioning sequence is known as the *tunnel sequence.* Here all the questions are of the same type – closed or nearly closed. Such a sequence only permits short answers from respondents (typically yes/no) and is used, e.g. by lawyers in court 'when they wish to direct a witness along a predetermined set of answers' (Hargie et al. 1994). Such questioning can be intimidating and unsettling and is often used deliberately to lead the respondent to a conclusion desired by the questioner or to catch the respondent out. Such questioning techniques are the means of interrogators and have no place in the consultation other than occasionally in short sequences of closed questions to help the patient when they are unclear what to say. For example:

Practitioner: 'Tell me about how your pain feels to you'.

Patient: 'Well it's just pain'.

Practitioner: 'I mean, is it hot or cold for instance?'

Patient: 'Neither really'.

Practitioner: 'Is it sharp or dull?'

Patient: 'Kind of sharp'.

Practitioner: 'Does it come in bouts or last for long periods?'

Patient: 'It's there all the time'.

Practitioner: 'Is it better in the morning or the evening?'

Patient: 'Evening'.

Even here the tendency for such questioning to be claustrophobic and intimidating should be noted and the practitioner above might have found alternative, more open ways, to ask her questions.

Regrettably, students are often taught tunnel sequencing when they learn the theory of how to explore a condition, and then have to discover open-to-closed questioning when in the training clinic. The following is what I mean by tunnel sequencing in this case:

- 'When did it start?'
- 'Where did it start?'
- 'How did it start?'
- 'What makes it better?'
- 'What makes it worse?'
- 'Where does it radiate to?'
- 'How has it been treated?'

A fourth type of questioning structure is the *erratic sequence* where the types of questions are varied rapidly and without a gradual flow or logical process. Such a technique is, again, used in interrogations – designed to confuse, disorientate and wrong foot the respondent. This type of questioning has no place in the consultation but often occurs in the early stages of student practice where there is a tendency to jump between open and closed questions erratically.

## Avoid leading questions

Leading questions are ones that direct the patient to answer in a way that is expected by the practitioner. Leading is generally undesirable in the consultation, as it diminishes the patient's autonomy, disables them from telling their own story, may yield misleading results and risks the omission of important information. Some types of leading question are also aggressively coercive. Although the practitioner cannot help playing a role in the formation of the patient's narrative that role should be as minimal as possible. Reliance on leading questions represents a maximal intervention in forming the patient's story and leads to the corruption or destruction of the patient's narrative. There are four types of leading questions: conversational leads; simple leads; implication leads; subtle leads (Hargie et al. 1994).

### Conversational leads

These tend to occur in social situations and include such examples as: 'It's bitterly cold today, isn't it?' The questioner expects the respondent to agree with her. Questions such as these engage the other person in conversation and help to foster relationships and social cohesion. The nature of these questions is usually uncontroversial and are easy for the respondent to 'go along with'. Practitioners may use conversational leads while greeting and settling the patient before beginning the consultation as such.

### Simple leads

These questions expect a particular response and tell the respondent what that response should be. The expected response may not be the one that the respondent would have freely given though, so that the respondent may feel under pressure to give an answer that they do not agree with, rather than risk causing 'a scene'. Simple leads are coercive in nature, tend to be judgemental and lead to unreliable answers and should therefore normally be avoided in the consultation. An example would be:

> 'Now I expect you exercise regularly, don't you?'

### Implication leads (also known as complicated leads)

This type of leading question puts the respondent under greater pressure than that applied by the simple lead. They direct the respondent to the expected answer but they also imply a negative judgement about the respondent if the respondent disagrees with the expected answer. There is no place for this type of questioning in the consultation. This type of question may be deliberately employed by politicians, for example. An illustration of this type of question is:

> 'Parents who really want the best for their children make the effort to ensure that they eat organic food, so I'm sure you'll make the effort for your child won't you?'

### Subtle leads (also known as directional questions)

These questions may not appear to be leading in nature at first sight and they may be posed unawares, with no intention to mislead. Nevertheless, they may direct the respondent to a particular type of answer. (Subtle leads can be, and are, used intentionally by some lawyers and police interrogators.)

Hargie et al. (1994) cited a study that purported to be conducting market research on headache products but was actually assessing the responses to two slightly different questions: 'Do you get headaches frequently, and if so, how often?' and 'Do you get headaches occasionally, and if so, how often?' The respondents in the 'frequently' group reported three times as many headaches per week than the respondents in the 'occasionally' group. Practitioners need to be particularly aware of their capacity to influence patient's responses by their choice of words.

### Non-verbal questions

Sometimes it is possible to ask questions without using words. For example, if the practitioner responds to a statement with a reaction of surprise or playful disbelief, the patient will read this as a request to justify their statement or provide further explanation.

## THE CONSULTATION ENVIRONMENT

Helman (2000) discusses two forms of context in which practitioner–patient relationships take place, and which influence the relationship:

- An *internal context* of the prior experience, expectations, cultural assumptions, explanatory models and prejudices (based on social, gender, religious or racial criteria) that each party brings to the encounter

- An *external context*, which includes the actual setting in which the encounter takes place ... and the wider social influences acting upon the two parties.

The setting of the clinical encounter in phytotherapy will normally be a consulting room in a CAM clinic of some type, or in the practitioner's or patient's home. Phytotherapists in the UK rarely work in medical environments such as GP surgeries or hospital-associated locations, although some do and more are likely to in the future. Phytotherapy consultations may take place in a number of other environments such as prisons. Whatever the setting, Helman (2000) directs us to become aware of the potency of symbols and what they communicate. Symbols include 'certain standardized objects, clothing, movements, gestures, words, sounds, songs, music and scents used in rituals, as well as the fixed order in which they appear'. Rituals are enacted in all forms of medical encounter and treatment – the consultation is one of them. Rituals are 'aggregates' of a number of symbols, with each symbol acting as a 'storage unit' containing and conveying information about 'values, norms, beliefs, sentiments, social roles and relationships'. Consulting environments tend to be laden with symbolic objects such as medical equipment, books, framed certificates, etc. Extremely loaded consulting rooms will have the potential to overwhelm and disconcert some patients and it is preferable that consulting spaces are uncluttered. Excessively clinical and excessively 'personal' spaces will tend to be off-putting and distracting.

It is worth sitting in your consulting room and asking what the symbols within it have to 'say'. The information they communicate may work for or against providing a setting that is conducive to the therapeutic relationship, although this may vary between patients, depending on how each reads the symbol. Consider what the following symbols on the desk, or on the wall above a consulting room desk (all of which I have seen but not on the same desk and wall I hasten to add!) might mean to different perceivers:

- An anatomical model of a knee
- A large pink crystal
- A set of surgical instruments
- Packs of acupuncture needles
- A dandelion head paperweight
- A human skull
- Chinese meridian charts
- A dream catcher
- Family photographs
- A collection of daggers
- A large, old, homeopathic *materia medica*
- A photograph of the practitioner in gown and mortarboard holding a scroll
- A pile of paperwork
- A large desktop computer
- African masks.

During home visits practitioners have the opportunity to see the patient's symbols and to gather information regarding their living circumstances. This may provide helpful information that is not captured in the clinic-based consult. Home visits place the practitioner in the patient's territory and therefore tend to alter the power balance towards the patient. Performing some physical examinations in the patient's home can require a degree of improvisation!

Basic requirements for a consulting environment that enables the phytotherapy consultation include:

- Natural light source and good but not harsh electric light
- A comfortable ambient temperature – warm enough for the patient to briefly undress to be examined
- Comfortable chairs
- A desk and examination couch
- Quiet
- Uncluttered space
- Neutral décor
- Absence of overtly clinical or 'personal' taste
- Child friendly and child safe.

Given these elements, any difficulties encountered in establishing a therapeutic relationship are unlikely to be significantly influenced by the consulting environment.

## CHILDREN

Keynotes for consultations with children include that they be conducted in a manner that is:

- *Child-centred:* the child is the patient and should remain at the centre of the consultation although it will be essential in all but the oldest children to gain information from key adults
- *Child-friendly:* the practitioner's attitude and conduct should be friendly and caring towards children; the consulting space should be suitable for children – not an intimidating clinical environment
- *Child-safe:* the consulting environment should be safe, especially for very young children.

Not all practitioners will be used to being with children outside of the clinic environment and some may feel awkward or unskilled in the presence of children. It is worth bearing in mind that children, like adults, dislike being patronized, talked down to or ignored and that they will, like adults, respond to warmth, gentleness, genuineness, encouragement and being valued as an individual. It is important never to underestimate children at any age and to bear in mind that, although a familiarity with children's development stages is helpful as a rough framework, there is considerable variation in the rates and ways that children mature. The practitioner needs to be careful with her use and choice of language as children tend to 'take everything in', even though they may not seem old enough to do so or may appear not to be listening.

While much of what is written in this chapter applies equally to children and adults, it is important to remember that children are not mini-adults and that the notion 'child' covers a wide spectrum reflecting distinct development stages at which children's abilities and needs differ. This is a major point and one not recognized in medicine until surprisingly recently as Armstrong (1979) shows (citing Catzel 1955):

> *Until the early years of the National Health Service paediatric teaching had begun 'with the assumption that the child is but a miniature version of the adult ... his diseases were the same as in adults but less severe ... his psychological make-up was similar to that of the adult but more innocent ... and that his treatment is identical except that it is scaled down to size'. (Note: The National Health Service in the UK was founded in 1948.)*

Armstrong relates how the delineation of child development stages was fundamental in providing a rationale to justify the differentness of children from adults and hence the necessity of considering children's health and illness specifically – as a territory not 'worked back' from adults but as deserving of attention and understanding in its own right and according to its own features. This shift was profound since it challenged ideas relating to normalcy in medicine:

> *Growth and development as active on-going processes were not consonant with the static ontology of the disease categories of clinical medicine. The traditional concept of disease was of a discrete pathology intervening in a state of normality ... However, on the basis of their growth and development, disease of children could not be based on a static model of normality: the normal child of three was different from the normal child of ten.*

Normal heart and respiratory rates and biochemical values differ widely and change rapidly especially during the early years of childhood. The child inhabits a dynamically altering body and experiences the world in a qualitatively and quantitatively different way from adults – what are seen as minor perturbations from an adult view can cause brief moments of extreme emotional upset in children; temporal perception is different, with a short period of time in adult eyes representing an eternity to a child. Children are popularly recognized to inhabit periods of change, to be 'going through a phase' and parents may ask 'I wondered if it was just a phase?' There is also a perception that transiting phases of change may be associated with disruption, both physical (e.g. 'growing pains') and psychoemotional ('he's a bit irritable at the moment but I think he's just going through a phase'). As children become older, adult tolerance of manifestations associated with change and development may decrease and even be seen as deviant (e.g. while babies' need for extended periods of sleep in order to enable growth and development is seen as normal, similar extended sleep periods in teenagers is not). As the child is seen to be approaching adulthood they are expected to behave more 'like an adult' but the notion and timing of the movement to adulthood is problematic. One of the little-examined correlates of the increase in longevity in developed countries over recent decades has been the stretching and extension of childhood. A number of other factors have shaped, and are shaping, the concepts of 'child' and 'adult' and the nature and timing of their differentiation, including the lengthening of time spent in 'education' as opposed to 'work'; socioeconomic conditions leading to changes in the ways and ages at which children separate their living space from that of their parents; popular disavowal of the need for adults to 'put away childish things', conveniently linked to the marketing of products and services so that activities previously associated with children (such as the consumption of 'toys') are now approved in adults (one modern stereotype of the adult who remains locked in teenage behaviours is the 'kidult'); and new-age exhortations to remain in touch with one's 'inner child' as a place of spontaneous creativity and unique feeling that remains with one throughout life so that one never ceases to be a child on some 'level'. A combination of the reconceptualizing and repackaging of the ideas 'child' and 'adult' within the context of political, cultural and socioeconomic change has led to an altered perspective on the ultimate defining act of an adult – that of becoming a parent oneself. Those having children at a younger age (late teens–early 20s; an age thought healthy and appropriate to have children until very recent times) may be socially stigmatized as opposed to those having children in their 30s (and beyond). The growing polarization between stigmatization of natural conception at a younger age and social approval of conception (increasingly technologically-aided) at an older age has implications for the children of both sets of parents.

Gill and O'Brien (1998) apply the following terms and figures to the stages of child development:

- Newborn, neonate: first month of life
- Infant: 1 month to 1 year
- Toddler: 1–3 years
- Preschool child: 3–5 years
- Schoolchild: 5–18 years
- Child: 0–18 years
- Adolescent – early: 10–14 years; late: 15–18 years.

By contrast, Swarz (2002) provides the following categorization:

- Newborn, neonate: birth to 1 week
- Infancy: 1 week to 1 year
- Early childhood: 1–5 years
- Late childhood: 6–12 years
- Adolescence: 12–18 years.

Gill and O'Brien's model is partly based on school stages, which vary between countries and are therefore more socioculturally specific than Swarz's, which is both simpler and more widely applicable. In either case there is clearly a very wide range of change occurring in the child between birth and age 18 years.

Children under the age of 16 are required to be accompanied by an adult according to the stipulations of professional bodies of phytotherapists and medical herbalists in the UK. Adults bringing the child to the consultation can include parents, grandparents, guardians and nannies. The dynamics of the accompanying adult/s need to be attended to. If two parents are present at the consultation they may provide helpful synergistic information and corroboration or they may correct and contradict each other – or a combination of the above.

If a grandparent is present alongside a parent, they may be supportive or they may be critical of the parent's account. The person accompanying the child may or may not know the child best; the person who knows the child best is not necessarily the parent (although it usually is) – it will tend to be the person who spends most waking time with the child. This could be a grandparent or nanny. Here, we will refer to the person who accompanies the child to the consultation and who has the most authority to speak on behalf of the child *in the consultation* as the key adult, since, although this is likely to be a parent, it is not necessarily so.

Silverman et al. (2005) describe some of the difficulties associated with working with all the parties involved in the paediatric consultation, an area about which very little research has been conducted, and some of the intricacies of what is required in working with children of different ages:

> *This triadic consultation, in which the doctor has to communicate with both parents and children at the same time, is particularly challenging as all parties will inevitably need individual attention ... Parents tend to interrupt their children ... They may disagree with their child's view of the problem, and it is useful to pick up cues from both parents and children when there is disagreement, particularly if the problem is a behavioural one. With teenagers, you may need to negotiate separate time with both the young person and their parents ... Engaging with toddlers and infants requires special skills, as they are naturally fearful of new environments and strangers. Older pre-adolescents can be very 'private' and self-conscious, and teenagers even more so.*

With very young children or children who are reluctant to speak, the history should be taken from the key adult in the same general ways as described above – working from open to closed questions, etc. Children from around the age of 5 years are usually able to give a large degree of their own case history with the key accompanying adult providing detail, corroboration and alternative perspectives. Younger children are able to add comments and these should be attended to. It is desirable to ask questions first of the child and then of the key adult, but only if the child is comfortable with this; if not, then the key adult should be questioned, drawing in the child as he shows interest and willingness to be involved. The manner in which you would like to conduct the consultation needs to be explained and set up before it begins, since the key adult will often expect to speak for the child unless directed otherwise. The subject can be broached in a form of words such as:

> *'What I'd like to do, if it's okay with both of you, is to ask most of my questions to Jack first and then get mum to add to what Jack says. Does that sound okay?'*

In order to facilitate working in this way, it is helpful to place the child in the priority chair (i.e. the 'patient's chair') with the key adult sitting next to the child but to one side of the practitioner's body direction (i.e. the home position should be directed at the child). The practitioner may need to adjust the home position between the child and the key adult as appropriate during the consultation. It is important to be relaxed and flexible in conducting child consults and to be willing to change the consultation if a child suddenly ceases to be interested in responding to questions for instance. Depending on age and preference the consultation may be taken with the child sitting on the key adult's lap, sitting on a chair, playing in the room, going in and out of the room – and a combination of these may occur during a given consultation. For example, a young child may begin giving a history sitting in a chair, then go and sit on mum's lap for a cuddle, then play in the room for a bit, then go out of the room for a while with another adult or older sibling, then come back – many permutations are possible! The practitioner needs to balance being flexible in going with the flow and ensuring that the information required is gathered. It may be desirable if possible for the child to leave the room with another adult (or on their own in the case of an older child) at some point/s in the consultation, so that sensitive issues can be discussed with the key adult without the child overhearing. Some subtlety and skill may be required on the part of the practitioner in managing this. Depending on the number of people in the room, their relationships (e.g. siblings tend to bicker with each other) and the degree of to-ing and fro-ing that goes on (e.g. visits to the loo), the consultation experience can be quite chaotic at times and the practitioner may need to gently manage the situation. Sometimes the practitioner may need to intervene to tell a child that a particular behaviour is unacceptable if the key adult has failed to do so – this should always be done carefully and with sensitivity. Timing needs to be tighter in consults involving young children, because if consultations go on for too long children can get bored and irritable, they may present challenging behaviour and adults can become stressed. Having age-appropriate toys and art materials available, and perhaps a small table to play on, will help a lot but only for so long. The key is to allow adequate time to do the job of the consultation well and thoroughly but to avoid stretching things out longer than is necessary. All parties concerned tend to appreciate time-efficiency in paediatric consultations.

Swarz (2002) has 'two simple rules in asking questions of children':

1. Don't ask too many questions too quickly.
2. Use simple language.

He observes that: 'Interviewers are often amazed by how well a child can respond to questions phrased according to these rules'. Children are sensitive to the practitioner's voice so that attention should be paid to talking calmly and soothingly.

Gill and O'Brien (1998) provide the following key points in child consultations:

- Mother is right until proved otherwise
- A good opening question is simply: 'Tell me about your baby/child'
- Things not to do:
  - Do not get the sex of the child wrong
  - Never refer to the child as 'it'
  - Do not speak derogatively in front of children
  - Do not use potentially worrying terms without explaining them
  - Do not misjudge the child's age – children are remarkably sensitive on this score
  - Do not disrespect the child's intrinsic modesty.

- Play with younger children as you work, tips for interaction include:
  - Tickle babies (tickles appear at 3 months)
  - Play peek-a-boo
  - Blow raspberries at babies
  - Blow on their faces ('they quite like this')
  - Give infants something to hold
  - Talk nonsense/rubbish to young children – 'they've quite a good sense of humour and may think you're a likeable idiot'!

Additional notes on child case history-taking:

- As with adults, children communicate in ways other than with words – be sensitive to non-verbal communication (e.g. facial expressions, noises such as crying, behaviour)
- When taking a case from a child you are inevitably exploring the whole family – to varying extents
- Be aware of the limits to your competence in dealing with family problems and psychological issues in children's disorders – refer to a family counsellor if appropriate
- Obtain both the child's and the key adult's perspective on each issue – starting with the child where possible then turning to the adult
- Open-to-closed questioning (as for adults) works well with older children but very young children may be unable or unwilling to provide responses to open questions, in which case closed questioning with options should be used – keeping options to a minimum to avoid confusion
- Plain and simple language should be used with younger children (but avoid patronizing), whereas older children can understand and use more sophisticated language. Bear in mind the wide range of individual differences, e.g. some 3-year-olds can be remarkably articulate
- Routine questions may include (depending on the child's age):
  - The mother's experience of being pregnant with the child (asked of the mother)
  - The labour and delivery and immediate postnatal experience of the mother
  - Early feeding – breastfed or otherwise
  - Who lives at home and what the relationships are
  - Previous childhood illness
  - Family history
  - Temperament of the child (ask of the key adult)
  - Mood, outlook
  - Response to illness (e.g. cold or hot picture)
  - Sleep
  - Appetite
  - Digestion
  - Diet – in detail
  - Allergies, sensitivities, intolerances
  - Drug history
  - Vaccination

- Whether anybody at home smokes
- Relationships – with parents, siblings, friends, at school, etc.
• Bear in mind that children (especially older children) may be reluctant to tell you certain things in front of their parents (e.g. regarding boyfriends/girlfriends, sexual activity, drug and alcohol use). It may be appropriate to negotiate spending some of the consultation talking to the child alone as the adult/s wait outside
• It is essential to be aware of the ways in which children may be abused and the evidence that suggests abuse, and to know how to proceed if you have suspicions (see Appendix 3).

## THE OLDER PATIENT

The notion of 'old' represents a concept in flux in countries where people are living longer. Retirement from employment used to label the movement into 'old age' (a socioeconomic definition) but this cannot hold in the light of changing expectations around ageing on the one hand and slippage around the notion of retirement on the other. On more solid ground, the fact of one's chronological age may not be in dispute but what the attainment of a particular age signifies is. Thoughts around what one should and should not do, and be capable of, at various ages are open to question. Chronological age, then, becomes a background detail that pales in significance compared with one's psychological age ('you're as old as you feel'; 'young mind, young body') and biological age (the state of the physical body determined by diet, exercise, smoking, alcohol, etc.). Alongside these perspectives, we have the idea of one's pathological age – as diagnosed by doctors ('you're as old as your arteries') and new scientific twists on one's potential age according to new readings of evolution and genetics, for example, so that the gerontologist and Reith lecturer, Tom Kirkwood (2001), can write:

> When we understand that we age because our ancestral genes programmed our survival but placed a limited priority on long-term maintenance and repair, we get some rather clear insights into the processes that lead to the frailty and illnesses of old age. The first and most encouraging message is that as soon as we recognise that we are programmed not to die, but to survive, we can see that the ageing process is malleable.

Ageing becomes a plastic thing that shifts from inevitable event to negotiable process – to the extent that some authors (e.g. Vijg & Campisis 2008) start to talk about 'a cure for ageing' (or more accurately, they re-engage with an ancient quest for the elixir of youth). A 'cure' presupposes a 'disease' of course as ageing is recast as a problem of pathology for science and medicine to solve as opposed to a natural part of human existence. The desire for a cure for ageing is partly about wishing to be healthier for longer and hence to maximize our enjoyment of our later years and reduce the infirmity and discomfort associated with old age, but it also provides a commentary on an attitude towards death. In the secular culture of science, the self is limited to a single finite incarnation so that it becomes imperative to preserve and extend the lifespan of the body. In extremis, the scientific urge begins to approximate the religious one, with the belief in everlasting life transposed from the spirit to the flesh. Where the inevitability of death is accepted, there remains a modern expectation that the final stages of ageing and dying will be managed so that they are comfortable and brief. Ironically, however, as a consequence of the prioritization of life and the enhanced technological ability to maintain it, the modern dying stage is often now longer, and longer-suffering, than it has ever been before.

For many people, the ideal death would be one that happens without a prolonged period of decline preceding it and free from pain: 'when the time comes I'd just like to go peacefully in my sleep' (is this an ancient wish or a vision made possible by the invention of anaesthesia?); 'I'd like to be well one day and gone the next' – such an abrupt death has the nature of an over-whelming traumatic event however, and these are generally far from peace-ful; for example a fatal myocardial infarction, car accident or being shot. Gentler deaths imply a period of diminishing bodily capacities gradually accumulating to an end-point.

Old age does not have to be seen as a transition phase (either toward death and salvation, or death and oblivion), it can be viewed as an important and integral period of existence in its own right – with its own particular qualities and characteristics, challenges and rewards. It is also a time of risk and uncertainty but such periods bring with them the potential for new insights and breakthroughs about our lives and their meaning, as Kleinman (2006) contends:

> We tend to think of dangers and uncertainties as anomalies in the continuum of life, or irruptions of unpredictable forces into a largely predictable world. I suggest the contrary: that dangers and uncertainties are an inescapable dimension of life. In fact ... they make life matter. They define what it means to be human.

In working with the older person, the phytotherapist needs to reflect on her own conceptions of, and prejudices about, ageing as well as her thoughts about death and dying. It is important to view old age as a normal life stage and not as an anomaly. Our later years are as fraught with potential as our younger years although the shift is from physical potentials to those arising along the emotional, mental and spiritual axes. The search for the self and for meaning remains in the patient, and remains to be supported by the practitioner.

Older patients have access to extensive narratives, a fund of stories that may need exploration over successive sessions; it may be both difficult and trivializing to attempt to take a 'full case history' in one session. The older patient may tell her stories with reference to a historical period that has features not known and therefore poorly appreciated by the practitioner – in which case clarification should be sought from the patient and/or personal research and reading. She may also speak of a time, and in a manner, that is out-of-step with current sociocultural norms, this may reveal opinions and biases no longer thought acceptable. In such instances the practitioner has to be careful to contextualize comments without reinforcing them.

Other considerations for the case history in the older patient are summa-rized below:

- Older people may experience isolation, loneliness and social exclusion. They may also have suffered much bereavement and other losses.

Remember the importance of human warmth, kindness, empathic listening and bearing witness in helping patients deal with sadness and loss but do not forget practical support and strategies in helping to improve the situation – including services available from other agencies. In dealing with other agencies and generally in seeking improved support the practitioner may become an advocate for the older patient.

- The patient may have impairments of hearing and speech so that it is essential for the practitioner to speak clearly and listen closely.
- Patients may be on multi-drug regimens that pose particular challenges for combining with herbal medicines. A detailed drug history should be obtained.
- Older patients may be accompanied to the consultation by a son or daughter or a friend. The dynamics of the inter-relationships between all those in the consulting room need to be appreciated and worked with but it is imperative to remember that the patient is central.
- Elder abuse does occur; just as with child abuse – it is essential to be aware of the ways in which the elderly may be abused and the evidence that suggests abuse, and to know how to proceed if you have suspicions (see Appendix 3).
- Non-specific symptoms are common and need careful exploration (e.g. 'fatigue'; 'indigestion').
- It is important not to jump too readily to ascribing symptoms to 'old age'.
- Sometimes patients will do this themselves, leading to under-reporting or under-playing of symptoms. Explore and challenge notions of 'that's just because I'm old'.
- Although decline in acuity and efficiency of many functions is common with ageing it is important to attempt to differentiate between a 'normal' diminishment and a pathological one, e.g. between forgetfulness and dementia.
- The experience of certain conditions may not be the same as that felt by younger patients; e.g. urinary tract infections may be free of dysuria but instead cause dizziness, fatigue or weakness. Careful individual assessment is required.

In reflecting on growing older, at the age of 75, the psychologist Carl Rogers (1995) spoke of the importance of engaging with uncertainty, similarly to Kleinman (above):

*I do feel physical deterioration. I notice it in many ways ... This slow deterioration, with various minor disorders of vision, heartbeat, and the like, informs me that the physical portion of what I call 'me' is not going to last forever ... So, I am well aware that I am obviously old. Yet from the inside I'm still the same person in many ways, neither old nor young ... Increasingly, I discover that being alive involves taking a chance, acting on less than certainty, engaging with life. All of this brings change and for me the process of change* is *life. I realize that if I were stable and steady and static, I would be living death. So I accept confusion and uncertainty and fear and emotional highs and lows because they are the price I willingly pay for a flowing, perplexing, exciting life.*

## USING INTUITION

We earlier referred to the use of deep listening when taking the history to help us 'read between the lines,' recognizing that sometimes we seem to immediately and easily grasp what underlies the patient's words. At other times, without consciously thinking about it or knowing how we did it, we suddenly perceive a diagnosis or know what to prescribe. These experiences are examples of intuition in action. Intuition is a slippery concept that can be considered a poor substitute for more 'credible' ways of knowing ('all I had to go on was intuition') or prized as the pinnacle of profound and effective perception. The *Collins English Dictionary* (2000) offers one definition as 'a hunch or unjustified belief', whereas a more accurate description of what it feels like in action would be: the instantaneous perception or understanding of a phenomenon without conscious awareness of the reasoning process that led to it.

Intuition derives from the Latin *intueri* (to gaze upon) and it is indeed implicit within the notion of the clinical gaze: in the history we look, speak, listen and seek to make sense of what is going on. In any given case, some phenomena may make little or no sense, others make sense upon conscious reflection and consideration, while others are immediately clear to us. This latter category is in the realm of the intuitive. Since the process underlying intuition is apparently elusive then, according to scientific rationalism, its conclusions must have the status of dubious knowledge. Yet practitioners seem to easily identify their use of intuition and value its contribution. In a study looking at Canadian family physicians' attitudes towards EBM, Tracy et al. (2003) found that: 'There was overwhelming agreement that intuition plays a vital role in the practice of family medicine. While the definitions varied from one physician to the next, a recurring element was that intuition has its origins in personal clinical experience. Even those participants who ... described themselves as evidence-based practitioners included intuition among the necessary tools for strong clinical decision-making. Indeed, EBM and intuition were perceived as complementary rather than opposing one another'.

Claxton's (2004) appreciation of intuition is particularly insightful and comprehensive and is worth citing at length, especially since he well describes elements of the case history-taking process:

> *Intuition refers to a loose-knit family of 'ways of knowing' which are less articulate and explicit than normal reasoning and discourse. This family has tended to be ignored, marginalized, romanticized or denigrated ... partly because of its historical association with claims for validity that seem grandiose or mystical ... The members of this family include the ability to function fluently and flexibly in complex domains without being able to describe or theorize one's expertise; to extract intricate patterns of information that are embedded in a range of seemingly disparate experiences ... to make subtle and accurate judgements based on experience without accompanying justification; to detect and extract the significance of small, incidental details of a situation that others may overlook ... Intuitions manifest in a variety of different ways: as emotions; as physical sensations; as impulses or attractions towards certain goals or courses of action; as images and fantasies; as faint hunches and inklings; and as aesthetic responses to situations. Intuitions are holistic*

*interpretations of situations based on analogies drawn from a largely unconscious experiential database ... The intuitive mental modes are not subversive of or antagonistic to more explicit, verbal, conscious ways of knowing; they complement and interact productively with them. People vary in their facility with intuition, their willingness to trust it, and in their ability to create both the inner and outer conditions which are conducive to it.*

Claxton sounds a warning, however, that intuition might 'also incorporate assumptions or beliefs that may be invalid or inappropriate' so that 'intuitions are instructive but fallible hypotheses which are valuable when taken as such'.

Commenting on Claxton, Eraut (2004) compares judgement as a 'deliberative process which draws mainly on explicit knowledge', with rapid decision-making as a 'largely intuitive process which draws almost entirely on tacit knowledge. Some of that tacit knowledge may be easily made explicit on later reflection, some with considerable difficulty and some not at all'. One of the great rewards for practitioners teaching clinical skills or having students observe them at work is that questioning from students helps to identify which types of activity fall into these three categories: the ones that are easy to instantly explain; the ones that take considerable effort to do so (but which one learns from immensely in the process of trying) and the ones that remain hard to pin down (which may be even more instructive in the long run). Eraut is helpful in describing the factors that enable rapid decision-making as 'first, the rapid reading of the situation with the aid of prior knowledge, and then, second, the rapid linkage of that situational understanding with an immediate course of action, using prior knowledge that has worked before and possibly adjusting it to take quickly recognized situational difference into account'. Intuition then, at least in the context of rapid decision-making, does not come from nowhere, it is grounded in and arises from the painstaking acquisition of knowledge and experience over years of living, studying and practising. As knowledge is gained and refined through testing, the practitioner is increasingly able to bypass previous conscious step-by-step plodding through the chains of association and is instead able to penetrate straight to the heart of the matter. The hard work pays off as processes that have previously, on multiple occasions, been laboriously thought-through are now internalized to the point of *simply happening*.

Eraut also refers to the involvement in assessment of 'metacognitive control of one's attention', which he illustrates by providing the example of a person 'picking up key features of a text when skim-reading, sensing which references to follow up and which to ignore when reading a journal article'. This involves the recognition of key words, phrases, patterns, juxtapositions and we can see how this easily transfers to the consultation where such recognition applies to stories, symptoms, behaviours, etc.

Several authors writing about intuition refer to Polanyi's notion of 'tacit knowledge'; Eraut (2004) defines it as 'knowledge (that) cannot be described or explained'. Gourlay (2003) correctly, in my view, points out that Polanyi has been largely misunderstood and, although he used the term 'tacit knowledge' he more frequently used, and *meant* 'tacit knowing' – the distinction being an important one in that 'knowledge' refers to a thing one possesses whereas 'knowing' indicates a process. It is worth going into this, since Gourlay's description of tacit knowing (drawing on various texts by Polanyi) beautifully describes the process of case history-taking, and it introduces an important related activity – imagination:

> *Tacit knowing, the 'power of perceiving coherence' among 'thousands of clues', is a 'fundamental power of the mind' whereby coherence is constructed and maintained by a 'mechanism of imagination-cum-intuition'.*

Gourlay argues that Polanyi was not interested so much in knowledge as a product as in the 'integrative process'. Phytotherapists must be interested in both the process and the products of the process such as diagnoses, prescriptions, advice and treatment plans so that practising results in concrete action. Intuition is a powerful means to arrive at such action when supplemented by imagination, which provides a creative dimension – imaginatively perceiving the connections that might exist between phenomena and constructing strategies so that these can then be tested.

Recommendations for developing intuition tend to refer to the central role of experience, e.g. Hogarth (2001):

> *I emphasize that intuition is largely the fruit of experience. Thus, in order to educate intuition, it is important to emphasize what you learn from experience and how you learn.*

Reflective practice would seem to be the most powerful and appropriate *how* for practitioners to use to tease and squeeze the maximum *what* from clinical experience. One becomes more intuitive the more one experiences, connects and learns. The most intuitive practitioner will be the one with the broadest frame of reference, the greatest diversity of interests, and the deepest and widest range of experience, combined with a synthetic and integrative propensity and well-honed critical faculties.

In ending this part of the chapter, let us mention three quotes attributed to Dr Johnson, which summarize the key ideas around intuition extremely well:

> *It is wonderful when a calculation is made, how little the mind is actually employed in the discharge of any profession.*

> *What we hope ever to do with ease, we must learn first to do with diligence.*

> *Those who attain to any excellence commonly spend life in some single pursuit, for excellence is not often gained upon easier terms.*

## ASSESSING THE FOUR ASPECTS OF BEING

In attempting to view the patient holistically and synthetically, we can propose the consideration, during history-taking, of four key overlapping and intermingling aspects, or realms, of being: the physical, emotional, mental and spiritual. It is artificial to separate these modes of being since they interpenetrate each other but, nonetheless, working with them as concepts can help to guide and inform practice. *As concepts,* each of these four aspects of being represent areas of contested knowledge, including (fundamentally), with regard to their location: the physical is identified with the substance of the body (i.e. it *is* the body); the emotional and mental aspects exist somewhere *within* the body; and the spiritual may be seen as somehow *infusing* the body but *extending* beyond it or entering it from without.

Seen from the perspective of a materialist culture, the physical is the least contentious of the four aspects, since it is the most tangible. The mental aspect is also credible, since it is associated with a physical organ – the brain. Yet mental activity (and the concept of 'mind') is elusive, since it does not necessarily 'feel' like it is located in the brain and mental activity is often seen as something that is extracted or abstracted from the body. Emotions are accepted phenomena but, while viewed as perturbations of the nervous system, their extension into the matter of the body can be so complete, and so deeply felt, that it is difficult to separate the physical body from the emotional body. The intangibility of the spiritual aspect contributes to rendering it the most contentious and the most suspect of the four aspects. Is what people term 'spiritual' no more than a mental construct – a way of mentally perceiving and interpreting the world as opposed to an 'entity'? If so, and if the foregoing also holds, then the body has only one concrete aspect – that of the physical body itself – but within the body the physical brain and nervous system generate and sense what we denote as mental, emotional and spiritual phenomena. This is a profane view of the body, distinct from the body known within the sacred worldview.

In his classic study on the nature of religion, Eliade (1959) distinguished between the way that the world is perceived in sacred and profane cultures. The sacred pertains in indigenous cultures, whereas the profane describes the modern secular worldview. The sacred world is pervaded by an awe-inspiring mystery (*mysterium tremendum*); an immanence that may be apprehended in hierophanies – moments when 'something sacred shows itself to us'. An 'abyss' of mutual incomprehension divides the sacred and profane worlds:

> For modern consciousness, a physiological act – eating, sex, and so on – is in sum only an organic phenomenon ... But for the primitive [sic], such an act is never simply physiological; it is, or can become, a sacrament, that is, a communion with the sacred.

In the sacred world, the person's dwelling is constructed as a microcosm so that it connects with, and shares the nature of, the sacred macrocosm. The same is true of the body so that there is a 'homology (between) house-body-cosmos', such that:

> ... in the last analysis, the body, like the cosmos, is a 'situation', a system of conditioning influences that the individual assumes ... man cosmicizes himself; in other words, he reproduces on the human scale the system of rhythmic and reciprocal conditioning influences that characterizes and constitutes a world, that, in short, defines any universe.

This correspondence and continuity between the person and the world needs to be professed and practised by an entire culture living in a sacred territory in order to attain coherence and power. Once the sacred worldview is separated from the sacred world (e.g. when indigenous people move from their homelands to modern cities) the 'religious experience is no longer open to the cosmos' and becomes 'a strictly private experience'.

Once the body is experienced as a private *thing*, disconnected from the world it inhabits, its physicality as an object is emphasized and becomes its primary defining feature. Mind, emotions and spirit must then be *contained within* the body and this retention inhibits the body's ability to extend out into the cosmos and to receive the cosmos into itself. The word spirit originates in Latin *spirare* 'breathe' and this is apt, since we can see spirituality as a form of respiration that flows between the world and the self, animating and sustaining the sacred. Spirit *moves* between heaven and earth, between individual and environment, but ceases to circulate when the body is withdrawn from nature in the transit from sacrality to profanity (the 'fall from grace with God'). The unity between person and cosmos is evinced in the ancient concept of *pneuma* (a Greek word for 'breath') as applied in Hippocratic medicine, here described by Kuriyama (1999):

> ... the Hippocratic treatise On Breaths *does draw distinctions:* pneuma *inside the body is called breath* (physa); *outside the body it is called air* (aēr); *and the flow of air is wind* (anemos). *But the very point of this work is to affirm the unity of outer and inner* pneuma, *of wind and breath, and to accuse disruptions in its flow as the cause of all disease. At the same time that it describes the afflictions arising from blocked breath within the body, the work waxes eloquent about how* pneuma *fills heaven and earth, brings summer and winter, guides the course of sun and stars.*

Quin (1994) shows how the notions of soul and pneuma as later described by Galen were eventually discarded in medicine, leaving in their place the brain and nervous system.

It is appropriate that herbal practitioners work in the realm of the spiritual since medicinal plants continue to represent, for us, a sign of the sacred nature of the universe. To work with plants is to expose oneself to the potential for hierophanies and to take a herbal medicine into the body can be a sacramental as well as a medicinal act – to partake of the sacred healing nature of the cosmos. Phytotherapy can certainly be practised as a profane science (reconceptualizing 'plants' as 'chemical complexes' and prescribing them in abstracted forms that deviate from their natural origins) and it is this profanity that some herbal practitioners object to. It retains its nature as a sacred art and its capacity to signify and engender sacrality, very simply, when the *actuality* of the plant as a healing life form is left to speak for itself – by which I mean when the patient apprehends the plant as a fact in nature.

Let us return to assert that all people possess physical, emotional, mental and spiritual dimensions and that wellness is engendered and supported when each of these aspects experiences appropriate activity and rest. Throughout the consultation, information can be noted that suggest whether, and to what extent, activity and rest may be taking place in these realms. We can note where there is an excess or deficiency of activity and where there is inadequate rest or lack of use. In doing so, we will soon realize that given activities or practices frequently overlap all four aspects, although they may be thought of as being focussed on one aspect in particular. For example: physical exercise such as swimming is clearly an activity residing in the physical aspect of the body but it may also provide an emotional release, clear the mind and help promote mental clarity, and be experienced as a spiritual at-oneing with the environment – a hierophany.

In assessing individuals with regard to the four aspects, we may find that there is a particular excess or deficiency of activity in one particular direction. For example, a patient may be experiencing an excess of physical or emotional activity/demand (requiring a movement to find rest or relaxation in each of those aspects) together with a deficiency of mental activity (no reflective thinking about the situation) and a lack of spiritual support or framing. In such a case it may be appropriate to recommend ways of aiding physical rest (e.g. taking relaxing baths or having massages); emotional release and relaxation (e.g. having a night out with a friend); mental focus (e.g. setting aside time to think about the current situation and make an action plan); and facilitating the opportunity for spiritual sustenance (such as learning meditation or spending time in nature). It is hard to be anything other than suggestive as regards this way of working since the potential patient predicaments and the number of enabling strategies are equally numerous.

Although everybody has all four aspects of being available to them at all times, a particular patient may be currently focussed primarily on one of them: stuck in an emotional reaction; fixated on physical experience or goals; concentrating on spiritual matters at the expense of the rest of the body; ploughing ahead with a mental decision while failing to take account of feelings. In the presence of such a situation, the practitioner can advise of the need to address other aspects of being and help the patient discover ways of doing so. This approach can be especially helpful in working with patients whose medical condition is not easy to apprehend or define (patients in the complex and chaos zones), since it is always open to consider which of the aspects of being the problem seems to be located within and going through this may suggest remedial strategies.

Although we have stated that many strategies have the potential to work across the four aspects of being, Table 5.1 makes some suggestions regarding those that might be considered to be primarily located in one particular realm.

## THE SIX NON-NATURALS AND THE PRIORITIZATION OF THE INDIVIDUAL

The case history is taken by the practitioner in the context of, and with reference to, her conceptions about which kinds of information are suggestive of health and which might indicate illness – with a particular accent on those that are potentially modifiable since these present treatment opportunities. Specific pieces of such information cluster around focal points that represent the key facets of wellbeing and which inform treatment regimes and preventive strategies. One set of these focal points is contained in the ancient medical concept of the 'six non-naturals' originating with Galen (*c.*CE129–216?). We will consider this as a basis for reflection on the reference points for case history questions because it continues to serve as an interesting model today.

Pormann and Savage-Smith (2007) explain that:

> *The term 'non-natural' was used for those circumstances which a person could in part control, while 'natural' referred to the system of humours, elements, qualities,*

**Table 5.1** *The four aspects of being and related strategies*

| | |
|---|---|
| **Spiritual activity and rest** | Spending time experiencing nature: the sea, woodland, sunset and sunrise, etc.<br>The arts: literature, theatre, music, etc.<br>Time spent talking and being with others.<br>Meditation.<br>Prayer. |
| **Mental activity and rest** | Games such as crosswords, chess.<br>Intellectual discussion and debate.<br>The arts: literature, theatre, music, etc.<br>Studying and educational activities. |
| **Emotional activity and rest** | The arts: literature, theatre, music, etc.<br>Time spent talking and being with others.<br>Conversation while sharing a meal.<br>Sensuality and sexual activity. |
| **Physical activity and rest** | Physical exercise: walking, dancing, swimming, etc.<br>Sensuality and sexual activity.<br>Eating.<br>Massage. |

*and other properties and forces (such as age) at work within the body itself ... humoral theory, combined with the 'six non-naturals', provided the explanatory basis for the cause and nature of illness as well as the theoretical framework within which it was to be treated.*

An additional area, completing a triad of natural-related phenomena, is that of the 'extra-natural things' (sometimes called the 'contra-naturals') which are 'the illnesses, their causes and their symptoms' (Ullmann 1978). 'Natural' things may be considered as relating to physiology; 'extra-natural' things to pathology and 'non-natural' things to health promotion, illness prevention (see Hill Curth 2003) and therapy (although they stand apart from other remedial strategies such as herbal medication). During the consultation, the phytotherapist needs to account for all three of these areas:

- Assessing the state of health as judged against notions of what constitutes normal or desirable function and behaviour
- Estimating whether and to what extent deviance from normative or optimal states of health is shown and the nature of this deviance (i.e. illness/disease)
- What opportunities are there for remediation, optimization and prevention?

The six non-naturals represent the general territories where such opportunities tend to lie and congregate so that, as Ullmann (1978) explains, if they are used: 'quantitatively and qualitatively in the right way and at the right time and in the right order, they preserve the "natural things" in their right condition'. Quantity and quality matter since: 'when a body deviates from the right proportion, a lifestyle must be followed which deviates from the right proportion in the same degree but in the opposite direction'. The lifestyle must therefore be oriented on the principle *'contraria contrariis'*. For example, if a patient is suffering from a lack of sleep it is insufficient for her to take on the amount of sleep that would be appropriate for a person who has a good normal balance between sleeping and waking, rather she must go through a period of time where she has more than the average normal amount of sleep.

The six non-naturals (using Ullmann's phrases) are:

1. 'The air around us': this refers to the air that is breathed (see discussion of *pneuma* above) but can be taken more generally to refer to the environment
2. 'Movement and rest': physical activity, exercise and rest
3. 'Eating and drinking': a primary focus looking at diet in great and subtle detail including the thermal and hydrational qualities of foods and their necessary seasonal variance. Choice of clothing material may also be included here since, like foods, this influences the body temperature
4. 'Sleeping and waking': the importance of sound sleep and the seasonal variation in length of time spent in sleep and wakefulness
5. 'Excretion and retention': the proper manner and degree of bathing, sexual activity and defecation, urination and menstruation
6. 'The soul's moods': This can be described as having to do with the passions or emotions; or the mental state. It is essential to address the emotional/mental state and peace of mind should be sought.

Ullmann concludes of the non-naturals that while: 'The explanations may seem to us naïve, the system may appear to us too scholastic', nonetheless, 'these rules for living are so sensible that they could be broadly accepted by the modern reader'. They were accepted and implemented as the basis for illness prevention, health promotion and illness remediation for over one and a half millennia. Cabre (2008) has pointed out that many of the actual activities relating to the six non-naturals (i.e. the work itself) have tended to fall to women within the domestic sphere: keeping the environment 'pure'; providing nurture in terms of food, clothing, nursing, emotional support, etc. Nutton (1995) describes the continuation of emphasis on the six non-naturals into the sixteenth century:

> *Medieval and Renaissance authors composed their books on diet (or, better, lifestyle … ) to take account of the non-naturals … Their medical counsels* (consilia), *thousands of which survive, mainly from the period after 1300 … dealt in turn with each of the six non-naturals, describing what foods, rest, ambience, evacuations (including one's sex life), exercise, and emotional state would best preserve or restore an individual's health' leading to 'a highly individualised form of therapy.*

Wear (1995) demonstrates that medical advice in the form of regimen based on the six non-naturals was the dominant mode of practice until 'well into the eighteenth century' and did not substantially shift until the 'bacteriological revolution' in the later nineteenth century: 'What was new was the way eighteenth-century medical men joined traditional ideas on health and the environment with a concern to reform the health of populations or groups in society; previously the emphasis was on reforming the health of the individual patient'.

A plethora of factors influenced the shift of focus from the health of the individual to that of groups including: Enlightenment values and ideas about the nature of science and society and how these should be applied to medicine; social problems associated with the Industrial Revolution; work within the social reform movement; population growth, concentration and urbanization; and the message implicit in the appreciation of contagion and the discovery of inoculation that the cause and cure of group diseases could be apprehended without giving consideration to the individual – in fact, by concentrating on the individual one might miss mass trends and the bigger picture of disease.

While public health initiatives may bring benefits to individuals, they are not *individualized* so that healthcare delivery that is based on central directives, standard operating procedures and approved treatment protocols cannot accommodate individuals if it is to hit its target figures for implementation. Medical 'care' based on central planning, which, in turn, is based on a corrupted take on EBM (i.e. one that keeps the 'research evidence' but ditches 'clinical experience' and 'patient values') is anti-individual. Popular and professional medical discourse refers to diseases and conditions as if they were entities in their own right, having an independent existence outside of the individual, recasting all disease in the light of germ theory so that each becomes a micro-organism to be taken on in the 'fight against' cancer, obesity, diabetes, asthma, etc. Real disease affects groups therefore we are all at risk; individual conditions are 'idiosyncratic' and therefore invalid. Fear of mass diseases and the discounting of individual deviances from group disease pictures and themes (i.e. 'classical presentations', or, more accurately, stereotypes) serves to further abstract the personal from the pathological.

There is a need to re-engage with the ancient and longstanding project of focussing on the unique personhood of the patient. Phytotherapists are well placed to give a lead in this renaissance since herbal practice has never completely dispensed with the approach exemplified by the six non-naturals. The retention of focus on the individual (enabled by the exclusion of herbal practitioners from mainstream medicine and therefore form the dictates of central planning) has, despite being considered archaic, ensured the survival of the discipline. There are always a significant number of people who have been inadequately perceived and served by the anonymizing nature of mainstream medicine and who stand in need of being comprehended as individuals. The emphasis in phytotherapy training on the importance of considering and advising on 'diet and lifestyle' provides a modern equivalent to the concepts of 'regimen' and the 'six non-naturals'. Wear (1995) defines regimen as 'the way to lead a healthy life' and providing suggestions and directions on how to do this is an essential part of the phytotherapy approach. The identification of where and how to place and style such advice is largely based on questioning around the territory of the six non-naturals. Such questions (and their equivalents in varying forms) can and should be asked at *every* consultation in order to provide an ongoing assessment of the key individual determinants and parameters of health and wellbeing. Such questions encompass the physical, emotional, mental and spiritual aspects we mentioned previously and concern the following areas of self-estimation by the patient:

- The sense of one's innate vitality accessed by questions such as: 'How does your energy level feel?'
- Mood, emotions, outlook: 'So tell me how you would describe your mood and how you are feeling emotionally'.
- Perception of being stressed: 'Tell me about how you would describe whether you were stressed or not at the moment'.
- Food and drink: 'Can you describe how your diet has been lately? Tell me about your diet'.
- Sleep: 'How has your sleep been?'
- Excretory function: 'How are your bowel movements? How is your digestion? What about passing water? How has your cycle been?'
- Home and work: 'How are things at home? How are things at work?'
- Physical activity: 'So tell me where you are at with exercise and physical activity at the moment'.
- Rest and relaxation: 'What's happening with regard to relaxation and rest right now? Tell me about rest and relaxation in your life'.
- Enjoyment and play: 'Tell me what's fun for you at the moment. What are you enjoying?'
- Prioritizing of the self: 'So what are you doing at the moment for *you*? So where are *you* in all that's going on at the moment?'
- Inspiration and mental stimulation: 'Tell me what's exciting you and inspiring you at the moment? Are you doing anything that is keeping your mind active at the moment?'
- Circulation and respiration: 'How has your temperature been? Have you felt especially hot or cold? How has your chest been? What about your breathing?'
- Immunity: 'Have you had any coughs, colds and so on?'
- Environment: 'How has the home environment been – in terms of things like temperature, noise and so on – anything there affecting you? What about your work environment?'
- Sexual interest/activity: 'How is your libido? How has your interest in sex been? How has sex felt to you? How has sex been?'

This collection of questions, coupled with a detailed exploration of current conditions/symptoms effectively constitutes the follow-up consultation and most of the initial consultation – the only thing to add in the latter case would be a more detailed systems review. I have asked the same individual patients these types of questions, posed in varying order and with slightly different wording, on multiple occasions (in some cases dozens of times) and have never heard an objection to their repetition (in fact if I omit one of them, patients often make a point of reporting on the missed area) and I have never personally perceived them as redundant because they are *perennially relevant*. From visit to visit such questions remain not only valid but *crucial*. Among the most crucial questions are the ones that openly invite the patient to speak of how they *really* feel, of how they are currently experiencing and seeing themselves at the most profound level. These questions are variations on the themes of:

*'So tell me how you are feeling in yourself'.*

*'How would you summarize where you are at; at the moment?'*

*'I would really like to know how you see your situation at this time'.*

Such questions, especially when asked for the first time or at particularly critical moments in the patient's life, frequently bring forth the patient's tears. These are extraordinarily profound questions because they permit the patient to access and to convey their own *felt and embodied reality*. They allow reality and genuine experience (the felt presence of the total body in the moment) to break through the constructs we place around connecting with our own *truth*. But the catch is: these questions only work properly, that is they only fulfil their potential to act as catalysts to the patient's self-perception, discovery, release and growth, if they are asked in the right way. The 'right way' has little to do with the actual form of words used and everything to do with timing and the practitioner's psychoemotional stance surrounding and underlying the action of posing the question – by which I mean that the practitioner must *really*, genuinely want to hear the answer and must *really*, genuinely feel love for the patient (or 'unconditional positive regard', if you prefer). If these qualities are lacking, then the potential for empathetic transcendence will also be absent.

It is also important to be aware that very simple questions may have the same effect when asked of people accompanying patients to consultations; this is especially the case for parents (or 'key adults') bringing children as patients. After finishing taking a child's case, if one turns to the parent and asks: 'So tell me about you, how are *you*?' the question is very commonly met with a deep emotional response that the practitioner does well to anticipate and allow time for.

## HISTORY FORMATS

### OPENING QUESTIONS

The consultation, whether a first visit or a follow-up, is formally initiated by posing the opening question. Foucault (1963) illustrates the shift in perspective between eighteenth-century medicine and modern biomedicine by discussing the change in style of asking this question from 'What is the matter with you?' (eighteenth-century) to 'Where does it hurt?' (modern biomedicine). The former question implies that the patient may have some insight into her own condition which she might be able to express, whereas the latter merely requires the location of the broken part that can then be handed over to the doctor to fix. In the phytotherapy consultation the key aim of the opening question is to empower patients to tell their own story.

The opening question is important since it can be used to enable a holistic exploration of the patient's predicament (or the opposite) and because it signals the way in which you wish to proceed and sets the tone for the rest of the consultation. In doing all this, the opening question can shape and affect further stages, and the eventual outcomes, of the consultation. Gafaranga and Britten (2003) showed evidence to support the assertion that: 'In relation to concordance, or shared decision making more generally … alignment or misalignment between participants will occur before any discussion about treatment options occurs'. The authors demonstrated that opening questions can serve to enable such alignment or to sow the seeds of misalignment.

The phrasing and articulation of the opening question provides information to the patient about whether their expectations are likely to be met or not; whether they can relax and trust the practitioner; what mood or state of mind the practitioner is in; whether the practitioner really wants to hear their story and what type of story they are going to be expected, or allowed, to tell. These perceptions apply at every consultation but are heightened at the first visit where the patient will be particularly sensitive to early cues given by the practitioner.

The overarching 'between-the-lines' message conveyed by the opening question should include the following sub- or co-messages:

- I really want to hear what you have to say.
- I am truly interested in what you have to say.
- I genuinely care about you.
- I am not prejudging you.
- I am poised to listen closely and carefully.
- I am open to hearing anything that you want to say.
- Please relax and take your time.
- It is safe to talk here.
- You can trust me.
- I will do my best to help.
- The floor is yours.

It may be hard to conceive that an opening line can possibly transmit such a wealth of information – but it can. Such a powerful 'message' (or collection of simultaneously articulated co-messages) can only be put across if it represents the genuine, embodied, viewpoint and stance of the practitioner – it cannot be simulated. The conduction and registering of the message can be facilitated and enhanced, however, by appropriate use of verbal and non-verbal activities such as:

- Looking directly at the patient
- Orienting the home position (i.e. the direction of the practitioner's lower body) towards the patient
- Leaning the upper body towards the patient
- Speaking relatively slowly, deeply and clearly
- Holding the gaze on the patient after asking the question
- Using open body language (e.g. keeping arms unfolded and hands unclenched).

Effective opening questions should be worded so that they are clear, open and unambiguous. A number of phrasings are possible and it is important to use or develop ones that suit your personal style. It is important to avoid flippancy (e.g. 'What's up?'); and questions that can easily be misread/misheard or which might suggest sarcastic replies even if these are not voiced (e.g. 'What brought you here today?' can be replied to as 'My car'. 'How can I help?' could engender, 'I don't know, why don't you tell me?'). 'So' can be used to introduce the question; to mark that a question is beginning that is formally starting the consultation. 'So' followed by a short pause can mark the transit from the initial exchange of pleasantries, or checking of personal details, to the actual business of the consultation.

Suggested opening lines for the first consultation include:

'So, tell me what's going on with you?'

'So, tell me what's happening with you?'

'So, tell me what it is that you would like help with?'

'So, tell me about what you would like help with?'

'So, tell me all about what it is that you would like help with?'

Follow-up consultations should also begin with a general open question. It is important not to assume that the patient is primarily concerned with the same key issue/s as at the last appointment since the picture may have changed – something may have got better or have been overtaken by a new development. Follow-up questions should not, then, begin with questions like: 'Tell me how your headache has been'. Certainly you can and should ask about the headache but not as your first question. Better opening questions for the follow-up visit are ones such as:

'So, how have you been since we last met?'

'So, how have things been since our last appointment?'

'So, tell me how things are with you?'

## OPENING ANSWERS

After posing the opening question, it is important to listen to the answer – closely and carefully – and to avoid interrupting the patient without good cause (the only good reasons to interrupt the answer to the opening question are usually: if the patient has strayed far from the subject; or if you are being overwhelmed with information and need to pause to take stock). Brief notes should be taken as unobtrusively as possible and these will serve to remind you of points that need to be developed or clarified later. Keep your body and your gaze directed to the patient.

Use 'tell me more' if the patient does not immediately provide a detailed response, e.g.

Practitioner: 'So, tell me what it is that you would like help with?'

Patient: 'Well, I have eczema'.

Practitioner: 'Tell me more about your eczema'.

Once the patient starts to give their full response, be careful to note, and be flexible in following, their order of priority. Listen for key sayings, even when these appear to be presented in an offhand way (heartfelt issues may often be first communicated in this manner), e.g. 'it's been a bit of a nightmare'; 'I'm sick and tired of it'; 'they wouldn't understand'; 'I don't want to worry them'. It is useful to write notes in the patient's actual words, using quote marks to indicate this. The tendency to translate patient stories into diagnoses or medical jargon should be resisted, for example, if the patient reports that they have a rash on their inner elbows that is itchy, write this up as 'rash, inner elbows, itchy' not 'eczema, antecubital fossa, pruritic', since the latter confers a diagnosis and medicalizes the patient in such a way that it might obstruct the practitioner from hearing new information that suggests a different interpretation later on. While taking the history, the practitioner needs to generate differential diagnoses but suspend final judgements.

In response to opening questions, patients may provide a huge range of information covering areas such as the circumstances surrounding the onset of the condition, its nature, precipitating and relieving factors, etc., saving the practitioner the job of raising separate questions about each of these aspects of the patient's situation. It is important to resist the urge to control and direct the structure and flow of the patient's narrative but rather to follow it. Once the patient has come to a pause it may be appropriate to say something to check that the patient has said as much as they want to, or can, for now, e.g.

> *'There's plenty for us to look at there but, before going on, is there anything to add or anything else you wanted to mention?'*

Or simply:

> *'Does that cover everything?'*

or

> *'Anything else to add?'*

It is worth going as far as one can to make sure that the patient has introduced everything that is going on with them in their opening answer/s. Providing the opportunity, and encouraging the patient to mention every last thing may occasionally yield a vital piece of information or encourage the patient to reveal something that is of consequence but which they had considered too small or silly to mention. A sample question in this area is:

> *'Before I ask you more about what you have said, tell me, is there anything else* at all *to add about your health and how you are feeling – no matter how small or silly it might sound?'*

Once you are clear that the opening question–answer period has concluded you can move on to asking further questions regarding what the patient has told you in order to clarify and gain detail where required.

## FOLLOW-UP CONSULTATIONS

We are starting with the follow-up consultation to emphasize its importance as the most frequently conducted type of consultation. In phytotherapy practice patients with chronic disorders may be treated for months or even years, accumulating multiple follow-up consultations with the same herbal practitioner (continuity of care with the same practitioner is the norm in herbal practice). Additionally, most clinical medicine texts pay scant regard to follow-up consults, leaving the reader with the highly misleading impression that practice is comprised of a succession of first visits. Having said this, it is worth noting Silverman et al's (2005) observation that: 'Follow-up visits have much more in common with new consultations than is often believed'. Certainly follow-ups may enter the mode of first consults as new conditions arise and are explored or when there has been a long gap since last seeing a patient, who returns with a new condition. On the whole, however, follow-up consultations are characterized by the practitioner and patient's prior knowledge of each other and the opportunity (not always exploited) for:

- Increased appreciation, by both practitioner and patient, of the richness and meaning of the patient's narrative
- Review of current healing strategies and generation of new hypotheses to test
- Innovation in modulating, or finding new forms of, support and treatment
- Growth in the therapeutic relationship.

These broad features relate to the aims of the follow-up consultation as seen by the practitioner, which include to:

- Check for change (improvement or deterioration) in the condition; or lack of change
- Consider changes in the light of expectations generated at the end of the previous consultation – are interventions (herbal medicine, dietary and lifestyle advice, etc.) meeting expectations?
- Decide whether specific interventions need to be scrapped, modulated or added to
- Check for new events or conditions
- Get to know the patient and their story better, in terms of quality and detail of understanding and appreciation of connections and influences. Returning to previous themes and detecting and exploring new ones
- Be alert to detecting emergent properties – which new ways of being or seeing are surfacing?
- Facilitate the patient's continuing project of self-reflection, discovery and development
- Aid the patient in perceiving significance and meaning in their predicament
- Maintain and deepen appreciation of the patient's context and situation within a wider network of influences (work, home, family, friends, culture, etc.)
- Provide ongoing support, caring, human warmth and positive regard.

## PREPARATION

It is essential to review the patient's notes *before* seeing her in order to re-familiarize yourself with her narrative, predicament and condition and your treatment and management plan. Attempting to check notes while the patient is in the room (i.e. alongside actually taking the follow-up visit) leads to awkward and mutually unsatisfactory consultations where opportunities for deeper appreciation and growth are diminished and the therapeutic relationship is adversely affected by the all-too-clear lack of preparedness (which may be read as a lack of care) on the part of the practitioner.

While reviewing the notes, it is very helpful to jot down key points for review and clarification in the margin of the sheet of paper you are going to use to record the follow-up history. This provides an *aide-memoir* that can be accessed with a quick glance rather than having to wade through larger amounts of text. It also means that brief comments can be written next to the key point while taking the history, so saving time spent on writing notes and thereby reducing time spent shifting your eyes from the patient.

Reviewing the case notes provides a golden opportunity for reflective practice. As you check the notes also check your reactions to, and perceptions about, the patient. How do you feel about this patient? Is there anything you overlooked last time? What new questions would you like to ask this time? If you have a 'heartsink' reaction to this patient you need to ask yourself why. Is there anything in the way you feel about or perceive the patient affecting your ability to help them? With chronic cases where progress is gradual, minimal or absent, it is important to be clear whether positive change is necessarily slow or whether you have ceased to be the right person to enable the patient's progress or, moreover, whether you may be obstructing the patient's progress or reinforcing a negative state. The latter scenarios call for a refreshed perspective and dynamic or a referral. In those chronic cases where change *is* necessarily very slow, and where the picture is stagnant but has potential for change (e.g. in those associated with chaos narratives), it is important for the practitioner to remain open to change in the patient. That is to say that the practitioner holds a frame of mind that allows rather than impedes the patient's change, based on the notion that 'energy follows thought'. This notion can be considered as an expression of intentionality, meant in the philosophical sense of a certain 'directedness' of thought. Put simply, if the practitioner's direction of thought is towards perceiving change in the patient, then change is more likely to be actually manifested/detected than if the practitioner holds a thought form that asserts that 'this patient does not change' (based on previous experience of the patient). The former open attitude of mind (or thought-directedness) can be self-generated by the practitioner, when required, by inwardly saying (and, more importantly, *truly meaning*) that: 'I am open to change in this person'. This pronouncement should be accompanied by the conscious setting to one side of previous experience and conceptions of this patient so that a fresh and re-energized approach can be taken.

## ENACTMENT

The opening question is asked, for example:

*'How have you been since we last met?'*

Then the opening answer is listened to – allowing plenty of time for the patient to fully express themselves and coaxing with 'tell me more' questions if the patient is not immediately forthcoming. It is important not to interrupt the patient and not to be too quick to jump to conclusions based on prior knowledge of the patient. It is also essential, in the opening exchanges, to set aside the issue that was dominant at the last meeting – in order to make space to hear new things. This is a crucial activity at the beginning of each follow-up consult – to seek and to hear what is new.

Once information has been gained regarding any new issues, themes and conditions, attention can shift to the agenda from the previous consult – using the prompt notes in the margin of your question sheet. These notes do not have to be followed in a linear fashion but they can serve as reminders and help to orient and focus questioning. Again, while working through previously identified issues, it is essential to remain open to receiving and hearing new information – whether negative or positive. Practitioners naturally tend to register information that supports their working hypothesis and exclude that which does not – unless the latter is so 'loud' that it cannot be avoided. The (difficult) key is to be open to hearing *all* information, regardless of whether it is 'loud' or 'quiet' and whether it initially appears to be positive or negative.

Following this, any routine questions assessing key general health parameters that have not yet been covered can (and *should*) be posed. By this I mean the types of questions directed at looking at the areas traditionally described as the six non-naturals, as discussed above. These can be briefly summarized, again, as having to do with assessing:

- The patient's sense of their innate vitality ('energy level')
- Mood, emotions, outlook
- Whether, and if so in what ways, the patient feels 'stressed'
- Dietary review
- Sleep
- Excretory function (GIT; US)
- Menstruation
- How things are at home and at work
- Physical activity (exercise)
- Rest and relaxation
- Enjoyment and play
- Prioritizing of the self
- Inspiration and mental stimulation
- Circulation and respiration
- Immunity
- Environment
- Sexual interest/activity.

Patients may answer routine questions with single words or short phrases: 'Fine. Okay. No change. Same as last time. Great'. Any replies that sound or feel ambiguous or uncertain should be queried to gain more information or clarification using 'tell me more' type questions or echo/repetition. An example of the latter type of questioning would be as follows:

Practitioner: 'How has sleeping been?'

Patient: 'Not bad'.

Practitioner: 'Not bad?'

Patient: 'Well it could be better but my son keeps waking early at the moment and he's been getting me up at about half five'.

At the end of the history it is always worth checking for completeness by asking:

*'Do you have anything else to add – anything at all?'*

*'Was there anything else you wanted to mention – anything at all?'*

This technique helps to catch:

- Any issues that might have arisen towards the end of the consultation but which the patient felt reluctant to introduce at such a late stage in the consult
- Other things the patient had been reluctant to divulge or had been holding to one side waiting for explicit permission to say it. *Note:* The emphasis on *'anything at all'* is important here.

## 'BY THE WAY …'

Thorough history-taking of this kind, including the final 'anything to add' question has the result that one rarely encounters the 'By the way …' situation. This is a scenario where, as the patient is walking across the room and is just about to leave following the end of the consultation, she turns (often in the doorway) and says, 'By the way …' followed by the description of one or more things that are still on her mind and which she has not had the opportunity to say. Regularly encountering the 'By the way …' phenomenon should trigger reflection on how effective one's case history-taking is.

## FOUR TERRITORIES

Above we have described four territories or zones of information available in the follow-up consultation:

1. New events, issues, themes
2. Previous issues and agenda
3. Routine questioning of key health-modulating factors
4. Anything to add?

These areas are not necessarily explored in the above linear sequence, and they usually combine and overlap to some extent. For example: information regarding new events, symptoms and issues may be disclosed at any point in the consultation; and the exploration of issues from the previous consultation/s usually significantly elides with routine questioning of key health areas. The above four territories merely serve as a reminder of the scope of the follow-up consult and as a framework to be creatively adapted in practice.

## CHANGE AND RECOLLECTION

As health issues improve, our memory of what they had been like previously varies in its acuity. Some conditions may be sharply and clearly remembered, and easily called to mind, whereas others are forgotten about or only give rise to the haziest of recollections. Additionally, when subtle and gradual improvements occur, we may accommodate to them and be unaware of the significant improvements that we have slowly accrued until we are stimulated to reflect on the issue.

These factors regarding the patient's recollection and judgement about change can act as confounding influences on follow-up consultations. When exploring symptoms and issues from previous consultations, the patient may contend that there has been little change and that little progress has been made. However, in comparing the current report with notes from prior consults, the practitioner may find that the degree of change appears to be greater than the patient perceives. In such cases, the practitioner needs to remind the patient about previous descriptions of the condition and test to see if these are accurate and, if they are, allow the patient to recognize the degree of change.

## THE INITIAL CONSULTATION

The first meeting between herbal practitioner and patient has the potential to be later regarded by the patient as a major life event. At the conclusion of the initial visit it is not uncommon for patients to remark on the distance that has been travelled and the depth of exploration that has taken place within the consultation. Comments noting the rare comprehensiveness of the encounter are frequently expressed: 'You know more about me than almost anybody now!' The practitioner is granted licence to ask the patient about anything that may be relevant to their predicament and is given access to information that the patient may only previously have divulged to one or two people, or indeed may never have told anybody before. Such intimate involvement is both an awesome privilege and a profound responsibility. It also has the capacity to be a healing engagement – when the consultation is skilfully conducted, the patient may gain a number of therapeutic benefits, many of which may remain unknown to the practitioner, such as:

- Crucial insights and perspectives regarding their predicament, including with regard to meaning and significance
- Enhanced sense of self-identity
- Reassurance that an issue is less dangerous than they had feared
- Release and recognition gained in the very act of speaking out their story, hopes and fears
- Relief at having been able to articulate their narrative to another person
- Gains associated with being heard, being taken seriously, not being judged
- Identification of key issues and themes for further work
- 'Sense-making' activity
- Feeling empowered.

Outside of healthcare related practice, it is rare for people to have the opportunity to hear the detailed narratives of the lives of other individuals (other than in books). In the course of a lifetime a person may only get to know a handful of other people in great depth. For a phytotherapist this cumulative experience may fit into each working day. This extraordinary fact should be noted: the business of the phytotherapist is to aid and accompany people in telling their life stories, being allowed a degree of access to their subject that literary biographers might dream of. The intensive nature of the consultation may have a profound effect on the patient but also has implications for the practitioner. Working at this level of concentration and focus can be emotionally draining and physically tiring – it is essential that the practitioner develops a sustainable style of practising and continually monitors and calibrates the balance between patient-care and self-care (see Appendix 2).

Students may be daunted by the technical and emotional challenges of the initial consultation but should be assured that facility will develop with sensitive and diligent practice, especially when this is supported by careful reflection on lessons learned from each encounter. Experienced practitioners, as they develop ease in case history-taking, may forget the momentous nature of the first consult for the patient and should constantly keep this in mind. The practitioner may wish to develop her own mantra to remind herself of the excitement and mystery of practice, to be spoken internally when preparing to take a new case, in the moments before the patient is brought into the room. For example: 'It is a great privilege to get to know another person and I relish this opportunity'.

The first consultation provides insight into episodes, issues and themes in a patient's life that are returned, and added to over the course of future visits. It is worth frequently revisiting the notes of the first consult as one sees a patient over time for a reminder of the initial story lines and to assess change but also to detect themes that may have subsequently been overlooked and stand in need of review.

Earlier, we mentioned that follow-up consultations have much in common with the first consultation; this is worth keeping in mind while reading the content below – much of which has relevance to follow-up visits.

## THE BLANK SHEET

Students will find it useful to use printed guide sheets that set out the structure of the first consultation and which prompt relevant questions. It is my opinion that such forms should be dispensed with as soon as the structure/questions have been internalized and at this point a blank sheet should be used instead. Set formats impose a linear structure on the consultation and limit flexibility, responsiveness and creativity. One tends to follow the form rather than the patient. Although we will, necessarily, follow a linear format in discussing the various territories of the first consult below, the suggestion is that these should be seen as movable and merge-able entities, which the practitioner can deploy spontaneously as required. For example, the 'family history' may arise within, or be spread between, the 'presenting complaint'; 'previous medical history' or/and 'social history'.

In using the blank sheet approach, widely recognized (as opposed to personally invented) acronyms can be jotted down to indicate the particular territory being explored, e.g. DH for 'drug history'. Even this is not always necessary since the realm under investigation will often be obvious from the notes recording the patient's responses. While it is important that notes accurately record information and are susceptible to being interpreted by another person these concerns should not give rise to the compiling of a legalistic text.

It can be helpful to keep a space at the bottom of each page or in the margin where you can make brief side notes, or *aides-memoire*, as you consult – these may refer to the names of herbs you are considering prescribing, dietary changes or other advice you wish to recommend, or issues you want to ask about later in the consultation. Such notes are often just single words, acronyms or brief sentences, e.g. 'work on liver'; 'adaptogens'; 'Centella'; '↑F&V' (increase fruit and vegetables); 'auscultate chest'. By recording then accessing these notes at relevant junctures, it is easier to keep track of key insights and ideas as they arise. Treatment and management notes can be brought together at the end of the consultation and used as the basis for formulating the prescription and management plan.

## TO BE CONTINUED ...

Although it is an aim of the first consultation to be as comprehensive as is practicable, it is never possible to get to know everything that might be relevant. It may not always be possible or appropriate to cover all the territories discussed below. The key is to focus on the areas for exploration that are most appropriate to the patient's predicament while ensuring that all questions essential to enabling well-informed and safe practice are posed; for example it is always necessary to enquire regarding the drug history. Other, less obviously critical areas can be explored during subsequent consultations.

Thorough exploration of the content zones pertaining to the first consultation as described below may need to be spread over several subsequent sessions. This is particularly the case when narratives are extensive (e.g. those of older patients), complex or chaotic.

## QUESTIONING PRIOR CONCEPTIONS

The patient may arrive for the first consultation with the phytotherapist following one or more consultations with one or more other practitioners addressing the same condition or predicament. This means that the patient can attend in possession of one or more diagnoses and/or assessments (conventional and/or non-conventional) and be following a single or mixed treatment/management plan. It is important that phytotherapists gather and evaluate the opinions, pronouncements and advice of other practitioners with an attitude of respectful scepticism. Respectful, because other practitioners may provide insights and advice that are helpful and 'correct' according to their own explanatory model; sceptical, because practitioners may provide assessments that are incomplete or faulty and advise treatments that are inadequate, irrelevant or even harmful. The phytotherapist, therefore, should never passively accept a diagnostic pronouncement or treatment directive but rather seek to question the accuracy and appropriateness of these key factors – to the extent that she is competent to do so.

The patient may express ideas about diagnosis, treatment and so forth that are self-generated and may be taking self-prescribed medication or applying other treatment interventions and lifestyle adaptations. These ideas and activities should also be met with respectful scepticism so that beneficial practices can be supported and partial, erroneous or harmful practices and beliefs can be appropriately challenged – assuming that judgements can be made that lead to the use of notions such as 'benefit', 'error' and 'harm'.

## RECOGNIZING LIMITATIONS

Practitioners must at all times be aware of the limitations to their competence in all areas of their work, but particularly with regard to diagnosis and treatment. It is my experience, and opinion, that patients are increasingly consulting herbal practitioners as a first port-of-call so that phytotherapists may be considered to be meeting at least part of one definition of what constitutes a primary care practitioner role. The definition I have in mind is that of Barbara Starfield who has explained that:

> *Primary care is not defined by who provides it. Rather it is a set of functions – first-contact care; person- (not disease-) focused care over time; comprehensiveness in attending to the needs of populations, subpopulations and patients; and coordination of care when services have to be received elsewhere or from others. Therefore, who best provides primary care is an empirical issue, not a theoretical one. What type of professional best achieves the functions? In most of the world, primary care providers – usually family physicians – are the providers of primary care, and thus physicians are generally considered as the 'gold standard'. But it does not have to be this way.*

Bodenheimer et al. (2008)

Phytotherapists can (and, I believe, increasingly *do*) meet the first of these criteria (serving as a point of first-contact care) and certainly meet the second – providing person-focussed care over time. Phytotherapists who are not also medical doctors almost always have no option but to operate outside of mainstream health delivery frameworks, such as the NHS in the UK, and therefore are excluded from the system that is required to deliver criteria three and four – comprehensiveness in meeting the needs of populations, subpopulations and patients; and coordination of care services. These areas are especially relevant where the patient has a condition that cannot be sufficiently appreciated, diagnosed or treated by phytotherapy alone or where phytotherapy is not the most effective choice (although it may remain the patient's preferred choice). The phytotherapist, then, must be alert to detecting when the patient should be advised to consult a primary care practitioner (normally a GP/family physician) who can fill the gaps in the herbal practitioner's primary care competency. Occasions for such advice include where there is a need for further investigation of the patient's condition and where additional or alternative treatment to that of phytotherapy is required.

Ominous ('red flag') scenarios should always be referred to practitioners (GPs or hospital doctors) working within mainstream healthcare, since this is the only system that is geared to provide rapid investigation, treatment and 'comprehensive' (the degree of comprehensiveness actually delivered is open to question in individual cases and is limited by the conventional medical model) institutional and community care for serious or severe conditions. While phytotherapy can and does play a role (sometimes a major role) in treating serious and severe disorders, it has to be acknowledged that there are practical limitations around when and how this role can be played, given that phytotherapy is excluded from mainstream medical services. This means that the requisite nursing, in-patient facilities and other means of support and care that are required to enable phytotherapy to fulfil its potential are simply not currently available.

## COMPLEXITY, NON-LINEARITY AND FLEXIBILITY

We have previously discussed that the consultation does not have to be conducted in a linear manner – in fact it should not, and generally *is not*, conducted in this way, since a rigid consultation structure and style obstructs the practitioner's goal of getting to know the patient. Flexibility, creativity and spontaneity are required in sympathetically responding to the patient's narrative. It is important to bear this in mind given that the way in which the questioning sequence is set out on the pages below cannot help but suggest a linear approach – this is not the case and the reader should constantly bear in mind that each section of the consultation outlined below will tend to overlap with others and that the sequence should be altered in response to the patient's lead. Additionally, 'bits' of sections may be explored in turn and mixed up, revisited and elided, so that the 'sections' set out below generally dissolve into new forms in practice. To aid ease of reading, the 'sections' approach has been retained below but the reader should just keep in mind the misleading nature of the enterprise – clarity and ease on the page do not translate to clarity and ease of application in the enacted consultation. It may have been more representative of actual practice to present the following sections in the manner of B.S. Johnson's (1969) novel *The Unfortunates* where the book is split into unbound sections that the reader can rearrange and read in any order they choose, apart from the first and last sections – which is very like the consultation.

## WELCOMING

Practitioners will develop and deploy their own individual style in meeting and greeting patients for the first time. Initial exchanges are important as these set the tone for how the consultation will be conducted and perceived. The message conveyed by the style of meeting and welcoming the patient should be to do with the expression of warmth, openness and friendliness.

It is recommended that the practitioner goes out to meet the patient in the waiting room rather than having her sent through to the consulting room. The waiting room represents relatively neutral territory that the patient has usually acclimatized to by the time the practitioner comes out to say hello. It therefore is likely to be a less intimidating space for the first meeting to occur.

By the act of going out to the waiting room to meet the patient, the practitioner can make a subtle but not insignificant statement about her willingness to work around the needs of the patient – 'I will come to meet you, rather than you having to come to meet me'. This act of consideration does not imply a submissive deference and it does not preclude the practitioner from later challenging the patient if appropriate – it merely indicates the practitioner's commitment to accommodate and focus on the patient. Additionally, standing up and getting out of the consulting room (no matter how briefly) between patients helps to move the practitioner's circulation and shift energy and to shift focus from one patient to the next.

In greeting the patient, it is common to use their name and to give your own in order to check that you are approaching the right person and to convey that the patient has connected with the right practitioner. By saying both the patient's and her own name, the practitioner is immediately beginning to make a firm mutual connection. How to use somebody's name is subject to a number of culturally specific rules and taboos. These may also be generation-specific, for example, patients who grew up in a more formal era or who are substantially older than the practitioner *may* prefer to be called Mr or Mrs. This is hard to estimate, however. The best policy is probably when in doubt to begin formally and then to ask permission to use a first name. An alternative strategy is simply to do what feels right to you and what is congruent to your style but to be sensitive to the reaction this has and modulate what you do accordingly. I tend to greet everyone by their first name but I vividly remember an older woman (let us call her Geraldine) who was affronted by my use of her forename and who responded witheringly: 'I am not *Geraldine*! I am *Mrs. DeVere*!'

A typical informal welcoming exchange would be along the following lines:

Practitioner: (approaches the patient) 'Is it David?'

Patient: 'Yes'.

Practitioner: 'I'm Peter. Good to meet you' (offers hand to shake).

Patient: 'Hello'.

Practitioner: 'Come through' (turning to lead the way to the consulting room).

Patient: 'Thank you'.

The patient is rather passive in this type of exchange and it is possible to structure meetings where the patient is more equally involved. To my mind, however, it is appropriate for the practitioner to lead the encounter at this stage. At this point, the normal codes of hospitality apply with the practitioner acting as host to the patient as guest, since the location of the meeting is in the practitioner's territory. Roles are reversed in this regard when the practitioner visits the patient at home.

It is not compulsory to shake hands but it has the benefit of establishing physical contact and signals the practitioner's comfort with the physicality of the patient. Handshakes are expressive (in both directions) and can indicate hesitancy, reluctance, nervousness, openness, enthusiasm and interest – as well as the state of peripheral circulation. If you do shake hands, make sure you are using your body in a way that communicates warm engagement and interest – this does not mean gripping tightly and shaking vigorously, rather that the shake is entered into with the full hand (partial giving of the hand – finger-shaking as opposed to hand-shaking – suggests disdain), making full contact.

The practitioner should hold the door open for the patient and indicate where the patient should sit, e.g. 'Would you like to take the seat by the window there?' I always provide the patient with a glass of water (important, especially since the patient will now be talking at length for over the course of an hour or so) and make a comment about this: 'There's some water for you, in case you need it'. As the patient is settling in (taking off their coat, sitting down, placing their bag on the ground, taking out a packet of medicines/prescription list/letter from the doctor/print out from the internet/pair of glasses, etc.), the patient and/or practitioner may make 'conversational leads', typically about the weather, travel to the clinic, finding the clinic and parking. No great effort needs to be made to initiate such exchanges – they are best left to arise naturally and spontaneously as the occasion affords.

At the end of this brief settling in period it is worth checking:

*'Are you comfortable? Do you have everything you need?'*

Practitioners will vary in how they proceed from here; my strategy is to begin the consultation as such by taking, or checking, the patient's personal details so that the formal opening line of the consultation is something like:

*'Now, can we begin by checking your details?'*

The articulation of 'now' is the signal that the consultation has commenced.

## PERSONAL DETAILS

It is usual to have a receptionist take at least some of the patient's personal details routinely as they book their first appointment and a form can be given to have the patient complete the details by themselves so that the practitioner need do no more than glance at the finished sheet. This represents a wasted opportunity however, since if the practitioner takes the details herself she can use the task to gently ease the patient into the consultation; to begin to build the therapeutic relationship and to gain an early insight into the patient's situation. Taking the personal details 'live' provides extra verbal and non-verbal information that words written into boxes on a form can never provide.

I normally copy the patient's name, address and telephone number onto a sheet before they arrive at the clinic and begin taking the personal details by checking that these are correct.

### Patient's name

It is important to make sure the patient's name is spelt correctly and that you are pronouncing it properly.

An example of extra information that checking the name may yield: A confirmation that the name is correct and then the patient volunteers: 'That's my married name, I've been meaning to change it back ... silly really ...'.

### Address

Again, check to ensure you have a full and accurate address. If you are going to send out medicines by post, it is particularly important to get the details right. It is also helpful to mention to the patient that you may send medicines to them by mail and whether they would prefer for the medicines to be sent to another address. Some people prefer to have medicines sent to work to avoid them ending up at the depot when no-one is at home. Once when I checked this, the patient said: 'Can I collect them from here? I don't want my husband to know that I'm coming here'.

Other examples of extra information that checking the address may yield:

*'I'm not sure of the postcode, we've only just moved in'.*

*'We're just about to move'.*

*'The house is on the market, we're having difficulty finding the right buyer – it's incredibly stressful'.*

If you know the area in which the address is located, this may be suggestive of socioeconomic and environmental influences. It is wise not to read too much into this, however.

### Preferred contact telephone number

Check that the telephone number you have is correct.

Example of extra information that checking the telephone number may yield:

*'I'd prefer that you don't call unless you absolutely have to'.*

*'I never answer the phone but you can leave a message'.*

*'I work nights so you'll be lucky to ever get hold of me!'*

### Date of birth

I normally take the date of birth, then ask the patient: 'So that makes you how old now?' I ask this partly to avoid making a mistake but mainly to gauge whether there is any reaction as the patient tells their age. Some people merely state the figure, whereas others may say things like:

*'Oh heck – I don't want to say it!'*

*'Older than I'd like to be'.*

*'Too old'.*

*'Old enough'.*

*'59 … coming up to the big one …' (or '79 … coming up to the big one …'; '29 … coming up to the big one …', etc.).*

Does the patient look their age? Older? Younger? A number of factors tend to 'age' patients, making them look older than they are, such as: smoking, heavy alcohol use, chronic stress, chronic lack of sleep.

Some conditions and transitions are associated with particular ages and stages of life, e.g. the menopause. Additionally, some diseases are unlikely to occur at certain ages.

## Gender

This is usually obvious and doesn't need to be asked. However, transsexual (or transgender) people and people who have had gender reassignment surgery will usually prefer to be classed in their 'target' sex (i.e. the sex they perceive themselves as, or have undergone surgery to become, rather than the sex they were born as, which is known as the 'assigned' sex). To be respectful towards the patient and to avoid confusion, the practitioner can record the patient's target sex as their definitive sex and then in brackets show the 'assigned-to-target' sexes so that for a person who was born male but who self-identifies as a female, the note would be: Female (male-to-female). This can be alternatively written as: F (M2F).

## Occupation

An 'occupation' can be construed as meaning a 'job or profession' or a 'way of spending one's time'. This personal detail is usually considered in the light of the former definition but can be extended to include the latter. When people are not in a full-time job, the way they spend their time may be quite varied and difficult to sum up in one or two words. It is not the aim to get a full description of how time is spent in this case, rather a general indication and further details can be gathered during the history-taking.

Enquiring as to a patient's occupation can be taken to imply that one *should* have an occupation, viewed in the sense of paid employment, or that paid employment is the superior mode with any other form of work or activity being of less worth. A common example of such an exchange is as follows:

Practitioner: 'Do you have a particular occupation?'

Patient: 'No, I'm just a housewife'.

It is hard to gauge what 'housewife' might mean without asking a clarifying question here:

Practitioner: 'Tell me about being a housewife'.

Patient: 'Oh you know, 24 hour unpaid job, ferrying the kids around, cooking, cleaning, that kind of thing'.

This is a substantial 'occupation' and one deserving of appreciation. It may be possible to account for a wider range of responses by phrasing the occupation question more broadly and inclusively, as follows:

Practitioner: 'Would you say that you have a particular occupation or a main way that you spend your time?'

Patient: 'Well most of my time is taken up with looking after everyone – kids, husband, the house ... the dogs! ... you know'.

The type of question posed by the practitioner in this case may be heard as being more open and less judgemental, and it may get the information you want more quickly. A question along these lines will work well in most circumstances but may feel less appropriate in an older person where one might ask: 'Should I assume that you are retired?' Such a phrasing leaves the patient free to contradict you, e.g. 'No, no, you shouldn't, I don't believe in retirement'. Being in the state of retirement does not mean that one is unoccupied however, e.g. retired people who are grandparents may be providing substantial amounts of unpaid childcare. If patients do class themselves as retired, it is still essential to appreciate how they spend their time – although it is acceptable to merely put 'retired' on the personal details sheet and seek more information during the case history itself. When a patient says they are retired they should be asked about what they did before they were retired and this should be noted: 'And did you have a particular occupation or type of work you did before you were retired?', or simply: 'What did you do before you retired?'

Some occupations carry particular risks or are associated with activities or pressures that may impact on a person's health. Details regarding these factors and others such as working hours, conditions and travel can be enquired about during the case history.

Other examples of extra information (from many possibilities) that asking about occupation may yield:

*'I haven't been able to work for years'.*

*'I can't work at the moment'.*

*'I can't do anything right now'.*

*'Yes, I'm a ..., more's the pity!'*

*'Yeah, got a great job, love it'.*

*'Yes, my work is my life'.*

*'Well, I'm trying to get work'.*

*'Yes, I do have a job – not sure for how much longer though'.*

*'I'm in the process of looking for a new job'.*

*'I spend most of my time trying to get well'.*

*'My health (or illness) is my job'.*

### Relationship status

It is important to ask about the patient's closest relationships, as these have such a large influence on a person's life and wellbeing. This particular personal detail is sometimes classed as 'marital status' and is enquired after by asking: 'Are you married?' This is unsatisfactory because it may be taken to imply that one *should* be married and that any alternative relationship has to be explained and justified. The question may therefore be seen as implying a judgement.

A more open and inclusive way of posing this question is:

*'May I ask whether you would describe yourself as single, married, with a partner ... ?'*

This question leaves the way open for the patient to reply in any way that they choose.

Responses to this question can be significant, e.g. a patient might reply: 'I am divorced' or 'I am widowed' rather than 'I am single'. When a patient describes herself as divorced but is still wearing a wedding ring, this might be taken to signal that she is not yet open to beginning a new relationship.

Other examples of extra information that enquiring about relationship status may yield:

*'Well last year was our Ruby Wedding anniversary'. (Ruby = married for 40 years.)*

*'I'm currently going through a rather messy divorce'.*

*'I've been alone for years'.*

*'I don't think anyone would want me while I'm like this'.*

*'I think they're going to run a mile when they hear I've got MS'.*

People may refer to being separated; in the midst of trial separation; having just got together or broken up with someone. If the issue is upsetting and recent or still raw, the patient may burst into tears in response to the question.

This personal detail is not structured to consider sexual orientation but, since this is central to relationship status, information regarding this may be implied or volunteered by the patient in defining their situation. Students often ask whether sexual orientation is a valid field for the consultation and question its 'clinical significance'. The point of the holistic consultation is not only to gather information that is clinically relevant but also to understand the person and their predicament in the broadest possible way. Since sexuality is a core dimension of human experience and identity it is a crucially valid area for the consultation. During the case history questions regarding libido and sexual activity, experience (e.g. whether sexual activity is comfortable or painful) and performance can be routinely asked as general questions assessing the patient's health and wellbeing. It is not common to routinely enquire with regard to a patient's sexual orientation and specific preferences unless these can be justified in relation to a particular line of clinical enquiry (arising during the taking of the history), since many patients will otherwise see such questions as intrusive, irrelevant and possibly offensive. The significance of sexual orientation may be viewed differently from various perspectives. While a person belonging in the dominant sexuality may not have had cause to consider it as part of their identity, a person in a socially spurned or minority group may experience things differently.

## Children

Regardless of how the adult patient has described their relationship status they can be asked whether they have any children. If they do, then the number, sex/es and age of the children should be enquired after. This provides you with a basic orientation with regard to the people who will be among the most significant in the patient's life. Children can be the source of great delight, anxiety and anguish for parents and will play a major role in influencing the patient's emotional and mental state.

Patients may report that they had a child who died; this is one of the most traumatic events that can happen to anyone and will obviously have a huge impact in shaping the rest of the patient's life. Such disclosure should be marked by an appropriate comment from the practitioner showing recognition of the profundity of the event, such as: 'I am very sorry to hear that', which will tend to close further immediate discussion of the issue, or: 'That must have been very difficult for you', which invites a reply.

Other examples of information that enquiring about children ('Do you have any children?') may yield:

'Well none yet but that's why I've come to see you'.

'Well we have three but they are all from my partner's previous relationship'.

'We have four but they are all from our previous relationships, we haven't had any children together'.

'I've got two but they live with their mother'.

'I wish I could say I had lots'.

'Unfortunately we don't have any'.

'I wasn't able to have children'.

'I don't think there's much chance of that now'.

'I never wanted them and I've been sterilized'.

'Oh yes – the source of all my problems'.

## Who lives at home?

It is important to establish who the patient shares a home with (either here in the personal details or later, e.g. under social history) since the person/s concerned will likely play a major role in the patient's life. If the patient lives alone it should not be assumed that they are unsupported or lonely (although they may be) and likewise if they live with a partner or children, etc., it should not be assumed that these people provide substantial support for the patient (although they may do). The nature of the home relationships may be enquired about in the history itself, although they may be hinted at in the reply to the general question being posed at this point.

Example replies to the question: 'May I ask if anyone lives at home with you?'

'My partner and all the children – it gets pretty crowded'.

'Just me … I wish I could say otherwise'.

'I've got three flatmates but one of them is making life hell actually'.

'My son moved out to go to university a couple of months ago, so it's just me now'.

'Just me and my wife – at long last!'

## GP details

It is standard practice to take the name and address (or at least the surgery name and general location) of the patient's doctor. This provides a point of contact should an occasion for communication between phytotherapist and doctor arise. I tend to just ask this question in a very basic way, since most patients are quite happy to provide their doctor's details: 'May I take your doctor's name for reference? And which surgery is that?'

Occasionally patients will ask why you want to know these details and how they will be used. A standard reply would be to explain that it is just in case you needed to raise a query with the doctor and that, in the normal course of events, you would ask the patient for permission to do so first, discussing the nature of your reason for contacting the doctor at the same time. Further discussion of the practical and ethical aspects of this issue is contained in Appendix 3.

If the patient can recite their doctor's full address and telephone number from memory, this suggests they have been frequent attenders, similarly if they are hazy about the doctor's name and the name or location of the surgery, then they are unlikely to have spent much time there. The patient's comments in response to querying this personal detail can be revealing about their attitude towards, and experience of, conventional medical care, and it is useful to ask about it for that reason alone, for example:

'I see Dr ..., who has been a great help'.

'I can't really say who my doctor is – you always see somebody different'.

'I try to keep away from doctors'.

'I don't know which doctors are there – I haven't been there for years'.

'I'm thinking of changing surgery, I don't like their attitude there'.

'My doctor is useless'.

'It was my doctor who suggested I might come to see you'.

'My doctor can't really deal with patients like me'.

'It's a very conventional practice – they don't really cater for me'.

Patients may disclose that they are not registered with a doctor, in which case the phytotherapist should encourage and help the patient to become registered if they wish to do so.

## 'How did you hear about me?'

It is useful to hear how patients come to know of us – most commonly this is on recommendation from another patient, in which case it is nice to have that patient's name in order to thank them. It is also useful to find out whether the patient has come as a result of promotional activity in order to gauge whether such activity is worth continuing. Additionally, it is good to know which other practitioners are making recommendations to you.

## PERSONAL DETAILS LEADING INTO THE HISTORY

Taking the personal details may be quite straightforward and provide a gentle transition into the more formal part of the history-taking. It also has the potential to raise an issue that could lead directly into the history itself, for example, during questioning about relationship status something like the following exchange may occur:

> Practitioner: 'May I ask whether you would describe yourself as single, married, with a partner ... ?'
>
> Patient: 'Well that's the reason behind why I'm here really, that's the major problem'.

The patient's response might be explained, for instance, by a recent break-up that is affecting sleep, mood, appetite, etc. In dealing with this response, the practitioner has two options:

1. Either to ask: 'Tell me more about that', leading directly into the case history and returning to complete the rest of the personal details at an appropriate juncture later, during, or at the end of the consultation.
2. Or to acknowledge the significance of the reply but ask for permission to delay exploring it until the personal details are completed: 'I can hear that this issue is very important but I'm going to ask if its okay for us to finish taking your details before I return to ask you more about it – is that okay?' In this case, the opening question of the presenting complaint section of the case history proper (see below) should begin with: 'So tell me more about what you said earlier when I asked you about your relationship'.

Option 1 follows the lead of the patient and may enable a more powerfully dynamic consultation to unfold, whereas option 2 is practitioner led but may have the benefit of providing a space for the patient to gather her/himself after introducing the general nature of the predicament before proceeding to its detail. The advanced practitioner may choose between these options depending on her intuitive reading of the particular case.

## PHYTOTHERAPY ORIENTATION

Following on from taking the personal details, it is advisable to check whether the patient has ever consulted a herbal practitioner before. If they have not you can give a brief explanation of what is going to take place. It is important to be aware that most new patients who have never experienced a herbal consultation before are unlikely to have a clear idea of what the process might be like and some may be nervous about it. A few words of explanation can help to alleviate any anxiety so that the consultation flows smoothly and is a pleasant experience for the patient. There is also an opportunity to orient the patient so that they are clear that you are open to hearing their full story and to encourage them to express themselves freely.

A sample explanation would be:

> 'We are going to allow plenty of time to talk about things in detail and I really want to hear your own thoughts and feelings and any questions you may have. Then we

will do any examinations that are relevant – just simple things like taking your pulse. After that, I'll tell you how I see things and what we might be able to do and you can see how that feels and we can discuss things from there. Does that sound okay?'

## THE PRESENTING COMPLAINT

We have discussed most of the points that are relevant in checking the presenting complaint previously in this chapter, so we will just briefly recap here.

Asking about the presenting complaint marks the formal start of the consultation in that we are now specifically asking: Why are you here? What is it that you would like help with? The specific reason for consulting may already have been revealed, however. This may have occurred during the preliminary exchanges or when taking the personal details or before the visit itself, perhaps in a preliminary phone or e-mail query. Additionally, some practitioners routinely ask receptionists to establish why the patient is consulting at the time of making their booking in order to prepare or orient themselves in advance of the meeting. I prefer *not* to do this since, to my mind, prior knowledge of 'the condition' can create unhelpful preconceptions in the practitioner's mind about 'the patient' that may inhibit the capacity to respond openly and creatively to their predicament. Whenever I do know of the patient's condition in advance of the first consultation, I try not to focus on it too much and when the patient comes I initiate the consultation by saying something along the lines of:

> 'I know we spoke previously on the phone and you told me a bit about your condition but I'd like to ask that we put that to one side and begin again so that you tell me now, as if we haven't talked before, what it is that you would like help with?'

This allows a fresh and spontaneous story to be told without the patient being tied to what they may have previously reported and to accommodate changes that may have occurred since that report was made.

Where these considerations are not relevant, the consultation may begin by asking something like:

> 'So ... tell me what it is that you would like help with?'

The emphasized 'So' followed by a brief pause indicates a shift from prior discussion and marks the formal beginning of the consultation.

When the question has been posed – simply (but deeply) listen. Do not interrupt the patient. If they are not spontaneously explaining their situation, ask 'Tell me more about ...'

## HISTORY OF THE PRESENTING COMPLAINT

When the patient has finished outlining their predicament, then, if they have not already covered the issues below (the likelihood is that they will have covered many of these factors without you directly asking about them) or if you require further information about them, then ask questions to clarify:

- The full dimensions of the predicament
- How it is affecting the daily life of the patient

- How it is making them feel
- When the situation or condition started
- What the pre-conditions or preceding circumstances were
- The detailed nature of the issue
- Exacerbating and relieving factors
- The patient's own views and beliefs (explanatory model) about the predicament with regard to its origins, perpetuating factors, significance and meaning
- How others are involved with and affected by the predicament
- Thoughts about the past, the present and the future
- Other, more minor or background concerns/details, beyond the major issue
- Whether anything else needs to be voiced – perhaps things the patient is unsure as to whether they may be important or is reluctant to say in case they seem trivial or silly (such elements will only be revealed if the practitioner explicitly invites disclosure of them).

The presenting complaint should naturally flow into the history of the presenting complaint so that they represent a continuum rather than distinctly separate parts of the history. By the time these two entwined factors have been fully explored you will normally have a good idea of what is going on and a working diagnosis. The combined 'presenting complaint/history of' is generally the most crucial part of the whole consultation, so adequate time and reflection should be dedicated to it.

## EXPECTATIONS I

Following on from the 'presenting complaint/history of' is a good point to check what the patient would like to get from the consultation. Asking, for example:

> 'Now that I know more about your situation I'm wondering what, especially, you would like to gain from herbal treatment and what you would like us to focus on?'
>
> or
>
> 'At this stage I'm interested to know what your goals are for this consultation – what you would really like to achieve?'

## PREVIOUS MEDICAL AND LIFE HISTORY: SENSITIVITY TO INITIAL CONDITIONS

It is likely that in exploring the history of the presenting complaint in a thorough manner, the consultation will already have covered some areas that would be classed as previous medical history. One way of beginning to check for other relevant events and details is to ask:

> 'Aside from all the things already mentioned have you ever had any other illnesses or medical conditions in the past that stand out in your memory?'
>
> 'Any serious medical problems?'

*'Any times in hospital?'*

*'Any, we might say, more minor conditions?'*

From here, one can proceed to looking at particular life stages:

*'Do you know how your mother's pregnancy was when she was carrying you?'*

*'Do you know how the birth was, when you were born?'*

*'Do you know if you were breast or bottle-fed?'*

*'And how was your health as a child?'*

*'What about when you were a teenager?'*

It is a convention to run through an inventory of certain conditions to check whether the patient has had those specifically, including:

- Epilepsy
- Jaundice
- Hepatitis
- Rheumatic fever
- Heart disease
- Atopy: asthma, eczema, hayfever.

This is rarely necessary when you have approached the previous medical history in the way just described, since there is plenty of opportunity for the patient to recall the conditions they have experienced. It is possible that something has been overlooked however, and running through a checklist may yield useful information. If the list is used it can be preceded by a few preparatory words such as:

*'Just for completeness can I ask whether you have ever had epilepsy? Have you ever been jaundiced, meaning that your skin has turned yellow?'*, etc.

The emphasis can then be shifted from the *medical* history to a general exploration of what the patient's life has been *like* – how they have experienced it. A sense of this may already have come through in the dialogue so far but can be further explored by asking questions such as:

*'How do you remember your childhood in general terms – what was it like for you?'*

*'What about your teenage years?'*

*'And as a young adult?'*

*'And since then?'*

Although very simply stated, these questions move the consultation from a medical to a life focus, permitting the patient to reflect broadly on everything that has shaped and impacted their life so far. This constitutes a profound invitation for deep exploration and may yield significant, complex and challenging results. The practitioner should be prepared for this.

In chaos and complexity theories, the emergent properties of a system are said to be 'sensitive to initial conditions', meaning that the relational interaction between earlier phenomena (starting, or foundational, phenomena) give rise to new phenomena (i.e. emergent properties). The patient's current predicament can be viewed as an emergent phenomenon (or, more appropriately, a collection of emergent phenomena) arising from the earlier phenomena and the relationships between those phenomena. The 'previous medical/life history', then, attempts to discern what those earlier phenomena were, appreciating them as causative or influencing factors shaping the current predicament. Such factors will always be multiple and can only ever be partially discernible but some may stand out as particularly significant (abuse, neglect, bereavement, etc.), while others may be considered more subtle (chronic low level stress, ambient anxiety, lack of sleep, etc.).

## ALLERGIES, INTOLERANCES OR SENSITIVITIES

This group of reactions needs to be explored at some point in the consultation to gain a perspective on the reactivity of the immune state and the patient's tolerance of foods and comfort with the environment. The pathophysiological differences between allergies, intolerances and sensitivities remain, to some degree, unclear and controversial. Allergic reactions are understood as immune-mediated hypersensitivity reactions that may cause severe and sometimes generalized disorders. 'Intolerance' is typically used to distinguish between food allergies and food intolerances, with the latter category showing not a classical hypersensitivity reaction but rather the involvement of enzymatic problems, pharmacological reactions or undefined reactions (Wuthrich 2009) leading to disorders that are generally less substantial and more localized than food allergies. 'Sensitivities' is a term typically applied to a pattern of reactivity to environmental factors such as low dose chemicals in conditions such as multiple chemical sensitivity (or idiopathic environmental intolerance) and opinions vary as to whether sensitivities have principally psychological or physiological origins (Bornschein et al. 2002; Caress & Steinemann 2003).

Although patients are unlikely to be aware of the intricacies of the debate contrasting this assortment of labels, there nonetheless appears to be a general lay sense of what they denote, with allergy being interpreted as a severe immune reaction; intolerance meaning a localized reaction to certain foods; and sensitivity meaning a tendency to be irritated by chemical factors in the environment. It is therefore worth presenting the patient with all three options to see how they interpret the question:

> 'Do you know, or do you feel that you might have particular allergies, intolerances or sensitivities to anything at all?'

This question can be followed up by posing specific closed questions, such as:

> 'For example, do you react to any particular ...
- foods?
- drugs or medications?
- or to cats, dogs, animals?
- or to wool or feathers?
- or soaps, perfumes, that kind of thing?'

## FAMILY HISTORY

Questions posed under the heading of 'previous medical and life history' are also likely to raise comment on family relationships and, specifically, the influence of family members on the patient.

The family history concerns an exploration of relationships and influences as well as an assessment of which (if any) medical conditions appear to be common in the family and therefore may impact on the patient.

This particular element of the consultation may begin by enquiring:

*'May I ask if your mother and father are still living?'*

A number of responses are possible here, in addition to clarification as to whether each parent is still alive, including the disclosure that the patient never knew one or either parent and does not know whether they are now living or dead.

If a parent is alive, one can ask:

*'How old is your mother/father?'*

*'How is her/his health?'*

If deceased:

*'How old was your mother/father when she/he died?'*

*'Do you know what she/he died of?'*

If a parent is deceased, this may be an emotional matter for the patient to discuss. If the patient is showing clear signs of upset the distress should be acknowledged and enquired about:

*'I can see that's emotional for you to think about ... Would you like to tell me more about how you're feeling?'*

It is not uncommon to see patients who are suffering considerable stress and guilt regarding an elderly parent who is still living but in a state that the patient feels is not of an acceptable level of engagement, comfort or wellness. One often hears such patients say: 'I know this is going to sound terrible but I just wish they would die – it would be such a release for all of us'. Being able to articulate such a taboo feeling may represent a powerful therapeutic event for the patient.

One can also enquire:

*'How is/was your relationship with your parents?'*

This question may conjure up strong memories, feelings and thoughts arising from both positive and negative recollections and experiences. Parent–child relationships are fundamental to human development and exploring this area can be one of the most significant zones of the consultation. As ever, the phytotherapist needs to be aware of the limits to her competence here and it is helpful to know a trusted psychological therapist to refer those patients to who need and wish to explore their family relationships and traumas in greater depth.

The ages, health and relationships with siblings can be questioned in the same way as above. This territory of the history can also be used to enquire about parents' relationship with their children and to ask after their children's health.

A question can also be posed regarding wider family relationships:

*'Do you know of any other conditions or issues that appear to be common in your family more generally – both on your mother's and your father's side?'*

If the patient has a perception that a particular condition (e.g. heart disease, osteoporosis) is common 'in the family' they may be carrying considerable, and perhaps unvoiced, anxiety regarding their own risk of developing the particular condition. Being able to voice fears around concerns of this type is important and the practitioner may be able to provide reassurance, explanation, advice on risk reduction and so forth that, once again, can represent a major therapeutic outcome to the consultation. *Note* that concerns may be expressed not only regarding the risk of physical disease but also around a family history of issues such as mental illness and alcoholism.

During this zone of the consultation, disclosure of family secrets, traumas and tragedies may take place and the practitioner needs to remember previous discussions in this book regarding the power of bearing witness, conveying love and positive regard for the patient and expressing human warmth and compassion – listening deeply and empathically so that the patient is 'heard'.

Negative mythology may be expressed in this zone and may need to be challenged in the patient's own interest. Listen for sayings such as: 'I'm just like my mother … That's just like my father … I have my mother's tendency to … Just like my father I never can …'

Families are complex systems and huge change has taken place in the conceptions and construction of families over recent decades. This complexity needs to be appreciated and anticipated by practitioners, e.g. the increase in the number of families where parents are not married; families with same-sex parents; families with parents who live apart; single-parent families; half-siblings, etc.

## DRUG AND TREATMENT HISTORY

While some parts of the initial consultation may be left over to explore at a future visit, time must always be found to enquire after the drug history. Herbal medicines are pharmacological entities and must never be prescribed in the absence of an appreciation of other medications that the patient is taking.

Questions with which to examine the drug history include:

*'Are you currently taking any medications prescribed by your doctor?'*

*'What are you taking? At which dose? How frequently? What has it been prescribed for? How long have you been taking it?'*

*'Have you taken any other medications over the last year?'*

*'Have you taken a particular medicine for long periods of time at any time in your life?'*

*'When did you last have antibiotics?'*

*'Are you taking any medicines you've prescribed for yourself?'*

*'Anything bought from the chemist?'*

*'Any nutritional supplements? Or herbs? Or homeopathic remedies?'*

*'Anything else that you take at all?'*

Some authorities recommend that you routinely enquire regarding specific commonly taken medicines and over-the-counter remedies such as: sleeping tablets, painkillers, antihistamines and antacids. This may not be necessary if the line of questioning above has been followed but it will help to make sure that you have covered things as fully as possible and sometimes patients may overlook mentioning medicines they have been taking for a long time (such as painkillers) unless specifically asked about them.

If patients are uncertain of the name or dosage of a medication, they can be asked to phone or e-mail the details to you and/or to bring the actual medication to the next appointment. It is a good policy to train receptionists, when making the first appointment, to request that patients bring their medication with them.

This zone of the consultation can also be used to find out about other treatments that the patient may be having, currently or recently:

*'Are you having treatment of any kind from another practitioner at the moment – things like acupuncture or osteopathy?'*

*'Have you had any other treatments over the last year?'*

Vaccinations can also be recorded here:

*'Were you vaccinated as a child?'*

*'Have you had any vaccinations or immunizations in recent times – perhaps related to work or travel?'*

## SOCIAL HISTORY

This zone covers information on the following areas:

- Smoking
- Alcohol
- Illicit drugs
- Exercise
- Relaxation
- Home life
- Working life
- Interests and pastimes.

These areas of exploration may arise naturally during the consultation at other junctures. They can also be redistributed into other sections of the history, e.g. alcohol intake and smoking may be incorporated into the dietary history.

Each area can be explored in the following ways:

## Smoking

*'Do you smoke?'*

If the answer is 'Yes', then continue:

*'Tell me about your smoking pattern'.*

*'How often do you smoke?'*

*'How many cigarettes do you smoke each day?'*

*'What do you smoke?'* (e.g. self-rolled or ready-rolled cigarettes).

The patient may volunteer that they smoke cannabis at this point, in which case questions can be asked to clarify which type, or preparation, of cannabis is used, how they take it, how often and how they feel it affects them.

Individuals may class themselves as non-smokers because they stopped smoking recently, but this cessation may have followed many years of heavy smoking. In order to establish the degree of past tobacco use, the following question should always be asked when a patient answers 'Do you smoke?' in the negative:

*'Have you ever smoked?'*

If so, it is appropriate to establish – when did they last smoke or when did they stop smoking; how long did they smoke for; and then establish the pattern and quantity of previous use as above.

If a patient is a smoker it is important to check their self-perception of their use to determine whether, and to what extent, they consider it to be a problem area or one that does not require attention:

*'May I ask how you view your own smoking – how you feel about it?'*

The patient might reply that they really want to stop but have had difficulty doing so (in which case support and advice can be offered as to how they may achieve this goal), or they may respond in other ways, for example:

*'I know its bad for me but it helps me cope with life'.*

*'I do want to give up – but this isn't the right time'.*

*'I enjoy smoking – I know what people say about it but I'm fine with it'.*

*'If I stopped smoking I'd have to start doing something worse'.*

I recall that one of my patients said:

*'It helps me cope with my husband, who is the most boring man on earth but we're too old to change – I won't be able to give up until he dies'.*

In response to the patient's confirmation that they are continuing smokers, however this may be explained or justified, the practitioner can point out the risks of smoking (although people are generally aware of these), challenge the patient's rationale for continuing to smoke and offer support and advice regarding stopping smoking but, ultimately, the patient's position must be respected. If the patient continues to smoke, their use should be checked at each follow-up visit so that the matter can be kept open to review.

## Alcohol

The pattern for asking about alcohol follows a format similar to that for smoking. Begin by asking:

*'Do you drink alcohol?'*

*'Tell me about your pattern of drinking?'*

Patients may drink every day; only a few times a year; not in the week, only at weekends; etc. This question can be followed by:

*'How often do you drink?'*

Responses such as: 'rarely'; 'only at odd times'; 'only socially'; 'not often'; 'once in a blue moon' or 'a lot'; 'too much'; 'probably more than I should do'; 'whenever I get the opportunity', etc. should always be clarified, e.g.

*'So tell me what you mean by 'rarely' – how often is that?'*

Where the patient is not readily specifying frequency, closed questions with options can be posed:

*'So would you say you have a drink every day, once a week, every few weeks … ?'*

The type of alcohol should be established:

*'What do you drink?'*

*'Always the same thing or different things?'*

And the quantity:

*'And can you give me an idea of how much you drink?'*

A number of supplementary questions may need to be asked here in order to get as clear an appreciation of quantity as possible. For example if a patient says they have 'a couple of glasses of wine a night', you can ask:

*'Does 'a couple' mean two or more than two?'*

*'Is that a small glass or a big glass?'*

*'In terms of a bottle of wine how much would that be?'*

*'Half a bottle? More? Less?'*

If a patient quantifies their drinking in units this needs to be queried since peoples' perceptions of what constitutes 'a unit' vary:

*'So can I just check what you understand a 'unit' to mean?'*

It is difficult for people to measure units precisely since they depend not only on glass size and alcohol type but also on the strength of the alcohol – patients will generally be able to describe the first two of these parameters but may not be able to clearly detail the final one. The UK government (based on advice from the Royal College of Physicians) recommends that men drink no more than 3–4 units of alcohol per day and that women drink no more than 2–3. Various studies have shown some benefits associated with light to moderate, regular alcohol use, including cardiovascular gains such as lowered risk of coronary artery disease (CAD), ischaemic stroke and CAD-related heart failure (Klatsky 2009). The beneficial, or at least low-risk, pattern of alcohol use would seem to include the following elements as rules of thumb:

- Light regular daily intake of alcohol is preferable to occasional heavy use ('binges')
- Light daily intake is in the region of 2–3 units for men and 1–2 units for women
- Alcohol should be taken in conjunction with food (alcohol can be absorbed through the stomach and having food in the stomach will modulate uptake)
- Each alcoholic drink should be followed by a drink of water
- Some types of alcohol are better than others, e.g. those containing antioxidants such as red wine
- The safe limit for pregnancy is not known, therefore the best advice is for pregnant women to avoid alcohol altogether.

A conventional approach would be to counsel all patients exceeding government usage guidelines about the risks of alcohol intake and to discuss the ways in which they might reduce it. However, the accuracy and reliability of the government unit guidelines is unclear and the Royal College of Physician's advice has been criticized as something: 'plucked out of the air … an intelligent guess' (Norfolk 2007). Certainly, individual tolerances of alcohol will vary in ways that may be hard to predict and estimate based on mediating factors such as the person's age, weight, general health, diet, exercise, etc. While counting units may be considered to provide a rough guide in the assessment of whether a given intake may cause, or is causing, harm, an additional approach is to consider whether alcohol use is already affecting the patient in a negative way in terms of alcohol dependence or alcohol abuse (harmful use). The most commonly used guidelines for establishing whether the patient is alcohol dependent or abusing alcohol are those given by the American Psychiatric Association in the *Diagnostic and Statistical Manual of Mental Disorders* (DSM) such as DSM-IV and the World Health Organization's *International Classification of Diseases* (ICD), such as ICD-10. While such guidelines tend to show strong reliability in determining alcohol dependence, they are generally considered less reliable in establishing the presence of alcohol abuse (Hasin 2003). The contrasting of alcohol dependence with alcohol abuse (harmful use) is important since dependence is not always associated with abuse (Hasin & Grant 2004) such that these two categories should not be considered to be interchangeable terms or concepts. Hasin and Grant (2004) suggest that:

> *Different biopsychosocial processes may give rise to the symptoms of alcohol dependence and abuse. For example, genes affecting alcohol reward, craving, or withdrawal (characterizing dependence) may differ from genes affecting novelty-seeking or behavioural undercontrol (characterizing abuse).*

According to DSM-IV (American Psychiatric Association 2000), substance dependence (including but not limited to alcohol) is:

*A maladaptive pattern of substance use, leading to clinically significant impairment or distress, as manifested by three (or more) of the following, occurring at any time in the same 12-month period:*

(1) Tolerance, as defined by either of the following:
   (a) A need for markedly increased amounts of the substance to achieve intoxication or desired effect
   (b) Markedly diminished effect with continued use of the same amount of the substance.
(2) Withdrawal, as manifested by either of the following:
   (a) The characteristic withdrawal syndrome for the substance …
   (b) The same (or a closely related) substance is taken to relieve or avoid withdrawal symptoms.
(3) The substance is often taken in larger amounts or over a longer period than was intended.
(4) There is a persistent desire or unsuccessful efforts to cut down or control substance use.
(5) A great deal of time is spent in activities necessary to obtain the substance … use the substance … or recover from its effects.
(6) Important social, occupational, or recreational activities are given up or reduced because of substance use.
(7) The substance use is continued despite knowledge of having a persistent or recurrent physiological or psychological problem that is likely to have been caused or exacerbated by the substance …

Whereas, substance abuse is defined as:

*A maladaptive pattern of substance use leading to clinically significant impairment or distress, as manifested by one (or more) of the following, occurring at any time in the same 12-month period:*

(1) Recurrent substance use resulting in a failure to fulfil major role obligations at work, school, or home …
(2) Recurrent substance use in situations in which it is physically hazardous …
(3) Recurrent substance-related legal problems …
(4) Continued substance use, despite having persistent or recurrent social or inter-personal problems caused or exacerbated by the effects of the substance.

The categorization of alcoholism as a mental disorder in the DSM schema underplays the physical symptoms of alcohol dependence and abuse, which vary depending on the extent of alcohol use and the physiological processes and body organs and systems affected. Additionally, the huge influence that the DSM enterprise now plays in determining and constructing 'mental disorders' has been challenged and criticized with regard to conceptual and philosophical viewpoints and with respect to the way that its conclusions are shaped by social, political and financial factors (Cooper 2005). When an alcohol-related problem is suspected, phytotherapists need to pose questions to discover whether adverse physical or psychological effects are being experienced as a consequence. Of course, such effects and symptoms may be the trigger to enquiring about alcohol in the first place, so that discussion of alcohol intake may take place earlier in the consultation (e.g. in discussing the presenting complaint), as opposed to being part of a routine screen under the social history.

Questions can be formulated to explore the various criteria of dependence and abuse as described above but in working with them it is important to keep in mind the need for an individualized, holistic and historical assessment, as Spanagel (2009) makes clear:

> *Alcohol-related diseases, especially alcoholism, are the result of cumulative responses to alcohol exposure, the genetic make-up of an individual, and ... environmental perturbations over time. This complex gene × environment interaction, which has to be seen in a life-span perspective, leads to a large heterogeneity among alcohol-dependent patients, in terms of both the symptom dimensions and the severity of [the] disorder.*

So that the best approach is one that attempts to gain:

> *... a systems-oriented perspective in which the interactions and dynamics of all endogenous and environmental factors involved are centrally integrated ...*

Phytotherapists can go a long way in taking such an approach but limitations of competence should always be borne in mind and patients should be advised of other sources of support that are available to them such as expert counselling services for alcoholism.

### Illicit substances

Querying the use of illicit substances must be done sensitively to avoid implying a negative judgement about the patient and in view of their nature as illegal materials. It may not always feel appropriate or necessary to ask about the use of these substances but the use of those such as cannabis is very common and may form a significant part of the patient's lifestyle and play a role in shaping the patient's self-identity and worldview. As such, quite apart from any specific health adaptation they may have, they are worth enquiring about.

Inquiry into this territory can begin with a question posed as part of a sequence of routine enquiry, following on from enquiring about smoking and alcohol use and within the same general arena of exploration:

> *'And may I ask about whether you take what are sometimes known as illicit drugs such as cannabis, cocaine and so on?'*

The response can be explored in the same general way as we have described for smoking and alcohol.

It should be borne in mind that though illicit drugs are prohibited, their use does not *necessarily* carry significant personal health risks and some have the potential to generate positive as well as negative experiences, see for example, Griffiths et al.'s (2006, 2008) research on the ability of psilocybin to enable the generation of 'substantial and sustained personal meaning and spiritual significance'. The fact that a substance is illegal does not mean that it is more harmful than legally permitted substances of abuse such as tobacco and alcohol. A House of Commons Science and Technology Committee (2006) report examining drug classification concluded that the UK's ABC system (where A represents the substances considered most dangerous and which are therefore most heavily controlled) was 'not fit for purpose', while the authors:

> ... identified significant anomalies in the classification of individual drugs and a regrettable lack of consistency in the rationale used to make classification decisions. In addition, we have expressed concern at the Government's proclivity for using the classification system as a means of 'sending out signals' to potential users and society at large – it is at odds with the stated objective of classifying drugs on the basis of harm and the Government has not made any attempt to develop an evidence base on which to draw in determining the 'signal' sent out.

A study by Levitt et al. (2006), commissioned by the House of Commons, examined the classification of several drugs and pointed out several issues, e.g. with regard to 'magic mushrooms' (a vague category including *Psilocybe* spp.) they said:

> The positioning of them in Class A does not seem to reflect any scientific evidence that they are of equivalent harm to other Class A drugs.

An evidence-based study by Nutt et al. (2007) classifying substances of potential misuse based on the harm they caused placed alcohol and tobacco above illegal drugs such as cannabis and several Class A drugs including 'ecstasy' (3,4-methylenedioxy-*N*-methylamphetamine – MDMA).

Practitioners need to be cognisant of the risks associated with individual prohibited drugs while bearing in mind that the category 'illicit drugs' is not a homogeneous one and that notions regarding their risks are influenced by social, political, cultural and media-generated views, opinions and biases which, in some cases, may have little congruence with the realities of risk of harm. Their use must be seen in the context of the individual – the risks associated with the particular substance(s) being taken and information pertaining to dosage, frequency of use, etc.; the reasons for use; the patient's perception of the benefits/harm arising from use; and any evidence of negative effects (symptoms of ill health) or dependency/abuse elicited by the practitioner.

### Exercise and relaxation

Consideration of exercise can be started by asking:

> 'Tell me about "exercise" in your life'.

or

> 'Do you take any particular form of exercise or physical activity?'

Some people may equate 'exercise' with formal physical activity taken in a gym for instance, rather than informal activity such as walking. If a patient says that they do not take exercise, then one can enquire:

> 'Are you physically active in other ways? Such as walking?'

The form, duration and regularity of exercise should be sought:

*'Tell me what kind of activity you do'.*

*'How long does each session last for?'*

*'How often do you do this?'*

The nature of exertion involved should be enquired after, e.g. there may be quite a difference between a gentle stroll and a brisk walk in terms of the impact on metabolism:

*'So when you are walking; how do you walk? Slowly or briskly?'*

Some forms of physical activity may be perceived as either 'exercise' or 'relaxation', for example yoga, tai chi and qi gong.

An opening question to ask specifically about relaxation is:

*'Are there particular things that you do in order to relax?'*

or

*'Tell me about "relaxation". Does that happen in your life?'*

'Relaxation' can be interpreted in different ways but the essence of this enquiry is to discover whether the patient has the time, space, opportunity and methods for resting while still being awake and releasing, or being free from, tension and anxiety. The end goal of rest, refreshment and release from tension may be obtained by various means which can be classed as modes of relaxation, such as:

- Relaxing exercise (yoga, tai chi, qi gong, walking, etc.)
- Meditation, chanting, etc.
- Bathing
- The arts (reading, writing poetry, watching a film, going to the theatre, listening to music, etc.)
- Receiving a massage, reflexology or aromatherapy treatment, etc.
- Having a meal with friends
- Gardening
- Knitting
- Playing games (crosswords, chess, bridge, etc.)
- Conversation
- Humour (comedy films and performances, laughter with friends, etc.)
- Being in nature (by the sea, in the woods, camping and trekking, etc.)

Some people may class 'exercise' as 'relaxation' if it provides them with a zone free from worries where they can let go of their cares and be in the moment. The issue here is to discern whether there is also a need to find space for *rest* as well as emotional peace.

In response to questions regarding exercise and relaxation, patients may say:

*'I don't have any time for it'.*

*'There's no space in my life for that'.*

*'I don't know how to relax'.*

*'I know I should make space for it but it's hard to'.*

*'I don't like exercise'.*

*'I can't do it, because …'.*

The practitioner can suggest methods of balancing activity and rest that meet the patient's own preferences and availability, e.g. going dancing as an alternative to the gym or joining a walking club such as The Ramblers if they prefer social interaction.

### Interests and pastimes

Forms of exercise and relaxation may be classed among the patient's interests and pastimes. It is worth asking after these, e.g. 'Do you have any particular interests or pastimes that you enjoy?', since the answer can tell you something about the patient's inclinations, temperament, activities and self-nurturing. Are they able to follow-up their interests? Or is there a reply such as this: 'I've been wanting to do an Italian class for years but there's never any time for me to do my things'?

### Home or/and working life

These essential areas are easily approached by asking:

*'Tell me about how things are at home/work'.*

or

*'Can you tell me about your home/work life?'*

Specific areas of interest are:

#### Home
- Who lives at home?
- If the person lives alone, how is that for them?
- What are the relationships between people at home like?
- How is the living environment?
- Are there any problems, for example with neighbours?
- What is the area in which the home is situated like?
- Are there any financial pressures or worries?

During exploration of these areas it may be suggested or disclosed that an abusive relationship is taking place involving the patient or another family member. The practitioner needs to be aware of how to advise the patient regarding the support that is available to them in such situations (see Appendices). Particular questions can be directed to explore issues suggested by the foregoing history perhaps regarding whether the home is adequately heated or ventilated; if it is damp or dusty; whether noise is a problem; how close to a main road it is; whether there are any smokers at home, and so forth.

#### Work
- Means of travel to work and how long it takes
- Whether work is enjoyed or otherwise
- Type of work and its nature
- Working hours

- Whether work is taken home
- Work environment
- Relationship with colleagues
- Support
- Workload
- Plans to change or develop the career.

The patient may take long working hours and a heavy workload for granted but this combination may be causing enormous pressure and health problems. Long travelling times may be exhausting and a lack of support or bullying in the workplace may be causing distress. The practitioner may be cast in the role of career counsellor at times – helping the patient think through ways in which the working life may be improved or changed, for example by:

- Negotiating a reduction in working hours or to work part of the week from home
- Studying (full- or part-time) or re-training for another career
- Looking at time and stress management techniques to lessen the burden of work
- Considering changes in lifestyle that might make a change of occupation possible.

## VITALITY

Western herbal medicine and naturopathy have traditionally worked with a belief in the *vis medicatrix naturae* – the healing power of nature. In this view, the body in optimum health, and in proper alignment with nature (which is actually the same thing), possesses a vital force or energy that enables self-healing. The practitioner's key responsibility is to help the patient stand in right-relationship with nature so that the self-healing vitality can be generated.

The body's vital capacity, its animating and restorative dynamic energy, can be strategically viewed as flowing in three overlaid dimensions:

- The general vitality of the body as a whole
- The vitality pertaining to specific body systems
- The vitality of particular organs (and of tissues that have the status of organs such as the skin, muscles and mucous membranes).

Vitality and integrity (in the sense of being whole, unified, consistent) are related concepts. In order to manifest integrity, the body and its systems and organs must be properly nurtured and utilized, with: appropriate diet, water, rest, activity and direction of thought (in other words with a fitting regime). The integral 'body' (successfully aligning its physical, emotional, mental and spiritual aspects) constitutes the vital organism. The patient's and the practitioner's estimations of the patient's vitality provide core insights into the patient's predicament and serve as key markers to figure progress in future consultations.

The subject of vitality can be broached with a question such as:

*'Tell me about your energy levels'.*

**Table 5.2** *Patient's vitality representations*

| Deficiency | Excess |
|---|---|
| Fatigue, tiredness, lassitude | The appearance of increased energy or stimulation (adrenalized) |
| Limited movement | Excessive movement |
| Passive appearance | Alert appearance |
| Slow to respond to stimuli | Quick to respond to stimuli |
| Blunted mood | Excitement, quick temper |
| Associated primarily with chronic disorders | Associated primarily with acute disorders or overactive conditions |

Most people seem to know what this means and give a range of responses indicating adequacy ('they seem OK'); deficiency ('I'm shattered'; 'I can't remember what energy is'); optimal levels ('great'; 'I feel fantastic'); or the appearance of excess ('I can't switch off'; 'I'm buzzing with it constantly'; 'it won't go away'). The concept of energy deficiency or excess is central to estimating the patient's vitality and the pictures representative of each state are represented in Table 5.2.

Critical fields to question in order to review and detect the factors involved in energy disruption include:

- Diet and digestion
- Activity and rest (exercise, relaxation, rest and sleep)
- Emotions and mental state.

Sleep is of prime importance and can be asked about by simply enquiring:

*'Tell me about your sleep'.*

Specific sleep-related questions include:

*'What time do you go to bed/wake up?'*

*'What do you do before you go to bed?'*

*'Do you get off to sleep okay?'*

*'How do you feel when you wake up?'*

*'How does the quality of your sleep feel to you?'*

If the patient wakes early:

*'What time(s) do you wake at?'*

*'How do you feel when you wake early? What's going on with you at that time?'*

*'What do you do when you wake up?'*

It may also be appropriate to ask about sleeping partners (e.g. do they snore or move about a lot?); what the patient eats or drinks before going

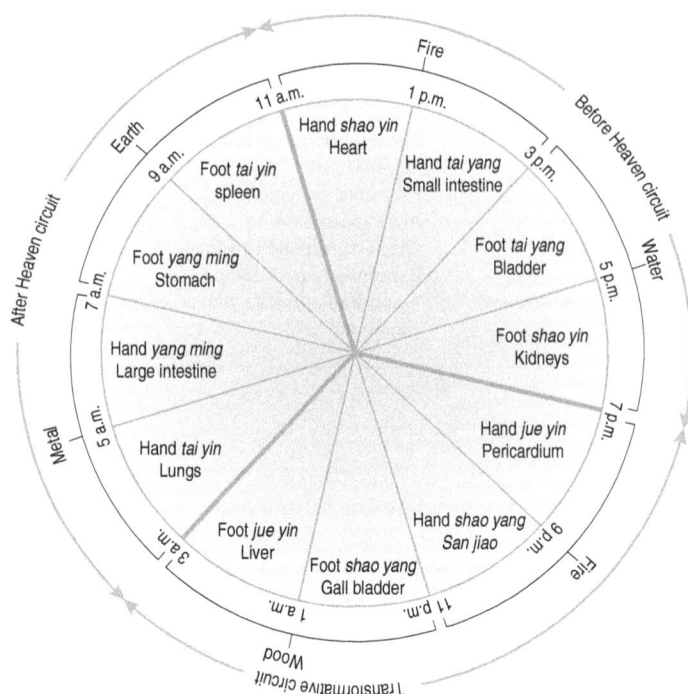

**Figure 5.2** Chinese body clock. *(Reproduced from Dowie 2009.)*

to bed (e.g. stimulants will tend to disrupt sleep); and what the patient has tried to help their sleep. The timing of early waking has significance with regard to the Chinese body clock (Fig. 5.2), which associates particular times of day with the activity of particular organs, e.g. waking between 1 a.m. and 3 a.m. is 'liver time' and waking between 3 a.m. and 5 a.m. is 'lung time'.

For patients whose sleep is disrupted because they have lots of things on their mind (they are always turning thoughts over in their heads, wake with 'mind racing', and feel they have too much to do or to remember) keeping a 'sleep journal' can be very useful. This is used, very simply, as follows:

1. While in bed, just before going to sleep, write down everything that is on your mind into a notebook (thoughts, ideas, to-do items, worries, etc.).
2. Close the notebook and place next to the bed; turn out the light.
3. If you wake in the night turn a low wattage light on and repeat writing down what is on your mind.
4. Repeat step 2.

Noise is a major obstruction to sleep and I have found in my practice that many women (particularly) suffer regular sleep disruption due to snoring by partners. Advice on how the sleeping partner's snoring might be controlled (by reducing alcohol and damp food intake – dairy, refined carbohydrates –

and losing weight if appropriate) will, if they can be followed, often be the best way of helping the patient herself sleep.

Darkness is important in the bedroom since it enhances melatonin secretion – the hormone crucially involved in sleep. A good duration and quality of sleep is essential to nurture vitality and to enable and enhance a number of central functions including: growth; tissue repair and regeneration; immune surveillance and deletion of aberrant cells; and psychological processing – all of which appear to be optimally deployed during sleep. Many of these functions involve melatonin, which also acts directly as a free-radical scavenger and modulator of apoptosis (Berra & Rizzo 2009).

Vitality is also reflected in mood (low mood, low vitality; good mood, enhanced vitality) so that the patient's interest in and engagement with life should be assessed in connection with perceptions of energy levels. In a similar way, appetite for food (as for life) is related to vitality – poor interest in food, poor vitality; healthy interest in food, good vitality.

Specific problems associated with disrupted vitality:

- Mood disorders (anxiety, depression) and emotional worries and distress
- Poor or disordered diet (e.g. high consumption of stimulant foods and drinks, lack of nourishing foods, missed meals, eating late at night).

## ENERGETIC ASSESSMENT

Ancient traditional medical systems such as Greek and Chinese medicine contain appreciations of the movement and play of energy (or gross and subtle *energies*) in the body – sometimes collectively referred to as 'energetics'. These notions derive from an appreciation of the dominant forces and elements apparent in nature and the ways in which they constitute and animate it, such as (in the Greek version):

- Earth
- Air (often best appreciated as 'wind'; a prime force of movement in nature)
- Water
- Fire.

These elements, and their combinations, possess or generate properties or qualities to do with, for example, temperature (fire is hot; earth is cold); hydration (water is wet; earth is dry) and motion (e.g. the movement associated with fire, water and air or wind). The elements and their properties constitute an energetic system that can be applied to the understanding of people, their bodies, and the various specific bodily states and conditions. For example, a person may be classed as constitutionally wet and cold, having a correlated phlegmatic temperament (introverted and stable, passive and thoughtful in Eysenck's classification, see Ch. 4), and being prone to wet/cold conditions such as chronic production of phlegm (a catarrhal tendency) and respiratory tract conditions. A particular condition can be accorded energetic properties, e.g. a specific type of diarrhoea may be classed as hot, wet and moving downwards. Additionally, a person or a condition can be classed as representing a deficiency picture (e.g. tiredness as a deficiency of vital energy) or excess picture (e.g. a fever as an excess of heat in the body). Although it has now become unfamiliar to the Western mind, the concept of energetics has nothing mysterious about it – it is an eminently sensible and practical notion and a way of seeing the world that remains common in many parts of it. For example, the thermal qualities of foods are basic common knowledge in many Eastern countries.

The appreciation of energetics leads to the ability to diagnose states and conditions and indicates appropriate treatment: the need for cooling remedies in hot conditions for instance, or the necessity of activities directed towards replenishment in pictures of deficiency. The approach is not always allopathic though – heat may need to be temporarily increased in a hot condition to bring it to fulfilment (e.g. in a fever); the downward movement of a diarrhoea may need to be encouraged in order to achieve full evacuation and guard against retention of the origins and products of disease. The detection and interpretation of energetic qualities may be easy to grasp and agree upon in gross instances (e.g. a living body is warm and mobile, whereas a dead body is cold and motionless) but inter-observer differences may appear in judging more subtle pictures where individual factors such as the exact degree of heat (is the phenomenon tepid, warm or hot?) and their complex relationships are open to qualitatively different readings. Chinese medicine recognizes additional layers of complexity represented by the concepts of 'true' heat/cold and 'false' (or 'illusionary') heat/cold and 'empty' or 'full' heat/cold, which are beyond our remit to discuss here but which permit a more nuanced and targeted treatment formulation.

In considering energetic factors in the history, account can be taken of all suggestions having to do with factors such as:

- Heat
- Cold
- Wetness (or damp)
- Dryness
- Movement of the phenomenon in the body (vertically and horizontally)
- Deficiency
- Excess.

These territories can be questioned directly (as we will see in a moment) but statements referring to them are made throughout the consultation – and can be perceived if the practitioner is alive to the possibility (e.g. features associated with an overactive state suggest heat, whereas those defining an underactive condition indicate cold). Suggestions of perturbations in these areas are also to be found during physical examination (e.g. pallor of complexion indicates cold and ruddiness indicates heat), and we will look at this dimension of energetic assessment in the next chapter. Table 5.3 gives examples of specific information that can help to diagnose hot or cold pictures.

Energetic information can thus be gathered throughout the consultation when one is oriented to energetic models and signs, with energetic aspects being discerned in the responses given to many (if not nearly all) questions.

**Table 5.3** *Patient information which can constitute hot and cold pictures*

| Hot | Cold |
| --- | --- |
| Reports feeling hot | Reports feeling cold |
| Dislike of heat | Dislike of cold |
| Prefers and seeks cold things (food, drink, baths, cold packs, etc.) | Prefers and seeks hot things (foods, drink, baths, hot water bottles, etc.) |
| Takes clothing off/wears less clothing | Puts clothing on/wears more clothing |
| Worse in hot weather/environments | Worse in cold weather/environments |
| Is overactive | Is underactive |
| Moves about/restless | Lies still/listless |

In this case the practitioner has an energetically disposed approach and will be alive to the energetic richness of the consultation as a whole. Such a practitioner will be able to extract the energetic juice from all relevant patient statements. Energetic information can also be sought by targeted questions. Such questioning can occur in a specific 'energetic assessment' section of the history, or as the occasion arises in following the patient's lead during the consultation, or as a combination of both. Examples of questions of this type include:

*'How would you describe your circulation?'*

The patient might refer here to the tendency to feel hot or cold. Other questions along this line:

*'Tell me about your sense of your own temperature'.*

*'Would you say that you were a 'hot' or a 'cold' person?'*

*'Do you generally prefer to sit in the sun or the shade?'*

*'How are you in cold/hot weather or environments?'*

*'When you get an infection like a cold, how does your body tend to react?'*

Additional closed questions with options may need to be posed to clarify the meaning of this question:

*'For example do you tend to get hot and be restless or to feel cold and prefer to lie still?'*

The tendency to get infections that come on acutely, strongly and with pronounced symptoms that clear quickly indicates a hot reactor, while a gradual, muted response that lingers suggests a cold reactor. (*Note*: Acute conditions are generally hot, whereas as chronic conditions are generally cold but may have hot phases, i.e. acute recurrences or exacerbations.)

*'Can you describe your skin, hair and nails to me – what are they like?'*

Dry, flakey (e.g. dandruff) skin and hair suggests dryness, while oily, greasy, sweaty skin/hair is indicative of wetness.

Patients can be asked about the direction of movement of a particular phenomenon, as is common in conventional practice in asking about the radiation of pain from a focal spot: 'Where does the pain spread to?'

Consideration of energetics in phytotherapy is a return to first principles: health and illness depend on an appropriate degree of circulation in the body as a whole and to specific organs and organ systems. The state of circulation of the blood is a fundamental factor determining the movement or stagnation of the body's 'energies' (which we can read as including cellular nutrition, respiration and metabolism). Herbal medicines are agents that can modulate and direct circulatory activity across a spectrum of activity – ranging across a spectrum of effects from the subtle to the pronounced: the complex phytochemistry of medicinal plants, singly or in combination, can bring a wide range of pharmacological influences to bear in the body that diversely and powerfully adapt physiological functioning. Although the energetic basis of Western herbal medicine is now poorly appreciated it remains, as Wood (2004) points out: 'inferred in the list of herbal "actions"'. During the evolution of Western medicine, the old energetic terms: hot, cold, damp and dry were dropped, and in their place, terms such as: stimulant (warming), refrigerant (cooling), mucilage (moistening) and astringent (drying) were adopted.

## TEMPERAMENT, PERSONALITY, MOOD AND OUTLOOK

'Temperament' can be construed to refer to the patient's nature, disposition, tendencies, behaviour, physiological type and emotional state and was formerly applied with regard to the patient's individual elemental (earth, air, water, fire) make-up and in relationship to their predominant humoural status (blood, phlegm, black and yellow bile) – giving the four temperaments as sanguine, phlegmatic, melancholic and choleric. Temperament now tends to be popularly conceived as more-or-less synonymous with 'personality', although it is common from a more technical perspective, to consider *temperament* as denoting the genetically-based portion of the personality with *character* having to do with the acquired dimensions (temperament playing nature to character's nurture). It is a term that continues to be used with a differentiated meaning in psychology, especially child psychology and development:

> *Temperament arises from our genetic endowment. It influences and is influenced by the experience of each individual, and one of its outcomes is the adult personality ... We have defined* temperament *as individual differences in reactivity and self-regulation assumed to have a constitutional basis ...*
>
> Rothbart et al. (2000)

This definition is consistent with the humoural tradition in implying a set of behavioural characteristics rooted in a particular physical typology (personal mixture, *crasis*, of the four elements) but shaped by external factors such as environment, occupation and so forth.

Numerous factors from the case history feed into forming an appreciation of the patient's temperament and personality including family history, and childhood and adult life experiences. Other specific areas include those pertaining to the patient's:

- Mood (psychoemotional state)
- Outlook (including views on the future)
- Self-view (and impressions of the views of others about the self)
- Sociability and comfort in solitude
- Worldview
- Personal beliefs and convictions
- Reactions in given situations.

Questioning and monitoring these areas can lead to the delineation of conditions, states or predicaments that require support, care and possibly treatment such as depression, anxiety, negative self-view, loneliness, severe emotional trauma, and so forth. As ever, the phytotherapist needs to remember the limits of her competence in dealing with these territories and to advise patients appropriately.

Below are examples of questions that may open up these subject areas.

- Mood (psychoemotional state):

A question of major utility is: 'Tell me how you are feeling in your self'. People tend to interpret this as an invitation to look at their inner feelings and emotional state and respond accordingly.

*'Could you tell me about your mood? How you feel emotionally?'*

- Outlook (including views on the future):

*'How would you describe your outlook on life?'*

*'How do you see your life at the moment?'*

*'How do you feel about the future?'*

*'How do you see the future?'*

*'If you think about the future, what thoughts do you have?'*

- Self-view (and impressions of the views of others about the self):

*'How would you describe your self?'*

*'If you had to describe your self as a person, what would you say?'*

*'How do you think other people see you, as a person?'*

*'How would people who know you well describe you?'*

- Sociability and comfort in solitude:

*'How do you get on with other people?'*

*'How are you in social situations?'*

*'How do you get on in the company of other people?'*

*'How do you get on with being by your self?'*

*'How is it for you when you are "in your own company"?'*

- Worldview:

  *'How would you summarize the way you see the world?'*

  *'Do you have a view on what the world is like? What its nature is?'*

- Personal beliefs and convictions:

  *'Do you have a personal view or belief about what life is about or what life is for?'*

  *'What is the purpose of life, as you see it?'*

  *'Do you have a particular spiritual or religious or other belief that helps you understand the world?'*

- Reactions in given situations, or to specific scenarios or ideas:

  This can be assessed throughout the consultation by gauging reactions to various questions and in the descriptions of reactions given in the patient's narrative. Pointed questions can also be formulated to assess this area:

  *'If you were in a situation where (describe scenario) – how would you deal with/ respond to/react to/cope with/ that?'*

## PERSONAL STYLE

This section proposes that, in getting to know the patient, it may be valuable to form an appreciation of their personal 'style', including with regard to their taste, preferences and way of being (i.e. manner of acting and presenting themselves). Such a view is compiled from virtually every territory of the case history (and via observation), with details provided by questions such as those to do with 'interests and pastimes', and areas such as the following:

- Regarding the arts:

  *'Do you enjoy any particular types of creative arts such as music, painting, theatre?'*

- If the patient specifies a particular form, e.g. music, one can ask:

  *'Which sorts of music do you like?'*

- The seasons:

  *'Which of the seasons do you like the best?'*

## DIET

Diet is a core focus area in the phytotherapy consultation with dietary adaptation constituting a key therapeutic strategy and zone of health promotion advice (a central part of 'regimen'). Dietary intake can be assessed in a number of ways and may be complemented by the use of diet diaries completed by the patient either in advance of, or subsequent to the first consultation. It is a region of continual return at follow-up visits.

A simple and open approach to exploring the diet is to ask: 'Tell me about your diet' and follow the patient's lead from there. A more formally structured exploration can follow or replace that initial question, or parts of it can be deployed to fill in the gaps in the patient's reportage. Even when a more formal protocol is used, such as that described below, it is helpful to begin by asking: 'Do you have any particular dietary preferences or do you follow a specific dietary approach?' In this way, you will tend to discover, e.g. whether the patient is currently undertaking a particular weight loss diet; whether they are vegetarian, vegan, etc; or whether they avoid wheat, dairy, etc.

The more formal method of investigation proposed here offers two related fields for exploration:

1. An opening survey of the patient's dietary intake and pattern of eating in terms of targeting what is eaten and when
2. A following general appreciation of factors influencing the patient's dietary choices and culinary capacities.

### Dietary intake and pattern of eating

This survey can be set up and explained in the following way:

*'I'd like to get an idea of what you typically eat by asking you what times you eat at and what you tend to have at those times. Is that okay?'*

The exploration begins by asking:

*'At about what time do you first eat during the day?'*

*'And what do you eat at that time?'*

The procedure then continues with repetition of the following questions until the dietary intake for the day is complete:

*'At what time do you next eat?'*

*'And what do you have then?'*

This approach has the advantage of allowing the patient to tell the times at which they eat rather than following an assumption made by the practitioner when terms like breakfast and lunch are used. This can be helpful since, for example, some people may take 'breakfast' at 5 a.m., while others eat it at noon. Avoidance of the words used to imply meal times and meal types can also help to avoid confusion, for example, while most people will agree that breakfast is the first meal of the day (although the timing of it may vary hugely), terms like 'dinner', 'tea' and 'supper' can mean different things to different people, e.g. one person's 'lunch' is another person's 'dinner'.

The pattern for this approach is then a repetition of the pairing: When do you eat? What do you eat? As the patient describes what they eat at each time in the day supplementary questions should be asked to clarify factors such as the quality and quantity of food eaten, e.g. if the patient says they have porridge at around a 7.15 each morning, the practitioner can ask:

*'What type of porridge is that? Is it instant oat flakes or whole oats?'*

*'How much do you have? Large bowl or small bowl?'*

*'Do you make it with milk or water?'*

*'Do you add anything to it? Sugar, salt, honey, etc?'*

This type of questioning provides the contrast between finding that the patient 'has porridge for breakfast' to discovering, for example, that they have 'a large bowl of instant oat cereal made with milk and topped with two or three spoons of sugar', so that the assumption that 'bowl of porridge equals a healthy breakfast' can be reconsidered.

Other queries along this line of approach include: when a patient says they have 'some toast' at about 11.30:

*'What kind of bread do you use?'*

*'What do you put on the toast?'*

*'How many slices do you have?'*

While assessing the diet the practitioner should suspend her notions of what constitutes an 'average' diet and remain open to the patient's individual story, as in all areas of the case history. Wide variations in dietary content and pattern or style do occur. For many people, the morning meal ('breakfast') is the least varying meal of the day, while the evening meal changes the most, but for some people this relationship is reversed. Some people follow a diet that is very limited in terms of food groups and specific food items, while others are incredibly diverse. It is important to have an approach that can discern and accommodate the patient's true dietary picture.

While reporting in response to 'what do you eat?' questions, the patient may include items such as drinks and snacks. If these items are not mentioned they should be asked about specifically, along with other factors that can modulate the diet such as restaurant and take-away meals. There are also key healthy food groups and types that should be enquired after specifically if they appear to be absent in the dietary history, such as fruit, vegetables, nuts and seeds.

*'So what about drinks? What do you drink during the day? When do you have it?'*

*'And snacks? Do you have any snacks throughout the day?'*

*'Do you eat out or order in take-away meals? How frequently? What do you have?'*

*'You haven't mentioned fruit. Does that have any place in your diet?'*

In concluding this zone of questioning, patients can be asked to what extent, and in which ways, the dietary regime described differs in response to such variables as weekdays as opposed to weekends, and home days as opposed to work or travel days. Incidentally, it may be worth saying that the commonly taken path to dietary assessment embodied in the question: 'Can you tell me about your typical diet, for instance what did you eat yesterday?' should be avoided, since, as a general rule, yesterday's diet is *never* typical, even if it can be remembered.

### General dietary factors

A wide range of questions can be put to get a sense of the patient's food attitudes, behaviours, preferences and practices, including:

*'Tell me how you feel about food?'*

*'How would you describe your attitude to food?'*

*'How would you describe your relationship with eating?'*

*'Do you enjoy eating?'*

This type of questioning can be asked routinely or in response to the patient showing signs of uneasiness in talking about food. Replies to questions in this area may be suggestive of an eating disorder, and as ever, the phytotherapist needs to be aware of the limits to her competence and be aware of when and how to recommend that a patient might also visit another practitioner (such as a psychological therapist) for additional support.

A group of questions can be asked to consider the patient's ability to prepare food and their access to the space and equipment required to do so. For example, people living in shared accommodation may have difficulty in accessing the kitchen at a time that suits them best, or for the duration of time that they would ideally like. Sample questions:

*'Do you know how to cook? Can you cook?'*

*'Do you have a place to cook?'*

*'Can you be left alone to cook in the way you like best?'*

If the patient does not know how to cook, the practitioner can recommend books and classes. Some phytotherapists may wish to offer wholefood cookery classes to groups of patients.

It is useful to explore the setting and manner in which the patient is eating, especially where a digestive condition is reported:

*'Could you tell me about the context in which you eat each of the main meals of the day? For example, where do you eat?'*

*'What's going on around you while you are eating?'*

*'Are you able to sit down and eat without interruption?'*

*'Do you do anything else while you are eating?'*

*'At work, do you eat at your desk or elsewhere?'*

*'Do you carry on working while you are eating?'*

*'Are meal times happy and relaxed times or can they be stressful?'*

*'What's going on when you are eating your breakfast/lunch/evening meal?'*

*'Do you eat standing up or sitting down?'*

*'Where do you eat your breakfast/lunch/evening meal?'*

*'Can you tell me about how you eat? For example, do you eat quickly or slowly?'*

*'Do you tend to chew your food or bolt it down?'*

*'Do you notice your food as you are eating it?'*

*'Do you savour your food or just "get it in there"?'*

*'What do you do after you eat your breakfast/lunch/evening meal?'*

A wide range of responses can be made to these questions, helping to build up a picture of the eating context and habits, especially with regard to whether the patient has time to eat, is able to focus on their food, and is having time to digest the food properly.

Food preferences, effects, attitudes, beliefs and influences can be explored with the following types of question:

*'Which foods do you particularly like?'*

*'Which foods do you dislike?'*

*'Do any foods upset or disagree with you?'*

*'Do you crave any particular foods?'*

*'How much experience do you have with different types of food?'*

*'How do you feel about trying new foods?'*

*'When you travel, do you eat the local food or try to find foods that are familiar?'*

*'Would you say that you were adventurous or conservative when it comes to food?'*

*'Do you have any opinions about organic versus non-organic food?'*

*'How often do you eat foods cooked from fresh ingredients?'*

*'How often do you have "ready-made" foods?'*

Two final categories can provide crucial information and opportunities for improving the diet.

### Food history

What were the patient's childhood experiences with food? What was the childhood diet like? Which kinds of messages about food were communicated in the family environment? For example, if the patient was pushed to always eat everything on her plate as a child, she may continue to do that throughout her life, even when her weight might benefit from eating less. Attitudes and behaviours around food, such as this example, can be challenged and alternative perspectives and practices can be offered and encouraged.

### Financial limitations

Are there any restrictions on food purchases imposed by scarce financial resources? If so, what form do the restrictions take? Where poor quality food is being eaten as a response to limited funds, the practitioner can advise on how a healthy diet might be achieved with the same budget by, for example, focussing on home cooked foods, fresh ingredients, vegetables and low-cost ingredients such as pulses. It may be appropriate to encourage the patient to grow some of their own food at home or on an allotment or to join a local community cooperative wholefood buyers group.

## SYSTEMS ENQUIRY

Where a thorough approach has been taken in the foregoing parts of the case history much, and probably most, of the information that may be considered to fall within the territory of the 'systems enquiry' will already have been explored. This will apply especially to the system, or systems, in which the presenting complaint/s are located. The systems enquiry can be viewed as a collection of mobile units of investigation, which can be brought forward and deployed wherever required, at any point during the consultation. For example, if a patient presents with a gynaecological disorder then most, if not all, of the questions contained within the notion of the 'reproductive system' can be posed within the 'history of the presenting complaint'. Discussion of the diet may lead naturally to questions regarding the functioning of the digestive system, and so forth. Familiarity with the systems enquiry is important in order to ensure that a good breadth and depth of examination within the relevant system can be undertaken whenever a phenomenon from that system comes into the clinical view.

The systems enquiry is best drawn upon as an *aide-memoire* at, or towards, the end of the consultation where the practitioner can briefly cast her mind over the systems list in order to check whether anything has been missed. A routine walk with the patient through the systems realm at the end of history-taking is often useful because it can suggest, or reveal, significant lines of investigation that had previously been overlooked.

A concise (but not exhaustive) guide to the key questions for each bodily 'system' is provided below. Each group of questions should be viewed as a potential treasure chest of golden information standing ready to be opened at any relevant juncture in the history-taking, with its contents being partially or entirely spent as required.

### Digestive system

- Open approach:

  *'Tell me about your digestion'.*

  *'How does your digestive system seem to you?'*

- More targeted, less open, questions:

  *'How would you describe your appetite?'*

  *'What about your bowel movements? How often do you have a motion? For example, do you pass a motion every day, every other day, every few days? Do you ever have difficulty passing motions? Is there ever any discomfort or pain? Do you ever get constipation or diarrhoea?'*

  *'What are your stools like? Is there anything that stands out about your stools? For example to do with colour or smell?'*

  *'Have you ever noticed blood in the stool? Or blood on the toilet paper after wiping?'*

  *'Have you ever had piles/haemorrhoids?'*

*'Do you ever get any abdominal upsets or discomfort?'*

*'Do you experience indigestion?'* If the answer is yes: *'What does "indigestion" involve for you?'*

*'Do you have any difficulties eating/chewing/swallowing?'*

*'Do you ever get a sore tongue/soreness or cracking at the corners of your mouth?'* (If affirmative, this suggests nutritional deficiency; the second part of the question refers to angular stomatitis).

*'Do you have any dental problems?'*

*'Do you ever have sore or bleeding gums?'*

*'Do you experience much flatulence or wind?'*

*'Do you ever pass a stool when you don't mean to? Do you ever lose control of your bowel movements?'*

### Urinary system

- Open approach:

  *'Tell me about passing water. How is that for you?'*

- More targeted, less open, questions:

  *'Do you have any problems passing water?'*

  *'How often do you pass water?'*

  *'Do you seem to pass a lot, a little or a normal amount?'*

  *'Is there anything that stands out about your urine? For example, to do with its colour or smell?'*

  *'Do you ever get any discomfort when passing water? Or bleeding?'*

  *'Do you get cystitis?'*

  *'Do you ever pass water when you don't mean to? Do you ever lose control of passing water?'*

  *'Do you ever have to get up at night to pass water?'*

Where men are experiencing changes in passing water which may be linked to prostate enlargement, they should be asked about frequency; starting and stopping; strength of flow; nocturia.

### Integumentary system (skin, hair and nails)

- Open approach:

  *'Tell me about your skin. What about your hair and nails?'*

- More targeted, less open, questions:

  *'Do you ever get any skin problems? Such as spots or rashes?'*

  *'Does your skin ever itch?'*

*'Would you describe your skin as oily, dry or normal? What about your hair?'*

*'Would you say you had sensitive skin?'*

*'Do your nails ever crack or go crumbly at the ends?'*

*'Do you bleed easily?'*

*'When you have a wound, how well would it tend to heal?'*

*'Does your skin react to anything?'*

*'Are there any fabrics you can't wear or that your skin doesn't like?'*

*'Are your nails strong or weak?'*

*'Do you cut your nails or bite them?'*

*'What kinds of products or treatments do you use on your skin/hair/nails?'*

*'How do you care for your skin/hair/nails?'*

*'How often do you wash? Do you bathe or shower? What products do you use?'*

## Musculoskeletal system

- Open approach:

    *'Tell me about your muscles and joints'.*

- More targeted, less open, questions:

    *'How do your muscles feel to you? For example, do they tend to feel tight or floppy?'*

    *'Do you have any problems gripping, holding, lifting – that kind of thing?'*

    *'Are you in any way impaired in using your body to do everyday tasks and to look after yourself? For example, cooking, dressing, doing up buttons?'*

    *'How is your mobility? Can you move your body as you want to? Do you have any difficulties getting around? For example, walking or driving?'*

    *'Do your muscles ever ache or do you get cramp?'*

    *'Do your joints ever feel stiff or loose? Is there any particular time of day when that happens?'*

    *'Do you get any back/hip/knee/hand/foot/shoulder/neck problems?'*

    *'Do you have any difficulty bending or kneeling? Are there any restrictions to the range of movement you have in any joint?'*

    *'Are your joints ever noisy when you move them? For example, do they ever, click, crunch, grind or pop?'*

    *'Do you get any pain in your joints?'*

    *'Do your joints ever get red or swollen? Do they ever get stuck or locked?'*

## Cardiovascular system

- Open approach:

    'Tell me about your circulation'.

- More targeted, less open, questions:

    'In terms of your circulation do you feel yourself to be a warm or a cold person?'

    'Do your hands and feet get particularly cold or hot?'

    'Do you ever get any tightness in your chest? Or pain?' If yes: 'Does it happen when you are active or at rest – or both?'

    'Do you ever have palpitations – feeling your heart beat rapidly or oddly?' (Note: It is worth spelling out what 'palpitations' means, as this is a word that might be interpreted differently by some patients.)

    'Are you ever breathless? Does it happen when you are active or resting – or both? Do you ever wake breathless in the night?'

    'Do you need to prop yourself up on pillows to help your breathing at night?'

    'Do you ever get any swelling – in your face, hands or ankles?'

    'Do you ever get discomfort or pain in your legs?'

    'Do your hands or fingers ever change colour or feel painful?'

    'Have you ever had your cholesterol levels checked?'

## Respiratory system

- Open approach:

    'Tell me about your breathing'.

- More targeted, less open, questions:

    'Do you ever get mucus or catarrh?'

    'Any sinus problems? What about your throat – any soreness?'

    'Do you get many coughs or colds – any more or less than other people?'

    'Do you cough? When do you cough? Do you bring anything up? What colour is the phlegm? Does it hurt to cough?'

    'Does your chest ever make noises? Such as wheezing or crackling?'

    'Do you ever get short of breath?'

    'Do you ever get discomfort or pain when you breathe in or bend over?'

## Immune system

- Open approach:

    'How would you describe your immune resistance?'

- More targeted, less open, questions:

    *'Do you ever get mouth ulcers?'*

    *'Do your lymph nodes ever enlarge? For example, lumps in your neck, under your arms or in your groin?'*

    *'How often do you get colds or other infections?'*

    *'Do you seem to catch infections easily, or the opposite?'*

    *'Do you have any persistent problems such as sore throat, snuffles, or cough?'*

### Nervous system

*'Would you say that you were clumsy or had good control over your movements?'*

*'Do you have any problems with balance?'*

*'Do you ever get tremors or shakiness?'*

*'Do you ever have headaches?'* If yes: *'Can you describe the pain to me? Where is the pain? Does anything else happen before or during the headache?'*

*'Do you have any problems with hearing or vision? What about taste, smell or touch?'*

*'Do you ever have any odd or unusual sensations anywhere in your body? For example, hot, cold, tingling or numb patches? In places such as your arms or legs?'*

Questions concerning sleep, mood, emotions and outlook can be placed in this section, as we already covered above.

Where the patient appears distant or disturbed, questions should be asked to check the psychoemotional state and basic orientation, starting with simple questions such as:

*'Do you know where you are?'*

*'Can you tell me why you are here?'*

*'Can you describe to me how you are feeling?'* or *'what you are experiencing?'*

### Reproductive system

- Open approach:

    *For women of reproductive age: 'Tell me about your cycle'.*

- More targeted, less open, questions:
    - Women:

    *'What age were you when your periods started?'*

    *'What was your period like for the first few years? How has it been since then?'*

    *'How frequently do you get your bleed? For example, every month, 28 to 30 days; or less; or more?'*

    *'How long do you bleed for?'*

*'How would you describe the flow of your bleed? For example, would you say it was heavy, light or normal?'*

If the flow is described as heavy: 'Do you use tampons or pads?' Women with menorrhagia often use both; 'What level of absorbency do you use? How often do you have to change your protection?' In menorrhagia, this can be up to every half hour. 'Do you have to wake in the night to change them?' In menorrhagia, the answer is often yes.

*'Do you get any pain with your bleed? Or at any other time in your cycle? For example, in mid-cycle?'*

*'Do you ever get any premenstrual symptoms? For example, breast tenderness, food cravings, bloating or emotional upset? How long before the bleed does this happen? Does it stop when the bleed starts?'*

*'Whereabouts in your cycle are you now?'*

*'Do you ever get an unusual discharge? Or thrush?'*

*'Do you ever get bleeding outside of your actual period?'*

It may already have been revealed that the woman is taking the contraceptive pill (e.g. under drug history) or using another form of contraception, but if not, ask: 'Are you using any particular form of contraception at present?'

The personal details are already likely to have established whether the woman has children but other pregnancies can be enquired after: 'I know you have two children but may I ask whether you have had any other pregnancies? And any terminations?'

- Women of menopausal or post-menopausal age:

*'When was your last period?'*

*If the woman is still having her period: 'Tell me about your last few periods'.*

*'Are you experiencing anything like flushes? Getting hot or sweating at night? Vaginal dryness or soreness? Mood changes or disruption? Dry skin, hair or nails?'*

- Men and women:

Asking about sexual interest and activity may be minimally or extensively questioned, depending on whether the patient has identified this as an area in need of investigation.
A routine question would be:

*'May I ask about your libido – your interest in sexual activity – how that has been recently?'*

Further basic questions include:

*'May I ask whether you have been having sex in recent times?'*

This question can be variously worded in the light, e.g. of whether the patient has previously described themselves as in a relationship or single, bearing in mind that somebody may class themselves as single, yet be having sexual relationships just as someone may be in a long-term relationship but not be sexually active.

*'Is sex pleasurable? Or is it ever uncomfortable or painful?'*

*'Are you happy with your sexual experiences and your performance?'*

## COMPREHENSIVE VERSUS COMPREHENSION

In every consultation, whether a first visit or a follow-up, the practitioner should aim to be as comprehensive as possible in covering all potentially relevant territory. However, it will commonly be difficult to achieve this goal, especially at first visits involving an extensive or complex narrative. The wealth of territories that we have just described in connection with the initial consultation can rarely be done justice in just a single appointment and the practitioner should not attempt to shoehorn every last item into one session. While *comprehensiveness* is an important target to aim for, an even more essential one is *comprehension* – appreciating the patient's predicament, hopes, fears and expectations; understanding the nature of their condition; or simply getting the gist of their situation, in order that work may begin towards achieving an enhanced position.

## EXPECTATIONS 2 AND TRANSITING TO THE PHYSICAL EXAMINATION

When the formal case history-taking section is coming to an end it is helpful to check whether the patient has anything they still wish to say or that has been left unexpressed:

*'Before we move on, do you have anything else to add?'*

*'Is there anything you wanted to discuss that we haven't yet covered?'*

Adding 'Anything at all?' to the end of these questions provides an extra encouragement and states that you really want to hear about even the smallest concern.

Extending a clear invitation to complete the history will help to ensure that the patient's key concerns and issues are noted, even if there is not enough time to discuss every one in detail at the first visit.

The end of formal history-taking is also a good time to review the patient's expectations and agenda, given that the profoundly reflective nature of the consultation in phytotherapy may have occasioned a shift in self-perception and a consequent reforming of wishes and expectations:

*'We've covered a lot of ground and I wonder at this stage what your priorities are for treatment and what else you would like to get from this consultation?'*

This provides an opportunity for the patient to take stock and reframe their initial agenda items. Examples of responses to this kind of question, at this point in the consultation, include:

*'I've realized that I need to work on my diet and I'd like us to focus on that'.*

*'I hadn't appreciated how bad my sleep has become and I really want to get that back to normal'.*

*'I still just want my skin to get better but I can see that there are things in my life that I can change to help it. I just don't know where to start though'.*

*'I'm not ready to stop smoking but I am ready to make other changes'.*

*'I just feel that I'm all over the place and I need a plan, something to follow to get me started'.*

*'More than ever I want to treat this naturally and I want to do everything I can, in every area that I need to'.*

*'I'm going to need some more time to think things through, to process all this'.*

The detailed response to these statements and requests will usually come right at the end of the consultation (after the physical examination) in the formulation and negotiation of the treatment and management plan. It is worth gathering this information now however, in order to bring the formal case history to a conclusion; to enable the patient to achieve a sense of completion regarding this major section of the consultation; and to prevent the feeling that the consultation is moving on too quickly or abruptly. For now, the practitioner can acknowledge the patient's words, indicate when these will be fully addressed and introduce the next part of the consultation – the physical examination:

*'Thank you for that. We are going to address everything you have said right at the end of the consultation. First of all though I want to do some physical examinations in order to see if we can gather any extra information that might be helpful. Is that okay?'*

As we suggested earlier, the physical examination does not have to be an entirely separate area of the consultation since parts of it can be incorporated into the case history at relevant points as phenomena are mentioned, e.g. looking at a skin rash or palpating a swelling. The patient may not wait to be invited to be examined and might, e.g. roll up their sleeve to reveal a skin rash as they are describing it. The practitioner can take the opportunity that has been presented in this way or ask to examine where indicated, as the consultation goes along.

In proceeding on from the formal case history, it should be remembered that the patient may continue to proffer new information, and the practitioner will continue to seek it, throughout the rest of the consultation so that history elements are still present within the physical examination and the negotiation of the treatment plan and case management. The consultation is a narrative event from beginning to end.

## REFERENCES

Ackerman D: *Deep play,* New York, 1999, Vintage.

American Psychiatric Association: *DSM-IV-TR: Diagnostic and statistical manual of mental disorders: text revision,* ed 4, Arlington, 2000, American Psychiatric Press.

Armstrong D: Child development and medical ontology, *Social Science and Medicine* 13:9–12, 1979.

Baron RJ: Medical hermeneutics: where is the 'text' we are interpreting? *Theoretical Medicine* 11(1):25–28, 1990.

Bean J, Ng D, Demirtas H, Guinan P: Medical students' attitudes towards torture, *Torture* 18(2):99–103, 2008.

Berra B, Rizzo AM: Melatonin: circadian rhythm regulator, chronobiotic, antioxidant and beyond, *Clinics in Dermatology* 27:202–209, 2009.

Bodenheimer T, Starfield B, Treadway K, et al: The future of primary care: the community responds, *New England Journal of Medicine* 359(25):2636–2639, 2008.

Bornschein S, Hausteiner C, Zilker T, et al: Psychiatric and somatic disorders and multiple chemical sensitivity (MCS) in 264 'environmental patients', *Psychological Medicine* 32(8):1387–1394, 2002.

Cabre M: Women or healers? Household practices and the categories of health care in late medieval Iberia, *Bulletin of the History of Medicine* 82:18–51, 2008.

Caress SM, Steinemann AC: A review of a two-phase population study of multiple chemical sensitivities, *Environmental Health Perspectives* 111(12):1490–1497, 2003.

Cassell EJ: *The nature of suffering: and the goals of medicine*, 2004, Oxford University Press.

Catzel P: Paediatrics, *British Medical Journal* 2:1028, 1955.

Churchill Livingstone: *Churchill's medical dictionary*, New York, 1989, Churchill Livingstone.

Churchill LR: Hermeneutics in science and medicine: a thesis understated, *Theoretical Medicine* 11:141–144, 1990.

Claxton G: The anatomy of intuition. In Atkinson T, Claxton G, editors: *The Intuitive Practitioner: on the value of not always knowing what one is doing*, Buckingham, 2004, Open University Press.

Collins: *Collins English dictionary*, London, 2000, HarperCollins.

Cooper R: *Classifying madness: a philosophical examination of the diagnostic and statistical manual of mental disorders*, Dordrecht, 2005, Springer.

Dowie S: *Acupuncture: an aid to differential diagnosis*, Edinburgh, 2009, Churchill Livingstone.

Eliade M: *The sacred and the profane: the nature of religion*, New York, 1959, Harcourt Brace Jovanovich.

Elwyn G, Gwyn R: Narrative based medicine: stories we hear and stories we tell: analysing talk in clinical practice, *British Medical Journal* 318:186–188, 1999.

Epstein O, Perkin GD, de Bono DP, et al: *Clinical examination*, ed 2, London, 1997, Mosby.

Eraut M: The intuitive practitioner: a critical overview. In Atkinson T, Claxton G, editors: *The Intuitive Practitioner: on the value of not always knowing what one is doing*. Buckingham, 2004, Open University Press.

Foucault M: *The birth of the clinic (first published 1963)*, London, 2007, Routledge.

Gadamer HG: *Truth and method*, London, 1989, Sheed & Ward.

Gafaranga J, Britten N: 'Fire away': the opening sequence in general practice consultations, *Family Practice* 20:242–247, 2003.

Gill D, O'Brien N: *Paediatric clinical examination*, London, 1998, Churchill Livingstone.

Gouk P, Hills H: Towards histories of emotions. In Gouk P, Hills H, editors: *Representing Emotions: new connections in the histories of art, music and medicine*, Aldershot, 2005, Ashgate.

Gourlay S: Knowing as semiosis: steps towards a reconceptualization of 'tacit knowledge'. In Tsoukas H, Mylonopoulos N, editors: *Organizations as knowledge systems: knowledge, learning and dynamic capabilities*, Basingstoke, 2003, Palgrave Macmillan.

Gray J: *Black Mass: apocalyptic religion and the death of utopia*, London, 2007, Allen Lane.

Greenberg M: Therapeutic play: developing humor in the nurse-patient relationship, *The Journal of the New York State Nurses Association* 34(1):25–31, 2003.

Griffiths RR, Richards WA, McCann U, et al: Psilocybin can occasion mystical-type experiences having substantial and sustained personal meaning and spiritual significance, *Psychopharmacology* 187:268–283, 2006.

Griffiths RR, Richards WA, Johnson MW, et al: Mystical-type experiences occasioned by psilocybin mediate the attribution of personal meaning and spiritual significance 14 months later, *Journal of Psychopharmacology* 22(6):621–632, 2008.

Hargie O, Saunders C, Dickson D: *Social skills in interpersonal communication*, ed 3, London, 1994, Routledge.

Hasin D: Classification of alcohol use disorders, *Alcohol Research and Health: the Journal of the National Institute on Alcohol Abuse and Alcoholism* 27(1):5–17, 2003.

Hasin DS, Grant BF: The co-occurrence of DSM-IV alcohol abuse in DSM-IV alcohol dependence: results of the National Epidemiological Survey on alcohol and related conditions on heterogeneity that differ by population subgroup, *Archives of General Psychiatry* 61:891–896, 2004.

Haskell R: *Deep listening: hidden meanings in everyday conversation*, Cambridge MA, 2001, Da Capo Press.

Helman CG: *Culture, health and illness*, London, 2000, Hodder Arnold.

Hill Curth L: Lessons from the past: preventive medicine in early modern England, *Medical Humanities* 29:16–20, 2003.

Hogarth RM: *Educating intuition*, 2001, University of Chicago Press.

House of Commons Science and Technology Committee: Drug classification: making a hash of it? Fifth Report of Session 2005–2006. London, 31 July 2006, The Stationery Office.

Hunter D, Bomford RR: *Hutchison's clinical methods*, London, 1956, Cassell.

Johnson BS: *The unfortunates*, London, 1969, Secker and Warburg.

Kaplan B: *The homeopathic conversation: the art of taking the case*, London, 2001, Natural Medicine Press.

Kirkwood T: *The end of age: why everything about ageing is changing*, London, 2001, BBC in association with Profile Books.

Klatsky AL: Alcohol and cardiovascular diseases, *Expert Review of Cardiovascular Therapy* 7(5):499–506, 2009.

Klein N: *The shock doctrine*, London, 2007, Allen Lane.

Kleinman A: *What really matters?* New York, 2006, Oxford University Press.

Kuriyama S: *The expressiveness of the body: and the divergence of Greek and Chinese medicine*, New York, 1999, Zone Books.

Leder D: Clinical interpretation: the hermeneutics of medicine, *Theoretical Medicine* 11(1):9–24, 1990.

Lenaerts M: Substances, relationships and the omnipresence of the body: an overview of Asheninka ethnomedicine (Western Amazonia), *Journal of Ethnobiology and Ethnomedicine* 2:49, 2006.

Levitt R, Nason E, Hallsworth M: The evidence base for the classification of drugs. Technical Report, Santa Monica CA, 2006, The RAND Corporation.

Lifton RJ: Doctors and torture, *New England Journal of Medicine* 351(5):415–416, 2004.

Macleod J: *Clinical examination: a textbook for students and doctors by teachers of the Edinburgh Medical School*, ed 2, Edinburgh, 1967, E. & S Livingstone Ltd.

Maio G: History of medical involvement in torture: then and now, *The Lancet* 357(9268):1609–1611, 2001.

Norfolk A: Drink limits 'useless', *The Times* 2007:20 October.

Nutt D, King LA, Saulsbury W, Blakemore C: Development of a rational scale to assess the harm of drugs of potential misuse, *The Lancet* 369(9566):1047–1053, 2007.

Nutton V: Medicine in Medieval and Western Europe, 1000–1500. In Conrad LI, Neve M, Nutton V, et al., editors: *The Western Medical Tradition: 800BC to 1800AD*, 1995, Cambridge University Press.

Nutton V: *Ancient medicine*, London, 2004, Routledge.

Penson RT, Partridge RA, Rudd P, et al: Laughter: the best medicine, *The Oncologist* 10:651–660, 2005.

Peterson MC, Holbrook JH, Von Hales D, et al: Contributions of the history, physical examination, and laboratory investigation in making medical diagnoses, *Western Journal of Medicine* 156(2):163–165, 1992.

Pormann PE, Savage-Smith E: *Medieval Islamic Medicine*, 2007, Edinburgh University Press.

Quin CE: The soul and the pneuma in the function of the nervous system after Galen, *Journal of the Royal Society of Medicine* 87:393–395, 1994.

Rogers C, Farson RE: Active listening. In Ferguson SD, Ferguson S, editors: *Organizational Communication*. New Brunswick, 1988, Transaction Publishers.

Rogers C: *A Way of Being*, New York, 1995, Houghton Mifflin.

Rothbart MK, Ahadi SA, Evans DE: Temperament and personality: origins and outcomes, *Journal of Personality and Social Psychology* 78(1):122–135, 2000.

Ruusuvuori J: Looking means listening: coordinating displays of engagement in doctor–patient interaction, *Social Science & Medicine* 52:1093–1108, 2001.

Sackett DL, Straus SE, Richardson WS, et al. *Evidence-based medicine*, Edinburgh, 2000, Churchill Livingstone.

Schechter GP, Blank LL, Godwain HA, et al: Refocusing on history-taking skills during internal medicine training, *American Journal of Medicine* 101(2): 210–216, 1996.

Silverman J, Kurtz S, Draper J: *Skills for communicating with patients*, ed 2, Oxford, 2005, Radcliffe Publishing.

Spanagel R: Alcoholism: a systems approach from molecular physiology to addictive behavior, *Physiological Reviews* 89:649–705, 2009.

Spiro HM: Empathy: an introduction. In: Spiro H, McCrea Curnen MG, Peschel E, et al., editors: *Empathy and the practice of medicine*, 1993, Yale University Press.

Swarz MH: *Textbook of physical diagnosis, history and examination*, London, 2002, Saunders.

Tracy CS, Dantas GC, Upshur RE: G. Evidence-based medicine in primary care: qualitative study of family physicians, *BMC Family Practice* 4(6), 2003.

Ullmann M: *Islamic surveys II: Islamic medicine*, 1978, Edinburgh University Press.

Upshur RE: If not evidence, then what? Or does medicine really need a base? *Journal of Evaluation in Clinical Practice* 8(2): 113–119, 2002.

Vijg J, Campisis J: Puzzles, promises and a cure for ageing, *Nature* 454:1056–1071, 2008.

Wear A: Medicine in early Modern Europe, 1500–1700. In: Conrad LI, Neve M, Nutton V, et al., editors: *The Western medical tradition: 800BC to 1800AD*, 1995, Cambridge University Press.

Wood M: *The practice of traditional Western herbalism: basic doctrine, energetics, and classification*, 2004, North Atlantic Books.

Wuthrich B: Food allergy, food intolerance or functional disorder? *Praxis* 98(7): 375–387, 2009.

# Physical examination and clinical investigation

Other ways of knowing

## CHAPTER CONTENTS

The nature of physical examination 323
Examination versus investigation 326
Evidence-based physical examination 330
Aims and potentials of physical examination 333
The varieties of the clinical gaze 334
Touching and knowing 335
'Energetic' assessment 338
General advice on examination technique 342
Investigation: the quest for certainty 343
Conclusion 348

This chapter provides a critical perspective on physical examination and clinical investigation and their role in the phytotherapy consultation.

## THE NATURE OF PHYSICAL EXAMINATION

Although physical examination is presented here as a distinct and separate section of this book, it is not necessarily enacted as a separate part of the consultation. We mentioned at the end of the last chapter that examination may occur at various points during the case history-taking, either because the practitioner asks permission to examine phenomena as they arise, or because the patient proffers part of the body to viewed, e.g. rolling up a trouser leg when describing their swollen ankles. Yet physical examination can be considered as extending beyond this into every moment of the encounter with the patient, beginning with the very first contact. This insight is gained when we consider an extended definition of physical examination as one having to do with the practitioner's use of her senses to comprehend the physical dimensions of the patient's being and expression. This is a process that is constantly in a state of play, although much of the value will be missed if the practitioner fails to attend to this fact. Examples of 'physical examination', seen from this orientation, include:

- *Hearing:* hoarseness in the patient's voice; a cough; laboured or altered breath sounds; or sniffing. All these phenomena could be detected in a

preliminary telephone consultation before seeing the patient for the first time
- *Seeing:* the patient's difficulty in rising from a chair; observing their posture and gait; tremor; skin tone and colouration. Such significant areas of examination can be noted from the time of first greeting a patient in the waiting room, to the moment they sit down in the consulting room
- *Touching:* the patient's hand when shaking it for the first time provides information regarding temperature and moisture or dryness; as well as strength or frailness; hesitancy or confidence
- *Smelling:* tobacco, alcohol, urine, etc., odour around patient; this can be one of the earliest and strongest sensory impressions.

In this view, 'physical examination' can be divided into two fields of activity: first, a general and continuous sense-awareness of the patient's physicality; and second, specific time-limited techniques of formal, explicit physical assessment. In each instance, the core work involves the practitioner's sensory engagement with the patient. To be regarded in this manner; that is, to be seen, heard, touched and smelled, can be a powerfully positive experience wherein the patient feels that they have been closely and carefully appreciated by the practitioner. It can also be an indifferent or unpleasant experience. Whether, and to what degree, the patient finds physical examination to possess positive or negative qualities will depend on a number of factors, including:

- The practitioner's approach to handling bodies – in general and in particular. There is a difference for example, between sensory and sensual engagement; and between an appropriately 'clinical' manner and objectification of the patient's body
- Whether the practitioner demonstrates positive regard or disregard for the patient
- Whether the patient is processed mechanically or tended organically
- Whether the reasons triggering formal examination have been clearly explained and justified
- The practitioner's skill and fluency
- The degree to which the patient's comfort is catered for and their modesty respected.

Physical examination yields both gross and subtle signs and these can be interpreted differently depending on the reference point/s of the practitioner. Phytotherapy courses tend to emphasize the biomedical approach to physical examination as a diagnostic means, yet phytotherapists are also usually interested in traditional approaches to this area and may integrate alternative perspectives (some of which are considered below), with the conventional model. In doing this, it is important that herbal practitioners are able to provide a coherent explanation of their approach and findings to patients.

The classical interpretation of the role of the physical examination is dual:

- To provide a means of testing hypotheses regarding differential diagnoses that have been generated during the case history (*directed examination*)

- To scrutinize the patient for additional new information regarding their condition (*general examination*, or routine screening, such as taking the pulse and blood pressure).

These represent entirely diagnostic goals, which do not fully account for the urge to examine. The predicaments and conditions of many patients (such as those classed as mood disorders) are not readily suggestive of the need for formal physical examination of any particular type, while many of the presentations that *do* indicate the involvement of a body system that is susceptible to examination fail to yield classical findings. In the latter case, either nothing of obvious consequence is found or the significance of the findings are unclear or deemed of poor legitimacy, e.g. generalized mild abdominal tenderness in the absence of other signs is conventionally read as indicating that, whatever the problem is, it probably isn't serious. While classical findings may be encountered relatively frequently in acute or severe pathology, they are rather rare in day-to-day practice outside of hospitals. Routine physical examination is typically similarly unproductive in generating clear evidence of pathology. The value of physical examination is brought into further question by the superior ability of many laboratory and technological techniques to see into the body and by the rise of evidence-based physical examination, which has highlighted the deficiencies of many examination techniques, as we will see shortly. Despite all this, however, physical examination continues to be taught as an essential facet of the consultation. In my view, Greaves (1996) critique of, and rationale for, the use of physical examination in conventional medicine could apply equally to herbal practitioners:

> *The physical examination, when it is carried out, is often restricted to just one or two simple procedures, such as taking the pulse, measuring the blood pressure or listening to the chest. Although these procedures may sometimes be of value for clinical purposes, their rather frequent and non-selective use cannot be explained solely in these terms. They would seem to have an additional significance: that of a symbolic routine, which may provide benefit to the patient and marks out the special content of the doctor's work over and above that of technical expertise. It allows the possibility of apparently straightforward clinical tasks embodying a personal quality which only gains meaning from the responsiveness of the patient in return, and so is shared by the doctor and the patient.*

Although significant (meaning 'disease indicating'), diagnostic clinical findings *are* sometimes discovered, the 'benefit to the patient' more frequently lies in other areas – especially in the very *absence* of 'significant' results. Physical examination represents a potent means of providing patients with reassurance regarding the nature of their condition. When the practitioner skilfully applies her senses to scrutinize the bodily area of concern and, following careful reflection, declares that all seems to be well, this may provide huge relief to the patient and restore confidence in the integrity of her own body to the extent that a 'significant' therapeutic influence has been exerted. The combination of laying-on of hands and reassurance can constitute an act of healing that the wise practitioner will be slow to spurn. This potential is lost when the examination is casual or perfunctory but is maximized when the ritual is performed solemnly, carefully and thoughtfully.

Once the healing potential of physical examination is recognized, the ways in which it can be applied need to undergo a review. The practitioner may decide, for example, to use physical examination with greater frequency and more serious attention. There may also be a new tendency to bring it to bear in circumstances where it would formerly have been dismissed as unlikely to be worth the effort or superfluous to requirements since the diagnosis has already been made on the history alone. Tension headache is an example where positive clinical findings (meaning definite physical signs of pathology) are rarely discovered on examination but it is a good example of a condition where careful physical examination can provide strong reassurance (patients with pronounced headache may secretly fear that they have brain tumours for instance), and *might* result in a lessening of symptoms. In such cases, physical examination presents a therapeutic opportunity more than a diagnostic one. To miss such an opportunity may actually lessen patient trust and adversely affect the therapeutic alliance. It is common to hear patients complain about seeing another practitioner, saying something along the lines of: 'I told her I had this pain and she didn't even touch me'. I remember explaining to one patient that this was probably because the practitioner thought it unlikely that she would find anything of clinical significance but the patient was unpersuaded: 'Yes, but she should still have tried'.

Greaves' highlighting of the personal nature of physical examination and the unique meaning dynamic of the patient–practitioner relationship in this part of the clinical encounter is important. Physical examination provides an opportunity for the practitioner to tangibly demonstrate care for the patient and to shift the consultation from an essentially cerebral dimension to a physical one. In making this shift, the patient is considered in a different way to that operating during the history taking and this may give rise to a sense of being considered more completely. While the history appears (deceptively) passive, the physical examination demonstrates clear action and may additionally provide a degree of release of psychological tension generated during the history-taking.

Physical examination therefore has to do with much more than diagnosis. Two of its key powers lie within its capacity to reassure and provide tangible personal care. It is a sensory means of knowing and relating that may dissipate tension and serve to 'earth' or ground the consultation. It may be therapeutically indicated even where it is not clinically so.

## EXAMINATION VERSUS INVESTIGATION

'Physical examination' is also known as 'physical diagnosis' and 'clinical examination'. It can be contrasted with 'clinical investigation', which refers to laboratory and other types of testing such as blood studies and imaging techniques. A group of differences between 'examination' and 'investigation' are implied here and are summarized in Table 6.1. The two key distinguishing features between these two notions have to do with the proximity of the practitioner to the patient, and with the means applied to make the assessment.

In *examination* the practitioner is present with the patient and assesses her at close quarters using her senses, with little equipment involved (and where

**Table 6.1** Summary of differences between physical examination and clinical investigation

| Examination | Investigation |
|---|---|
| Performed by the practitioner | Performed by another |
| Embedded in the consultation | Occurring outside of the consultation |
| Human | Mechanical |
| Sensory | Technological |
| Personal | Abstract |
| 'Soft' evidence | 'Hard' evidence |
| Considered subjective | Considered objective |
| Immediate results | Mostly delayed results |
| Generally non-invasive | More likely to be invasive |
| Very low to no risk of adverse effects | Adverse effects more likely |

it is used, it is rudimentary, e.g. the stethoscope) – the practitioner is the active generator of findings. *Investigation* normally takes place in the absence of the practitioner (i.e. is performed by another person), and relies upon technical equipment – the practitioner is the passive recipient of results. While examination arises and takes place within the consultation and makes information available immediately, investigation takes place removed from the consultation and there may be a time lag of weeks between a test being ordered and the results being delivered. Patients' thoughts and feelings about these two modes of exploration can vary, for example patients *may* consider investigations to offer more definitive results than examination but can be more anxious about undergoing investigations, especially where these are invasive.

Physical examination is an attempt to conjecture from manifestations appearing on the surface of the body about what may be taking place inside of it. Ancient systems of medicine developed sophisticated schemas of interpretation around key examination areas such as those of the pulse and tongue to the extent that these were relied upon to provide definitive accounts of the patient's condition. (Previously, we quoted Kuriyama 1999: 'In the second century B.C.E., in the earliest case histories of China, the sick summon Chunyu Yi not with vague pleas for succor, but with the specific wish that he come and feel their pulse'.) The pulse remains a 'vital sign' in biomedicine but it is not *felt* anymore – rather it is *counted* or transmogrified into a line on an ECG trace, the varied and multiplied forms of which suggest the outlines of mountains in early Chinese landscape art.

In Chinese medicine, the pulse is categorized with words such as: floating, deep, empty, slippery, choppy, soggy, hollow, scattered, wiry, overflowing, knotted, hasty; words which relate to natural phenomena and qualities drawing on such reference points as the properties and activities of water. Pulses are further described and taught in terms that relate to the natural world, for example, regarding the 'slippery' pulse: 'In ancient times, it was described as feeling like 'pearls rolling in a basin' or 'raindrops rolling on a lotus leaf'" (Maciocia 2004). In contemporary biomedicine the lexicon relating to the pulse retains some connection with the natural world (fast, slow, full, empty, bounding, collapsing) but is primarily concerned with the number of beats and their rhythm. The music of beats and rhythms is considered to be 'heard' better by machines so that heart monitoring, such as by the ECG, is taken as the ultimate authority on the patient's situation. The technical language associated with this type of investigative scrutiny is accorded greater credibility than the nature-terms used in examination – the precision of identifying a 'variable PR interval' is preferred to physical detection of an 'irregularly irregular' pulse.

In ancient and traditional medicine, the ultimate diagnostic authority is the practitioner and the key reference point is nature, whereas in biomedicine, technology has become both authority and reference point. This is unsurprising given that the internal geography of the body can be exquisitely revealed by technology that penetrates more deeply than the human senses. MRI scanners can display the no-longer-hidden body in fine slices of digital meat. In the face of such astonishing capacities, continuing to bend the human senses to dimly perceive what the machine can so lucidly expose may seem not even quaint but wilfully perverse, and perhaps irresponsible. Yet the risks and costs of high-tech investigative techniques prohibit their widespread use to varying degrees depending on the affluence, healthcare politics and level of techno-centrism of particular cultures. Physical examination remains, in conventional medicine, at least as a handmaiden to clinical investigation, used (along with the case history) to screen and decide whether the risks, inconvenience and costs of investigation should be borne.

The shift of the locus of authority and reference in medicine from practitioner/nature to technology is part of such a movement in cultures generally. Innovations in technology shape the way in which the body is discussed and perceived, moving away from organic metaphors to mechanical ones (e.g. that the eye is like a camera or that the brain is like a computer). The increasing familiarity with, and emphasis on, technology does not represent a smooth and linear transition from the natural to the technical however, rather there is interplay between the two themes as opposed to a straightforward rejection of one in favour of the other. The history of what is known as the 'annual physical examination' or 'periodic health examination' provided to adults in America reflects the complexity of this relationship (and the complex relationships between case-taking, physical examination and clinical investigation).

The idea of providing periodic health examinations to 'apparently healthy persons' (Dodson 1925) crystallized in the 1920s and began to be variably implemented from that time. The format of the examination differed across America at the outset and has never been universally standardized. An early example of a 'Guide Card' for the examination is shown in Figure 6.1. This shows that the 'examination' combined history-taking (including focus on diet and work-related issues) with a mix of physical examinations and minimal reference to 'laboratory tests' 'when indicated' (Thomson 1925).

Prochazka et al. (2005) showed that the annual physical examination is today based largely on a range of blood tests (such as lipid panel, liver function tests, thyroid and complete blood count) and urinalysis as well as

**MEDICAL SOCIETY OF THE COUNTY OF NEW YORK**
Periodic Health Examination
## GUIDE CARD FOR HEALTH EXAMINATION

| Under Heading of: | MAKE SPECIAL INQUIRY ABOUT: | |
|---|---|---|
| OCCUPATION: | **Character of work performed?** (Manager or Steno. for example.) <br> **Nature of industry?** (Steel Foundry, Lead Works or Mercantile.) | |
| FAMILY HISTORY: | **Relationship of affected persons?** <br> **Hereditary factors?** e.g. Vascular or Cardio-Renal Disease Tendency: Note causes of death which might have a bearing on applicant's condition. | |
| PREVIOUS HISTORY: | Infectious Diseases: | Scarlet fever, diphtheria, whooping cough, etc.? Syphilis, gonorrhea, tuberculosis. |
| | Vaccination: | Smallpox. |
| | Immunizations: | Typhoid fever, diphtheria, scarlet fever. |
| | Other Diseases: | Rheumatism, tonsilitis, pleurisy, hemoptysis, frequent colds, migraine, nervous breakdowns. |
| | Menstrual: | Irregularity, abnormal flow, backache, etc. |
| | Obstetrical: | Miscarriages, stillbirths, number of pregnancies, character of labor. |
| HABITS: | Food: | Regular hours? Home cooking, restaurants, or lunch counter? Hurried meals? Moderate or hearty eater? Excess of meats, eggs, pastry, sweets, delicatessen, condiments or seasoning, fried or roasted foods? <br> *Proportions:* Carbohydrates, protein and fats, suited to applicant? |
| | Sleep: | Sufficient number of hours? Disturbing factors (noise, especially if night worker)? Ventilated bedroom? Feel rested on rising? |
| | Alcohol: | Specify average number of glasses of various types of liquor taken per day? |
| WORKING CONDITIONS: | Hazardous substances: | Poisonous gases, vapors, fumes or dust with which applicant may regularly or occasionally come in contact? Character of dust? |
| | Sanitary Conditions: | Defects of ventilation, lighting, heating, moisture, or posture? |
| | Mental or Physical Strain: | Factors causing monotony or extreme mental tension or physical strain should be especially noted in so far as they may cause *fatigue*. Overtime ditto. |
| PRESENT CONDITION: | Respiratory System (Cardio-Vascular): | Cough, shortness of breath, pain (pleuritic or precordial, etc.). |
| | Nervous and Mental: | Signs of maladjustment, nervous breakdown, psychoses, or organic nervous disease. |
| | Gastro-Intestinal: | Nausea, vomiting, pain (time of occurrence), location and character, etc. |
| PHYSICAL EXAMINATION: | Nutrition: | Undernourished or overweight? |
| | Eyes: | Note exophthalmos; infections of conjunctivæ; other pathologic states; examine eye-grounds when necessary. |
| | Throat: | Note conditions of tonsils and pharynx. Larynx when indicated. |
| | Teeth: | Note caries, pyorrhea or other condition requiring dental care. |
| | Genitalia: | Genito-urinary disease? |
| | Orthopedic Defects: | Note spinal curvature, flatfoot or postural defect or skeletal pathology. |
| | Glandular Disturbance: | Presence of enlarged glands in special localities, or general. Also, any abnormality of thyroid, thymus or pituitary glands. |
| | Reflexes: | Pupillary reflexes, knee jerks, etc. |
| | Gynecological: | Infections, lacerations, displacements, etc. |
| LABORATORY TESTS: | | Wassermann test and also other laboratory examinations when indicated. (X-ray, blood examinations, sputum, feces, gastric contents, etc., etc.). |

WEIGHT AND HEIGHT CHART ON OTHER SIDE

**Figure 6.1** Guide card for health examination. *(Reproduced from Thomson 1925, with permission.)*

height, weight and blood pressure measurements and cervical smears and mammograms in women, with these ingredients being variously combined. Investigation has moved from an optional extra in the 1920s to occupy centre stage in the early twenty-first century. The authors questioned public and practitioner attitudes towards the examination and contrasted their background understanding that: 'Current evidence does not support an annual screening physical examination', with their study findings that 'a relatively high percentage of the general public desired an annual physical examination' and that most primary care physicians believe that such an examination 'detects subclinical illness'. Interestingly, while 63% of physicians believed that the examination was of proven value (contrary to the evidence), '94% believed that an annual physical examination improved the physician–patient relationship and provided valuable time for counselling on preventive health behaviours'. This latter belief returns us to Greaves' insight that, beyond diagnosis, physical examination 'would seem to have an additional significance' and adds to our earlier discussion of the extra dimensions of the examination.

Following a personal reflection on the issues surrounding the annual physical examination Laine (2002) concludes that:

*The regular laying-on of hands and stethoscope (and maybe phlebotomy needle, too) is not a needless ritual if it fosters trusting clinical relationships and ensures that patients receive effective counselling and preventive interventions.*

In an accusation that could be levelled more generally at the change in emphasis of conventional medicine as a whole over the course of the twentieth century, Han (1997) contends that the American annual physical examination has changed:

*... from a comprehensive fact-finding exercise aimed at detecting physical defects and amassing the available techniques of history-taking, physical examination, and laboratory technology into a parsimonious collection of tests for the early diagnosis of disease.*

He gives two perspectives on the reasons for this change, a 'conventional view' and an 'alternative argument'. The conventional take accounts for the change as reflecting: 'a positive evolutionary advance in knowledge – a replacement of naïve enthusiasm with scientific scepticism'. Whereas the alternative perspective argues that: 'shifts in the acceptance and content of the periodic health examination were tied to fundamental changes in the objectives that the examination served'. These objectives have included: 'scientific knowledge, economic savings, professional empowerment, the physician-patient relationship, data collection, satisfaction of patient demand, and administrative efficiency'. The appreciation and practice of the consultation, in all its aspects, continues to be shaped by these influences.

## EVIDENCE-BASED PHYSICAL EXAMINATION

Perhaps surprisingly, Reilly (2003) was able to observe that:

*Little is known about the clinical importance of skilled physical examination in the care of patients in hospital.*

Even less is known about the same issue in contemporary herbal practice, although this fact is possibly less surprising given the very small size of the profession and the lack of a research culture in herbal medicine as in other modalities classed within the CAM bracket.

In response to research suggesting that there are 'widespread deficits in the physical examination skills of practising physicians', Ortiz-Neu et al.

(2001) investigated the competency of 3rd-year medical students in conducting cardiovascular examination in eight medical schools, concluding that their results suggested: 'fundamental inadequacies in the current paradigm for teaching physical examination skills'. Other authors (such as Bordage 1995) have expressed concern regarding the decline of the emphasis on, and competence in, physical examination skills on the part of medical students and physicians. My experience, as a teacher and examiner working with herbal medicine students and practitioners suggests that physical examination skills are often inadequately taught (teaching is frequently partial, rushed, with insufficient time allowed for practise); that a desirable level of examination-related knowledge and fluency is rarely achieved by the time of the final clinical examination; and that herbal practitioners soon reduce their use of physical examination techniques to a narrow base when in practice.

The level of competence in physical examination skills is therefore a concern in both conventional medicine and phytotherapy but addressing this is hampered by further concerns that call into question the reliability and validity of physical examination in the first place. If physical examination is unreliable, then why should efforts be made to improve the teaching and practice of it?

Physical examination is a largely subjective art and a number of papers have found poor interexaminer (or 'interrater') reliability in conducting particular examination techniques (such as Yen et al. 2005, looking at abdominal examination of children), while others have found a good degree of reliability (such as Weiner et al. 2006, studying examination of chronic lower back pain). One issue here has to do with the degree of expertise possessed by the examiner. For example, a skilled examiner who is able to help patients relax and who uses 'reinforcement' (a technique that causes momentary relaxation of the body part being examined) in testing reflexes is more likely to be able to elicit them.

A further concern regarding the value of physical examination is raised by studies that have shown certain investigative techniques to be superior to examination techniques in particular cases. For example: Kolb et al. (2002) found that combined mammography and ultrasound was superior to palpation in detecting small breast cancers; Spencer et al. (2001) showed that the use of a portable echocardiography device was more effective than physical examination in assessing the heart in cardiovascular patients; Wipf et al. (1999) showed that chest examination was unable to confirm or exclude the diagnosis of pneumonia and that X-rays provided the best diagnostic test. None of these studies called for the abandonment of physical examination however, some (e.g. Spencer et al. 2001) have drawn attention to the areas of strength as well as weakness for examination techniques, but all have suggested the need to become more aware of the accuracy and reliability of physical examination. Other studies have clarified the value of examination. For example, in a small study, Nardone et al. (1990) explored the value of physical examination in suggesting whether patients had anaemia. They looked at pallor in the conjunctivae, face, nails, palms and palmar creases and concluded that 'the absence of pallor does not rule out anaemia'; that examination of nailbeds and palmar creases was of no value in assessing anaemia;

and that if combined pallor of the conjunctivae, face and palms was found this did indicate the presence of anaemia.

In the foregoing discussion, we have drawn on the developing evidence base for physical examination, which has both raised and addressed concerns regarding the credibility of this part of the consultation. An influential paper in developing the notion of evidence-based physical examination was that of Sackett and Rennie (1992), which justified and introduced a series of articles in the *Journal of the American Medical Association* (*JAMA*) that scrutinized examination methods. The authors first noted the value of physical examination in:

- Frequently providing 'everything we need to clinch a diagnosis' (ruling in)
- Permitting 'us to rule out diagnostic hypotheses' (ruling out)
- 'Developing rapport with, and understanding of, our patients'
- 'Expressing our respect for them and their predicaments'.

'But' they cautioned, 'there is a science to this art of medicine', and the time had come for a more rigorous evaluation of physical examination to take place. The old physical examinations should be treated in a way similar to the new diagnostic procedures, where:

> ... it is now commonplace to see the advocacy of (such) procedures supported by their repeated, independent, blind comparisons with reference or 'gold' standards ... No laboratory or physiologic test deserves adoption until it has been so tested.

Physical examination then, was like a dusty old attic where treasures might be discovered among a lot of rubbish; it stood in need of a good sorting out. *JAMA* was to undertake this task by publishing 'regular reviews of the precision and accuracy of specific elements of the clinical examination', despite the risk that, in doing so: 'Some hallowed elements ... justified by time and authority, may go down in flames ... Many more ... will be placed on probation because their precision and accuracy are simply unknown ...'.

Subsequent *JAMA* articles appeared under the banner of 'rational clinical examination', eventually leading to the publication of a book with that title (Simel & Rennie 2009). An earlier attempt at providing a manual of *Evidence-based physical diagnosis* was made by McGee (2001). The work done by these authors in increasing the scrutiny applied to physical examination amounts to an effort to save it, as if it were an endangered species, in the face of a movement that considers, as McGee put it: 'that physical diagnosis has little to offer the modern clinician and that traditional signs, although interesting, cannot compete with the accuracy of our more technologic diagnostic tools'.

Phytotherapists need to engage critically with the revision of the physical examination repertoire that is taking place via the evidence-based approach – taking its lessons and insights on board but challenging it where it reduces physical examination to a merely diagnostic act. The human dimensions of the examination need to be remembered.

## AIMS AND POTENTIALS OF PHYSICAL EXAMINATION

We have now reached a point where it might be useful to summarize the possibilities and opportunities offered by physical examination, arising from the foregoing discussion, and to introduce others that have not yet been made explicit.

Aims and potentials of physical examination:

- Diagnosis of medical conditions (ruling in)
- Exclusion of diagnoses (ruling out)
- Providing reassurance
- Monitoring the response to treatment and healing progress/decline
- Determining the energetic characteristics of the patient
- Early detection of conditions (e.g. hypertension)
- Estimating the need for referral for investigation
- Avoidance of the need for more invasive testing
- Cost-saving (as opposed to use of more expensive investigations)
- Provision of care and expression of human warmth and consideration
- Enhancing the therapeutic relationship
- An opportunity for counselling and discussion of preventive health strategies
- Meeting patient expectations (and thereby avoiding patient dissatisfaction with not being examined – 'I went with this pain over my heart and he never even looked at my chest').

Two capacities of the physical examination listed above that we have not previously touched upon need to be highlighted:

1. Monitoring of the response to treatment and healing progress/decline
2. Determining the energetic characteristics of the patient.

The first of these has to do with the repeated use of physical examination in follow-up visits with the same patient in order to determine whether improvements, stasis or deterioration in the condition are occurring. For example, a series of musculoskeletal assessments can determine whether range of movement is increasing at the shoulder or hip; repeated auscultation can determine whether abnormal breath sounds are persisting or diminishing; repeated sphygmomanometry will show changes in blood pressure, and so forth. This ability to track and monitor is one of the most useful attributes of physical examination but is, strangely, rarely emphasized.

The second relates to traditional diagnosis around such pivotal issues as whether the patient's condition is hot or cold in nature, or whether it represents a pattern of excess or deficiency. We will explore this idea in more detail below.

Taken together, the full list of the aims and potential of physical examination provided here makes clear the substantial usefulness of this means of engaging with the patient. Physical examination is far from outmoded; rather it remains a crucial and wide-ranging domain of the consultation. Given the form and nature of the phytotherapy consultation (its extended length; its focus on the individual, etc.) herbal practitioners are well placed to maximally exploit the potential of the physical examination and it is to be hoped that a fuller appreciation of the dimensions of this territory will be developed in herbal education – in both initial and continuing forms.

## THE VARIETIES OF THE CLINICAL GAZE

*The clinical gaze is not that of an intellectual eye that is able to perceive the unalterable purity of essences beneath phenomena. It is a gaze of the concrete sensibility, a gaze that travels from body to body, and whose trajectory is situated in the space of sensible manifestation.*

Foucault (2007)

The approach to physical examination – how it is to be done, what its findings signify – is culturally shaped. The radial pulse described by an ancient Chinese medicine practitioner is not the same radial pulse felt by the ancient Greeks and Romans. In these contrasting cases, both the techniques used and the conclusions drawn may differ dramatically. There are multiple ways in which the body can be viewed – each according to its own internal logic and placed within a broader conceptual framework or understanding of the nature of the world.

Kuriyama (1995) explores 'visual knowledge' in ancient medicine, asking the question: 'What is it, exactly, that the eyes can know?' The predominant answer in Greek medicine has to do with 'form', while in Chinese medicine, the reply is 'colour', so that Kuriyama can state:

*If the eyes of the Hellenistic dissector were trained on structures, the Han dynasty physician fixed on hues.*

Kuriyama provides examples of the use of colour in Chinese medical diagnosis:

*A face tinged with yellow or red, the* Neijing *teaches, signals fever; white means cold; and green and black, pain. In fevers of the liver, redness first appears on the left cheek; in fevers of the lung, on the right cheek; in cardiac fevers, on the forehead.*

As Kuriyama points out, recourse to observing and interpreting colour in diagnosis is not perplexing – after all, contemporary biomedicine still takes notice of changes in skin colour (e.g. in jaundice, or the malar flush), rather: 'What puzzles is that colours should be judged paramount ...'. The reason for this emphasis connects with the meaning of colours within a grander scheme of perception and understanding, whereby they possess 'cosmic as well as somatic significance':

*Each of the five basic colours of green, red, yellow, white and black corresponded to one of the five phases (wuxing = wood, fire, earth, metal and water) of cosmic change. By observing the hues tingeing a patient's face, the physician could determine the phase governing the patient's condition. A florid countenance, for instance, bespoke the dominance of fire; a visage with yellowish tints, the waxing of the earth. Nuances of shade, differences in when and where various hues appeared, and the indications of other senses could add practical complexities; but the principle was simple: to see was to see colour, because the five colours linked the eye to the five-fold transformations pacing the cosmos.*

The way we perceive the body arises from the way we see the world, which derives from what we have been taught and what we believe. Herbal practitioners trained in the western tradition in the UK, at least, tend to combine a biomedical rationale for the working of the body with a variable range of other explanatory models such as those associated with notions of holism, vitalism, naturopathy, Hippocratism and with vestiges of specific herbal movements such as Physiomedicalism and Eclecticism. As regards physical examination, the tendency appears to be to learn conventional diagnostic examination but then to implement it to only a very limited extent in practice. This lack of utilization may be due to a number of factors, in addition to issues around the quality of teaching previously mentioned, such as:

- Low diagnostic need (where patients have already been medically diagnosed)
- Lack of awareness of the non-diagnostic dimensions of physical examination (as listed above)
- Lack of a sense of congruency between conventional examination techniques and the practitioner's personal conception of herbal medicine
- Substitution with alternative examination techniques that possess greater congruency.

Where examination strategies have reduced to a small core the capacity to apply the senses to apprehend the patient is similarly diminished and the range of potential routes to knowing the patient is narrowed. This is regrettable when seen in light of the benefits that physical examination has to offer both practitioner and patient. One means of re-energizing interest in physical examination (aside from promoting a fuller realization of its capacities) lies in the potential for integrating conventional and traditional techniques. A critical comparison of the various types of examination used in medical traditions from around the world represents a fascinating project, implying as it does, a cross-cultural analysis that leads to the very roots of perception in medicine. The scope of phytotherapy is broad enough to engage in this task – on the one hand appreciating the focussing obtained by the lens of evidence-based physical diagnosis and on the other, learning from the expansive cosmic insights afforded by traditional diagnosis.

## TOUCHING AND KNOWING

Let us return to the work of Shigehisa Kuriyama in following on from the last section, since he has offered us one of the best examples of a comparison between traditional ways of perceiving the patient that we have yet had, in his work on ancient Greek and Chinese medicine (Kuriyama 1999). He has highlighted the profound nature of such a project in that:

... *differing ways of touching and seeing the body were bound up with different ways of* being *bodies.*

In contrasting varied approaches to physical examination, we stand to gain in appreciation, not just of diagnosis, but also of how people *are*, how they understand and experience the world. The role of sensory experience as a means to understanding is emphasized by Kuriyama:

> *This is the primary lesson that I want to stress: when we study conceptions of the body, we are examining constructions not just in the mind, but also in the senses.*

Physical examination is a sensory engagement with the patient, that is conditioned by training and honed with practice. While some phenomena will be obvious even to the untutored (e.g. a marked deformity or gross restriction of movement), others require prior orientation in order to be detected (e.g. fine distinctions between heart sounds). Even when a sign is obvious, its significance may not be, however. The construction of meaning in biomedicine is based on an appreciation of the anatomical body and it conditions the way in which the senses are used in the physical examination. Sensory perception has to be formed and directed by repeated acts of creative imagination before many phenomena can be registered. The mind has to learn the heart cycle and the range of sounds that can be associated with it *before* they can be *heard*. Even then the actual act of comprehending needs to be repeatedly imagined before it actually occurs. This is demonstrated each time a skilled clinician points out what they perceive as a clear finding to a student who is unable to discern it. The finer points of physical examination have to be believed before they can be seen.

Biomedical physical examination is based on apprehending 'the body *as* the body', divorced from a wider network of global associations (as in the Chinese cosmology–somatology relationship) but also lacking an internal web of connections (of the kind for instance that enables the Chinese practitioner to see evidence of heart pathology manifesting, quite literally, on the very tip of the tongue in the tongue's 'heart area'). Abstracted from the cosmos and lacking internal coherence, the body is reduced to a collection of isolated parts which, although they must be examined *in situ*, are essentially disconnected from the rest of the body when viewed in the examiner's mind's eye. This habit of thought arises from the way that the body is conceptualized in biomedicine, which in turn derives from the primary means used to form that perception, namely dissection. To think of 'the body' in biomedical terms is to imagine its innards – as the liver is examined the clinician is oriented, not to its function or network of associations and meanings; not to its significance, but rather to its *location*. While the anatomical way of perceiving the body may seem like the most natural, indeed the *only legitimate*, way of apprehending the body to those inducted into this particular school of perception, it has not seemed like that in every medical culture. Indeed historically, as Kuriyama points out, 'anatomy is an anomaly' since:

> *Major medical traditions such as the Egyptian, Ayurvedic, and Chinese all flourished for thousands of years without privileging the inspection of corpses. For that matter even the treatises of Hippocrates, the reputed source of Western medical wisdom, manifest scarce interest in anatomical enquiry.*

What we perceive the body to *be* affects the manner in which it is examined and the way we interpret the significance or meaning of 'findings'. The anatomical body is approached as a collection of parts that the examiner-as-mechanic can assess for soundness as regards: location, size, shape, juxtaposition with other parts, signs of wear or features suggesting aberrant changes (e.g. the four cardinal signs of inflammation). Findings are related to diagnostic models that represent 'diseases' – where there is good correlation between findings and the disease template, then a diagnosis can be made. Where no clear correlation is evident yet the patient is experiencing some degree of discomfort or disruption of function (a very common situation) then there is an absence of meaning. Where the degree of disruption, nonetheless, is considered substantial the patient may be referred for investigations to see if the powers of technology can explain what the human senses cannot (or at least that the sensory deployment based on the anatomical model cannot). If the degree of disruption is considered minor or 'unlikely to be serious', then the patient may be commended to surrender to the healing power of temporality, in other words 'to wait and see' what happens.

Kuriyama describes how: 'Greek pulse theory ... sought strictly to segregate what a pulse is from how it feels, fact from perception'. This is an operating condition still firmly set in the biomedical mind as the body is examined. When perception does not supply the necessary information required to diagnose a fact, however, the patient is left without an explanation for their suffering. This is a result that is usually unacceptable to both patient and practitioner, yet the practitioner may not feel competent to provide, or justified in providing, a rationale. The patient is left with doubt, a lack of meaning, and the suggestion that her predicament is not credible and therefore invalid – this is a state of mind that is not merely unsatisfactory but potentially nocebogenic (see Ch. 2). 'Good' clinicians know or sense this and will attempt to provide some rationale or explanation, even in the absence of concrete findings, but, lacking the certainty associated with the detection of a 'fact' they may be insufficient to meet the patient's desire to understand their situation.

Alternative ways of seeing and reading the body may offer explanation where the anatomy-based model cannot. These may lack the specificity prized in biomedicine but their capacity to generate global rationales offers the very thing that conventional medicine is deficient in providing. For example, a Chinese medicine practitioner might see a coherent picture in a combination of signs that are considered inconclusive, uncertain, incidental or insignificant by the biomedical practitioner. The presence of a geographical tongue or a pale tongue with scalloped edges, along with general pallor, cool skin, lack of tone and general listlessness could be diagnosed as a pattern of 'yin deficiency' and appropriate remedial measures advised, perhaps (depending on the individual case) including: rest, a special diet, sexual abstinence and particular physical exercises. The conventional practitioner has no immediate diagnosis for this picture but may refer for tests, though if these come back as negative (e.g. thyroid is okay, no anaemia) he will have to rely on explanations such as 'I think you're probably just a bit run down'. This hazy non-diagnosis may actually result in advice being given that is similar to that given by the Chinese practitioner. The key difference then lies in the nature of the Chinese diagnosis, especially that, in comparison with the conventional diagnosis, it:

- Is given more rapidly
- Is made with greater confidence
- Is more certain and coherent
- Is a diagnosis of preference rather than as a last resort
- Fully, rather than partially, explains the situation
- Leads to better targeted advice
- Usually leads to the provision of treatment strategies (particularly herbal medicine in this case) that are not available in conventional medicine, such as the use of 'tonics' (herbal adaptogens).

Whichever model is used, however, the provision of a coherent explanation for the patient's predicament may not be associated with the prospect of 'cure'. In the face of this knowledge, it is important to remember that, regardless of the examination philosophy or set of techniques used, it is always possible to apply them in a way that conveys care, attempts to find meaning, and bears witness to the patient's suffering so that physical examination contributes to the patient's 'healing' if not to their 'curing'. We can recall here the distinction between these two modes of activity given earlier, where healing was described as being:

> ... directed at addressing and resolving the existential predicament of the person who is ill – at relieving (to the extent possible) the perceived lived body disruption which the illness engenders.
>
> (Toombs 1993)

## 'ENERGETIC' ASSESSMENT

Since it appears to be desirable for practitioners to bring more than one interpretive model to bear on the physical examination, in order to combine the advantages and to compensate for the deficiencies of each, we need to ask to what extent is it possible to do so? To what extent can one combine different ways of seeing the world without having to reject one in favour of another – or without becoming confused? Individual practitioners need to answer this question for themselves but I have argued throughout this book for a pluralist approach to medicine. This can apply as regards physical examination as in any other zone of the consultation. There is no need for phytotherapists to reject the orientation and techniques of biomedicine but rather to realize its biases and limitations and to remain open to the potential of other models to provide additional means of appreciating the patient.

A number of authors (e.g. Holmes 1989; Tierra 1989; Kenner & Requena 2001; Ross 2003) have attempted to explore the relationship, and forge links, between Western herbal and medical rationales and those of Eastern medical systems. Others have called for a refreshed awareness and use of the diagnostic and classification methods traditionally used in Western herbal medicine from Galen to the nineteenth century schools such as the physiomedicalists (Wood 2004). Discourse in these areas tends to be coloured by an insistence on the need for, and validity of, an 'energetic' appreciation of both patient and plant. We began a discussion of the meaning of energetics in the previous chapter but let us continue it here. Although much used, the term 'energetic' appears to be hard to define. We gave a perspective on this in the last chapter but we might also think of it as denoting a *desire* on the part of Western herbal practitioners to reconnect with their vitalist origins in the face of the biomedicalization of herbal practice. Traditional medicine systems such as Chinese medicine and Ayurveda, as well as the Western tradition understood as a Hippocratic humoral system, are held up as examples of 'energetic medical systems'. The quest to rediscover, develop or integrate energetic approaches can be seen as an attempt to remedy a perceived lack of a defining philosophy in contemporary Western herbal practice. It is perhaps best understood, however, as a cry for prioritizing the phenomenological mode of being – for the primacy of sensory experience and of 'feeling'. Weary (and wary) of the abstractive mode of positivist science that places a distance between the herbal practitioner and her patients/plants; and cognisant of environmental imperatives that require us to draw closer to nature; the herbal practitioner's call for an energetic stance may be understood to be driven by a (frequently unrealized) political urge that has to do with the ecological need for human beings to experience 'the felt presence of the body in the moment'. The energetic position looks for feelings not facts, for connection not abstraction, and for the 'realness' of immediate felt experience. Identified as an eco-spiritual sensibility, we can see how the notion of 'energetics' may be seen as both crucial and controversial. For the purposes of this chapter, we can focus on providing an insight into what 'energetic physical examination' might look like by considering its role in traditional medicine. Before doing so, let us note that it can be argued that physical examination of any type tends by nature to be energetic if we go ahead and define 'energetic' as having to do with phenomenological perception – in this interpretation the examiner has only to open her senses in the presence of the patient for the energetic information to come through.

Physical examination techniques are widely used in traditional systems of medicine. In Chinese medicine, a sophisticated approach is well documented (e.g. Maciocia 2004); including pulse and tongue diagnosis. Ayurveda also uses a number of detailed observational techniques such as pulse diagnosis, the benefits of which are described below:

*Pulse diagnosis allows one to retrieve detailed information about the internal functioning of the body and its organs through signals present in the radial pulse. This information involves not only the cardiovascular system, but the other bodily systems as well. From the pulse, the diagnostician learns to gain information about the functioning of the bodily tissues, the state of the* doshas *and aggravation of the* doshas, *and much more, including ... early stages of imbalance that precede full-blown symptoms*

Sharma & Clark (2002)

Current conventional diagnostic practice sees little in the radial (or any other pulse) beyond cardiovascular signs. Traditional pulse-taking includes the four modalities known in conventional medicine: the rate, rhythm, volume and character – but has a more extensive range of pictures that variously

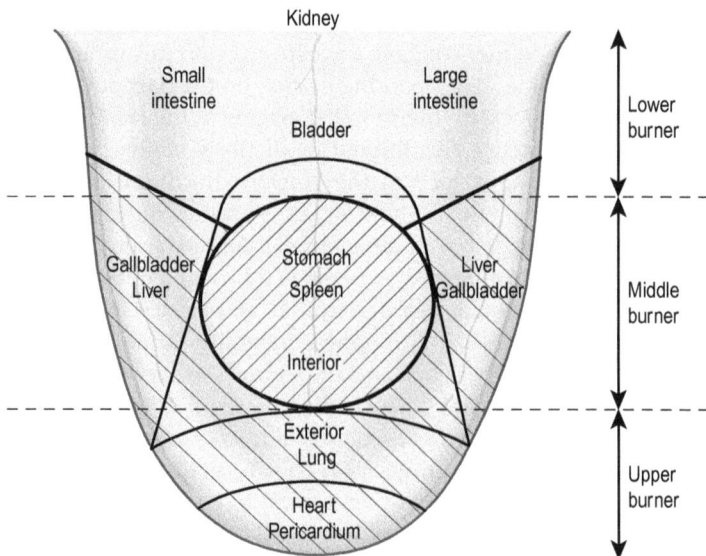

**Figure 6.2** Diagram of tongue diagnosis. *(After Dowie 2009.)*

combine these factors. Certainly, the traditional approach has a more complex and global understanding of what is meant by 'character', which can be considered as referring to how the pulse literally feels under the clinician's fingers – its shape or tangible waveform.

Chinese tongue diagnosis includes representation of body organs and systems on the surface of the tongue (Fig. 6.2). In addition to the clues provided by the positioning of phenomena on the tongue, the characteristics of the phenomena are also significant, e.g. colour and coating. These latter phenomena are also attended to in conventional medicine, but they are read differently. In conventional medicine, a white coating of the tongue may be interpreted as a yeast infection (Candidiasis), whereas in Chinese medicine it may be seen as a sign of 'damp'. The conventional reading links the phenomenon with an external cause (yeast/fungus) and a named disease (oral thrush) whereas the Chinese interpretation identifies an internal bodily state or predisposition – the condition of being damp. Such apparently different readings are not necessarily incompatible; in fact they may complement and inform each other. The 'damp' state may be read, for example, as indicating an underlying weakness of the immune system that has provided the environment in which a fungal infection can take hold. A practitioner versed in both ways of seeing may be able to say: 'Ah, you have a fungal infection due to an excess of damp'. Treatment of the damp state with herbs and dietary advice (e.g. avoiding damp foods such as cheese, bananas and salad) may clear the fungal infection and prevent recurrence by altering the damp disposition. This may represent deeper and more effective treatment than the conventional option.

Kim et al. (2008), in common with other researchers, showed a low level of inter- and intra-practitioner agreement on the diagnosis of tongue presentations between Traditional Chinese Medicine practitioners, indicating low reliability for this method. It has been suggested that such lack of consensus is in part due to differences in interpretive models and there is some evidence to suggest that when a standard diagnostic model is used, agreement levels increase (Zhang et al. 2008). This may not be the right way to go about understanding traditional diagnosis however, appreciating each practitioner–patient encounter instead as a unique and variable phenomenological event with traditional diagnostic schemas providing general orientation points as opposed to strict rules.

Tongue 'indications' are provided by Finley Ellingwood (1919), a herbal doctor of the Eclectic school, under the heading '*A summary and comparison of the liver remedies*', as a guide to selecting which particular herb is most suited to the patient's picture. These are summarized below:

- *Leptandra virginica:* Tongue pale, coated uniformly white, or greyish-white and moist; bitter taste in the mouth
- *Iris versicolor:* Is indicated when the tongue is narrow, pointed, somewhat red, with thin edges, especially if coated in the centre with a yellowish coat
- *Chionanthus virginica:* Tongue flabby, broad, coated white or yellowish, edges indented
- *Chelidonium majus:* Tongue flabby, full and broad, pale, irregularly coated, mucous membrane pale, free mucous secretion.

It is hard for most UK phytotherapists today to imagine working with such specific and detailed information linking herbs and indications. Practitioners of Chinese herbal medicine, however, are likely to say: 'this is how we work!'

Perhaps the most accessible and fundamental energetic approach has to do with distinguishing between hot and cold pictures. In terms of the physical examination, we can distinguish between these poles in ways that include those listed in Table 6.2.

One response to Table 6.2 might be that the correspondences are *obvious*, which is really the point. Energetic classification systems are based on direct and straightforward interpretation of readily perceptible phenomena. At the most fundamental level, they represent associations that practitioners could easily discover by themselves. The implication of taking an energetic approach to the physical examination, however, is that one can follow it through with related treatment and advice. For example, if a hot picture is detected, then

**Table 6.2** *Distinguishing between hot and cold pictures*

| Hot picture | Cold picture |
| --- | --- |
| Patient is warm to the touch | Patient is cool to the touch |
| Erythema: of nail beds, tongue, etc. | Pallor: of nail beds, tongue, etc. |
| Increased reflexes | Decreased reflexes |
| Dry tongue | Wet tongue |
| Tongue: no coat or yellow coat | Tongue: white coat |

one needs to know which herbs, foods and behaviours will have an appropriately cooling effect. In this manner, originating in sensory experience, whole systems of medicine have been developed.

## GENERAL ADVICE ON EXAMINATION TECHNIQUE

A few practical pointers:

- Focus on developing confident touch: patients can feel your confidence, caring and knowledge through your hands as you touch them. Hesitancy or casual technique may be read as evidence of uncertainty and undermine the patient's confidence in you
- Focus on warmth: warm attitude, warm hands, warm (but not excessively so) room
- If you have cold hands wash them with warm water before examining and dry vigorously with a towel. If they are still cold, do not apologize for them, as this introduces a negative message into the examination. Better to be positive: 'now, my hands are a little cold but they'll warm up as we go along'.
- Show on yourself and then do to the patient: as you explain what you want to do, use simple positive language and keep it brief; use your hands to mime over your own body what you will do – do not wave your hands over the patient as they will not be able to see properly and are likely to become confused
- Be careful with language, especially of words or phrases that may alarm the patient (e.g. when assessing reflexes say 'tap' not 'hit')
- Attend to the patient's comfort and dignity – imagine yourself in the patient's position; how would you like to be treated?
- As you examine, remember to pay attention to the patient's non-verbal responses, it is especially important to keep glancing at the patient's face for signs of discomfort or anxiety
- Children may find it easier to point to where the problem is than to talk about it
- Be careful in talking to children during the examination. Swartz's (2009) advice is sound: 'one of the best ways to make a child feel comfortable is through praise. When one is talking to a child, it is useful to say, "thank you for holding still. That makes the examination easier". The use of "you're a good boy" or "you are such a sweet girl" should be kept to a minimum, because this may produce embarrassment. Therefore praise should be given for a child's behaviour and not for his or her personality'.
- Be aware of the reactions of others who may be in the room. For example, with children, Butler (1995) has described the 'maternal grimace sign' derived from experiences where: 'a mother's dramatic grimace during the gentle examination of a comfortable child alerted the clinician to parental anxiety disproportionate to the child's illness. Addressing parental anxiety proved fruitful [and] made it easy for the clinician to avoid inappropriate treatment and investigation of the children …'

## INVESTIGATION: THE QUEST FOR CERTAINTY

In his book on Native American medicine, Virgil Vogel (1970) quotes George Bird Grinnell in attempting to provide an understanding of the definition of what constitutes 'medicine' in indigenous thought:

*All these things which we speak of as medicine the Indian calls mysterious, and when he calls them mysterious this only means that they are beyond his power to account for ... We say that the Indian calls whisky 'medicine water'. He really calls it mysterious water – that is, water which acts in a way that he cannot understand ... All Indian languages have words which are the equivalent of our word medicine, sometimes with curative properties; but the Indian's translation of 'medicine', used in the sense of magical or supernatural, would be mysterious, inexplicable, unaccountable.*

We can explain the development of ever more penetrating forms of technological investigative techniques as part of a continuing quest to achieve certainty and control in the practice of medicine. Ancient indigenous cultures have attempted to transcend the diagnostic and prognostic limits imposed by human capacities by recourse to 'magic' and shamanic journeying in the spirit world, whereas modern biomedicine has done so by developing technological instruments and processes. We earlier identified 'certainty' as one of the practitioner qualities most associated with the power to catalyse healing effects in the patient. Even when dealing with cases where no effective treatment could be provided, it has always been possible for a practitioner to create a strong positive reputation through their ability to explain the nature and cause of the patient's predicament and to accurately predict its course. Facility in diagnosis and prognosis engenders confidence and trust on the part of patients and is the basis of the practitioner's authority.

Parsons (1951) discussed the 'strain' placed on practitioners by the 'general effect of the existence of large factors of known impossibility and of uncertainty' in the practice of medicine. Uncertainty (which Parsons also termed 'indefiniteness') exists not only at the 'physiological-biochemical levels of analysis' but also with regard to the 'psychic factor in disease' and it is prone to generate non-rational solutions since:

*... magical beliefs and practices tend to cluster about situations where there is an important uncertainty factor and where there are strong emotional interests in the success of action.*

A state of uncertainty calls for interpretation in order to change it into a condition that is 'known' and understood. Investigative techniques replace magical explanations and processes in bringing about this transformation – the shaman's ceremonial space becomes a gleaming laboratory and vision is induced by means of the MRI-scanner in place of the botanical 'hallucinogen'.

Helman (2000) suggests that medical diagnostic technology: 'can be seen as an extension of the human senses' in the same way that Marshall McCluhan described media technology (radio, television, etc.) as extensions of the central nervous system – as a means of amplifying or exaggerating capacities for listening and looking. Related to this idea, technology can also be interpreted as an attempt to compensate for sensory capacities that were lost or left behind in some previous Golden Age. In his study of notions of the body in Restoration England, Schaffer (1998) describes how:

> *Many held that human senses were defective because when Paradise was lost, so was the perfectly knowing body. Humanity could not now attain the prelapsarian certainties of Adam, first of natural philosophers.*

However, the development of technology such as the microscope provided instruments that were: 'close analogues of prelapsarian capacities'. Schaffer quotes Henry Power, a Yorkshire physician, as writing in 1664 that: 'with the relevant "Engines" the "faculties of the soul of our Primitive Father Adam" might be reproduced and surpassed'. Schaffer also cites Robert Hooke (author of *Micrographia*, 1665) as saying that microscopes were 'artificial organs added to the natural' which extended the 'domain of the senses'. Schaffer concludes:

> *Instrument makers could restore men to Eden. At this conjuncture of political and moral Restoration, the incapacities of the human body were therefore simultaneously the reason why instruments were needed, the source of understanding of the way these instruments worked, and the subject at which experimental investigation should be directed.*

For some at least, technological innovation could be considered not merely friendly but almost divine.

Greaves (1996) provides a different exploration of the development of diagnostic investigations categorized in two phases, with the first starting in the nineteenth century, when: 'the focus of medical attention changed from the patients' description of their illnesses to the doctors' description of disease'. This shift was enabled by developments in medical technology such as Laennec's introduction of the stethoscope in 1816, which emphasized the detection of pathological signs and altered the practitioner–patient relationship, since:

> *The stethoscope gave the doctor more intimate knowledge of the patient's body, and simultaneously distanced him from the patient.*

Whereas previously patients had possessed definitive knowledge about the state of their own bodies, now the practitioner was able to detect phenomena that patients themselves could not discern – this privileged access increased the authority of the practitioner at a cost to the patient's self-conception. While physicians had always had some degree of access of this type and trained powers of perception that were unknown to the laity (such as those to do with the complex reading of the pulse), the use of instruments represented new, more potent and more abstracted ways of perceiving the patient. Previously, although lacking training in detection and interpretation, the patient could, nonetheless, look at their own tongue in a mirror or palpate their own pulse in an attempt to verify the practitioner's findings. Now the patient lacked the resources (i.e. the investigative instruments themselves) as well as the skills to check what had been pronounced, calling for greater levels of trust in the practitioner than ever before and reducing patient autonomy.

Greaves explains that as the instruments and techniques of investigation became more sophisticated, so the gap between patient and practitioner widened until eventually instruments became so advanced that they required their own operators – such as the X-ray machine presented by Roentgen in 1895. This constitutes Greaves' 'second phase' of investigative development, accelerating throughout the twentieth century. While phase one was characterized by the use of instruments that *enhanced* 'the doctor's own sensory powers' at the expense of opening a gap between practitioner and patient; phase two added to or *took over* from those powers, further increasing the practitioner–patient gap but now also creating a gap between the practitioner and 'his own clinical experience'.

Greaves' analysis, then, reveals two phases of development in investigative technology associated with two stages of separation between patient and practitioner. The first phase of change, bringing in what Greaves has called 'soft' technology (such as the stethoscope) may appear rather trivial when judged from the perspective of modern high-technology culture. Indeed we now include the use of such instruments within the context of physical examination and do not consider them as representing formal investigative strategies. Nonetheless, they provided an intermediate step in the construction of 'hard' investigative technology such as the various imaging machines.

In the process just described, the locus of authority regarding the patient's body in conventional medicine shifted from the patient himself, to the doctor and then to the 'technology'; the investigative process or machine. This direction of travel ultimately disempowers both patient and practitioner, since both lose authority to pronounce on the status of the body. Greaves cites Reiser (1978), who observes that:

> *Many modern physicians thus seem to order the value of medical evidence in a hierarchy: facts obtained through complex scientific procedures they regard as more accurate and germane to diagnosis than facts they detect with their own senses, which in turn, they value more than facts disclosed by the patient's statement.*

Jewson (1976) sees the process of change leading to the explanatory dominance of investigative techniques as one that moves through three distinct approaches to medicine (or 'medical cosmologies') over the course of the late eighteenth century and on through the nineteenth. These are: Bedside Medicine; Hospital Medicine; and Laboratory Medicine and their key characteristics are summarized in Table 6.3. For Jewson, the 'eclipse' of Bedside Medicine by the latter two approaches, in sequence, constituted 'a shift away from a person orientated toward an object orientated cosmology'. Hospital Medicine first 'dissolved the integrated vision of the whole man into a network of anatomical structures' before Laboratory Medicine 'by focusing attention on the fundamental particles of organic matter, went still further in eradicating the person of the patient from medical discourse'.

The results and implications of technological investigations, whether a leucocyte count or chest X-ray, only possess meaning and make sense when viewed with regard to an explanatory frame of reference and in the context of an individual patient. A number of variables pertaining to these categories, i.e. having to do with technical frames of reference and patient uniqueness,

Table 6.3  Medical cosmologies, 1770–1870

|  | Bedside Medicine | Hospital Medicine | Laboratory Medicine |
|---|---|---|---|
| Perception of the patient as: | Person | Case | Cell complex |
| Conceptualization of illness as: | Total psychosomatic disturbance | Organic lesion | Biochemical process |
| Task of the medical investigator: | Prognosis and therapy | Diagnosis and classification | Analysis and explanation |
| Subject matter of nosology: | Total symptom complex | Internal organic events | Cellular function |
| Research methods: | Speculation and inference | Statistically oriented clinical observation | Laboratory experiment according to scientific method |
| Diagnostic technique: | Qualitative judgement | Physical examination before and after death | Microscopic examination and chemical tests |
| Mind/body relation: | Integrated: psyche and soma seen as part of same system of pathology | Differentiated: psychiatry a specialized area of clinical studies | Differentiated: psychology a separate scientific discipline |

Adapted from Jewson (1976).

tend to puncture the illusion of 'certainty' that an MRI film or liver function test chart, as an artefact, may appear to possess. The information provided still has to be interpreted and this may not be straightforward. Even in a well accepted and widely used test such as the lipid profile a wide range of questions and doubts surround its clinical application, such as:

- How confident can we be that following the 'normal range' of parameters for each component of the test is relevant for the particular patient at hand?
- How sure are we that the 'normal range' is valid in general terms?
- How high is too high for this particular case?
- And how low is too low? By fixating on the elevation of total cholesterol, may we risk lowering it excessively? What are the risks of excessive lowering?
- Could there be reasons why this particular test might be unreliable? For example: Did the patient actually follow the pre-test fasting advice properly?
- What else do we need to know to decide whether this result is more or less significant for this particular patient? For example: What is the family history of cardiovascular disease and is this likely to be relevant or not?
- Assuming action needs to be taken, what is the best form? How would the patient prefer to proceed? Medication, diet, exercise, weight loss,

CAM therapies? A combination of these? If medication is used, might it cause adverse effects? What is the risk–benefit ratio in this particular patient?

The accuracy and relevance of tests cannot be taken for granted; they are subject to uncertainty just as in every other area of medicine. Overemphasis of the authority of investigation and of its accuracy, reliability and sensitivity can have a deeply negative impact on patients when their suffering fails to be detected by tests. Rhodes et al. (2002) in their study of the use of imaging tests for diagnosing chronic back pain found that:

*The hope invested in testing is a two-edged sword. When physicians cannot locate the problem, or express doubt about the possibility of solution, patients feel that their pain is disconfirmed. To feel 'deligitimized' is, in fact to experience a series of negative consequences, from not being seen, to not being heard, to a sense of deficiency and shame.*

At the very least, practitioners need to have alternative ways of helping patients find an explanation and meaning when tests fail to provide them, otherwise the patient is left to draw the conclusion that their predicament is inexplicable and *meaning-less*. Herbal practitioners and others in the CAM bracket are well used to encountering patients who are seeking new and better-fitting stories.

None of the above detracts from the fact that investigative techniques are frequently useful and often essential, rather it points out the need for all practitioners who purport to work in a patient-centred manner to be aware that it is in the nature of investigative techniques to move the focus away from the patient, unless the techniques are carefully marshalled and approached critically. Investigations are not sufficiently subtle or comprehensive as to be helpful in all situations. A commonly encountered example is the patient who has a clear clinical picture of a thyroid disorder but who is discovered on investigation to be within normal parameters. Prioritizing the results over the patient's experience in such a situation is to miss an opportunity to relieve suffering and prevent further deterioration. Many doctors are as critical as CAM therapists of the limitations of investigative technology and the warping effect it tends to exert on the consultation, e.g. Dixon and Sweeney (2000) state that:

*Our intention is to challenge the dogma of modern technological medicine that ignores both the therapeutic effect of the doctor and the self-healing powers of the patient ... Western medicine is now facing a crisis. Modern technology, its very life blood, is failing to deliver the goods.*

Some varieties of phytotherapy, generally those arising within or developing out of conventional medicine, are more comfortable with investigation. The 'neuroendocrine' or 'endobiogenic' phytotherapy of Duraffourd and Lapraz (2002), for example, has developed a panel of indices calculated from standard blood tests (the 'Biology of Functions') that is integral to their approach. This reflects the tendency that French medical holism has shown, as Weisz puts it, to be: 'at once antireductionist and deeply reductionist', influenced by: 'terrain holism, which did not shrink from defining individuals in terms of pH or hormonal balances or cellular perturbations, all constructed by the laboratory'.

Herbal practitioners who are not doctors have been excluded from Hospital Medicine and do not have privileged access to Laboratory Medicine. In essence, we are still at the stage of Bedside Medicine – perhaps not such a bad place to be after all.

## CONCLUSION

Over time, the focus of conventional medicine has adjusted so that: 'the sick person's body has gradually replaced his or her narrative' (Pilloud & Louis-Courvoisier 2003). Ever-greater emphasis on the body's interior microarchitecture, analysed by increasingly sophisticated technology (from the stethoscope to genetic testing) has obscured the macroscopic picture and muffled the patient's authentic voice. Perhaps the greatest contribution that herbal practitioners have to offer to the consultation in the light of this circumstance is our insistence on hearing the patient's story in the telling of the case history. Yet, physical examination and investigation are important additional means of coming to know the patient and of assisting healing – they need not be territories of abstraction. On the contrary, physical examination at least provides substantial opportunity to deepen the therapeutic relationship between practitioner and patient. Investigation, meanwhile, has extraordinary capacities to render the body transparent, amplifying the practitioner's senses to the point of conveying the powers of a super-hero, yet such awesome abilities must be kept strictly as servants and never allowed to become masters.

*Technology* has its origins in Greek *tekhne* meaning 'art, craft or skill' and is paired with *episteme* usually translated as 'knowledge'. The relationship between epistemology and technology can be considered as that between (theoretical) knowledge and (practical) experience – each informing the other. Both of these are at play in the consultation and stand to be appreciated and integrated.

Leder and Krucoff (2008) have discussed the deficiencies associated with the 'objectifying touch' of physical examination and the 'absent touch' of technological investigation, in calling for greater awareness of the potential for 'healing touch' in the clinical encounter. This is touch that is applied with skill and expertise but which contains and communicates attention, care and compassion such that it has: 'impactful meaning, demonstrating reciprocity, vulnerability, and the intent to help'. Many patients are crying out to be treated in this way.

## REFERENCES

Bordage G: Where are the history and the physical? *Canadian Medical Association Journal* 152(10):1595–1598, 1995.

Butler CC: The 'maternal grimace' sign, *Archives of Family Medicine* 4:273–275, 1995.

Dixon M, Sweeney K: *The human effect in medicine: theory, research and practice*, Oxford, 2000, Radcliffe Medical Press.

Dodson JM: The American Medical Association and periodic health examination, *American Journal of Public Health* January:599–601, 1925.

Dowie S: *Acupuncture: an aid to differential diagnosis*, Edinburgh, 2009, Churchill Livingstone.

Duraffourd C, Lapraz JC: *Traité de phytothérapie clinique: endobiogénie et médecine*, Paris, 2002, Editions Masson.

Ellingwood F: *American Materia Medica: therapeutics and pharmacognosy*, Portland, 1919, Eclectic Medical Publications.

Foucault M: *The birth of the clinic*, (first published 1963), London, 2007, Routledge.

Greaves D: *Mystery in Western medicine*, Aldershot, 1996, Avebury.

Han PKJ: Historical changes in the objectives of the periodic health examination, *Annals of Internal Medicine* 127(10):910–917, 1997.

Helman CG: *Culture, health and illness*, ed 4, London, 2000, Hodder Arnold.

Holmes P: *The energetics of Western herbs: integrating Western and Oriental herbal medicine traditions*, Vol. 1, Boulder, 1989, Artemis Press.

Jewson ND: The disappearance of the sick man from medical cosmology 1770–1870. In Beattie A, Gott M, Jones L, et al, editors: *Health and wellbeing: a reader*, 1976, Basingstoke, 1993, Macmillan/Open University.

Kenner D, Requena Y: *Botanical medicine: a European professional perspective*, New York, 2001, Paradigm Publications.

Kim M, Cobbin D, Zaslawski C: Traditional Chinese medicine tongue inspection: an examination of the inter- and intrapractitioner reliability for specific tongue characteristics, *Journal of Alternative and Complementary Medicine* 14(5):527–536, 2008.

Kolb TM, Lichy J, Newhouse JH: Comparison of the performance of screening mammography, physical examination, and breast US and evaluation of factors that influence them: an analysis of 27,825 patient evaluations, *Radiology* 225:165–175, 2002.

Kuriyama S: Visual knowledge in classical Chinese medicine. In Bates D, editor: *Knowledge and the Scholarly Medical Traditions*, 1995, Cambridge University Press.

Kuriyama S: *The Expressiveness of the body: and the divergence of Greek and Chinese medicine*, New York, 1999, Zone Books.

Laine C: The annual physical examination: needless ritual or necessary routine? *Annals of Internal Medicine* 136(9):701–703, 2002.

Leder D, Krucoff MW: The touch that heals: the uses and meanings of touch in the clinical encounter, *Journal of Alternative and Complementary Medicine* 14(3):321–327, 2008.

Maciocia G: *Diagnosis in Chinese medicine: a comprehensive guide*, Edinburgh, 2004, Churchill Livingstone.

McGee S: *Evidence-based physical diagnosis*, London, 2001, Saunders.

Nardone DA, Roth KM, Mazur DJ, et al: Usefulness of physical examination in detecting the presence or absence of anaemia, *Archives of Internal Medicine* 150(1):201–204, 1990.

Ortiz-Neu C, Walters CA, Tenenbaum J, et al: Error patterns of 3rd-year medical students on the cardiovascular physical examination, *Teaching and Learning in Medicine* 3(13):161–166, 2001.

Parsons T: *The social system*, London, 1951, Routledge & Kegan Paul Ltd.

Pilloud S, Louis-Courvoisier M: The intimate experience of the body in the eighteenth century: between interiority and exteriority, *Medical History* 47: 451–472, 2003.

Prochazka AV, Lundahl K, Pearson W, et al: Support of evidence-based guidelines for the annual physical examination: a survey of primary care providers, *Archives of Internal Medicine* 165:1347–1352, 2005.

Reilly BM: Physical examination in the care of medical inpatients: an observational study, *The Lancet* 9390(362):1100–1105, 2003.

Reiser SJ: *Medicine and the reign of technology*, 1978, Cambridge University Press.

Rhodes LA, McPhillips-Tangum CA, Markham C, et al: The power of the visible: the meaning of diagnostic tests in chronic back pain. In Nettleton S, Gustafsson U, editors: *The sociology of health and illness reader*, Cambridge, 2002, Polity.

Ross J: *Combining Western herbs and Chinese Medicine: principles, practice and materia medica*, New York, 2003, Greenfields Press.

Sackett D, Rennie D: The science of the art of the clinical examination, *Journal of the American Medical Association* 267(19): 2650–2652, 1992.

Schaffer S: Regeneration: the body of natural philosophers in Restoration England. In Lawrence C, Shapin S, editors: *Science Incarnate: historical embodiments of natural knowledge*, 1998, University of Chicago Press.

Sharma H, Clark C: *Contemporary Ayurveda: medicine and research in Maharishi Ayur-veda*, Edinburgh, 2002, Churchill Livingstone.

Simel DL, Rennie D: *The rational clinical examination: evidence-based clinical diagnosis*, New York, 2009, McGraw-Hill.

Spencer KT, Anderson AS, Bhargava A, et al: Physician-performed point-of-care echocardiography using a laptop platform compared with physical examination in the cardiovascular patient, *Journal of the American College of Cardiology* 37(8):2013–2018, 2001.

Swartz MH: *Textbook of physical diagnosis history and examination*, London, 2009, Saunders.

Thomson AN: A survey of the present status of the periodic health examination, *American Journal of Public Health* January:599–601, 1925.

Tierra M: *Planetary herbology*, London, 1989, Lotus Press.

Toombs SK: *The meaning of illness: a phenomenological account of the different perspectives of physician and patient*, London, 1993, Kluwer Academic.

Vogel VJ: *American Indian medicine*, 1970, University of Oklahoma Press.

Weiner DK, Sakamoto S, Perera S, et al: Chronic low back pain in older adults: prevalence, reliability, and validity of physical examination findings, *Journal of the American Geriatrics Society* 54(1):11–20, 2006.

Wipf JE, Lipsky BA, Hirschmann JV, et al: Diagnosing pneumonia by physical examination: relevant or relic? *Archives of Internal Medicine* 159:1082–1087, 1999.

Wood M: *The practice of traditional Western herbalism: basic doctrine, energetics, and classification*, Berkeley, 2004, North Atlantic Books.

Yen K, Karpas A, Pinkerton HJ, et al: Interexaminer reliability in physical examination of pediatric patients with abdominal pain, *Archives of Pediatrics and Adolescent Medicine* 159:373–376, 2005.

Zhang GG, Singh B, Lee W, et al: Improvement of agreement in TCM diagnosis among TCM practitioners for persons with the conventional diagnosis of rheumatoid arthritis: effects of training, *Journal of Alternative and Complementary Medicine* 14(4):381–386, 2008.

# Concluding the consultation and providing ongoing care

## Coherence and continuity

7

**CHAPTER CONTENTS**

**Introduction** 352
**Moving towards a conclusion** 352
**Aims and strategies in closing** 353
  Coherence and understanding 353
    *Awareness of placebo and nocebo effects: facilitating the meaning response* 355
    *Giving advice* 356
    *Referral: involving others* 357
    *Aids to providing information* 358
    *Aids to memory* 358
    *Low literacy* 358
**Talking about herbal medicines** 359
  The nature of herbal medicines 360
**The practitioner as leader and manager** 360
  Facilitative leadership 362
  Servant leadership 363
  Shared leadership 363
**Returning to the practitioner as teacher** 364
**Shared decision-making and co-planning** 368
**Regimen: the treatment plan** 374
**Closing the consultation** 375
**Continuity of care** 377
  *To be continued ...* 380
  *Keeping promises* 380
  *A lot can happen between consultations* 380
  *Recognition* 380
  *Being available* 380
  *Rapid responses* 380
  *Additional charges* 381
  *Modes of communication* 381
  *Re-scheduling visits* 381
  *Additional prescriptions* 381
  *Frequency of visits* 381
  *Changing nature of the patient's predicament* 382
  *Involving and working with others* 382
**Reflective practice and research** 382

## INTRODUCTION

The final stage of the consultation, following on from history-taking and examination, is concerned with coming to conclusions to do with interpreting the patient's predicament, clarifying diagnosis, and deciding upon the best forms of treatment and advice. It involves summing up 'where we are now' and asking 'what do we do next?'

It is common for this section of the consultation to be delivered in a rather compressed and hurried manner, yet it is as important and as deserving of due space and attention as any other part of the consultation. Indeed, it is crucial that the concluding phase is handled well or the patient may leave the encounter feeling confused to the extent that the good work done in earlier parts of the consultation may be undermined.

When skillfully conducted, the closing stage of the consultation can help both patient and practitioner gain a sense of coherence and completion that enables each party to end the encounter feeling satisfied. The aim of this chapter is to help practitioners achieve that goal. Phytotherapists see many patients who require ongoing care within a continuing relationship with the practitioner, and this is addressed at the end of this chapter.

## MOVING TOWARDS A CONCLUSION

The boundary between the closing part of the consultation and the foregoing ones may be somewhat hazy. As the practitioner attempts to draw things together and establish conclusions, new issues relating to the history may emerge. For example, by presenting a summary of her thoughts, the practitioner may trigger the patient to provide more information and reflections pertaining to the history. This is fine but may present a time pressure. If the practitioner has been summarizing, reflecting back and clarifying throughout the history, then major new avenues are less likely to open up during the final stage of the consult. Even so, the concluding section is still likely to be, and should be, a continuing active engagement and discussion where new discoveries can be made – especially with regard to matters such as patient preferences around treatment and in connection with advice.

It is essential to allow adequate time for conclusions to be discussed and negotiated – one of the less-mentioned practitioner skills is the ability to fully engage with the patient while maintaining a non-obvious focus on the clock. In order to provide sufficient time it may be useful, and is sometimes necessary, to formally bring the foregoing consultation to a close and announce the need to move to the territory of conclusions by saying something like:

> 'I'm going to suggest we stop at this point so that we have enough space to summarize where we've got to and what we might do in terms of treatment and so on. Are you happy to move on to doing that now?'

Getting to conclusions may mean that another area of discussion has to be delayed until the next visit. Patients can be reassured that you recognize the need to return the deferred topic and that you will make time for it in the following consultation. One might say, for instance:

*'I'm aware that we need to review your diet but I'm going to suggest that we do that at the next appointment because I want to make sure we have enough time today to draw everything together and discuss treatment. Is that okay?'*

It is important to make a note so that you remember to keep this type of promise and it may be helpful to make the note-writing explicit in order to enhance patient confidence that you will not forget: 'I'm going to write that down now so that I won't forget'.

The final section of the consultation involves providing explanations; giving advice and reassurance; and discussing the prescription. These elements unpack to disclose a wide range of sub-topics and related issues, which we will explore under the next heading. Before moving on, however, let us briefly underline the importance of these general subject areas. It is essential to draw the consultation to a point of focussed attention and action in order to realize the potential of the phytotherapy approach and of the herbal prescription. If the practitioner has power to activate the medicine, then this capacity is perhaps at its strongest in the concluding stages of the consultation. If the patient leaves feeling confident about the treatment and with a clear understanding of what it will do, they are likely to gain maximal benefits from it. In the opposite scenario (confused about the treatment, not sure what it is supposed to do), results, not to mention compliance, are likely to be poorer.

## AIMS AND STRATEGIES IN CLOSING

### COHERENCE AND UNDERSTANDING

We have identified the key elements of the consultation's conclusion as being: explanations, advice, reassurance and treatment (the prescription). All of these may also arise during the foregoing consultation; they are not discreet entities that can only appear after the consultation has been constructed, rather they are modes of being or themes that can occur throughout the consultation. By the time the closing section of the consultation is entered several explanations may already have been provided; a range of advice given; multiple reassurances conveyed and treatment options mentioned and discussed. The core task for the practitioner at the end of the consultation is to draw these together, emphasize the most important and introduce any other perspectives that have not previously been mentioned.

The phytotherapy consultation is generally broad (in scope), long (in duration) and complex (in nature) and is therefore characteristically wide-ranging, non-linear and information rich. In order to keep track and to retain focus on comprehension and action, it is helpful for herbal practitioners to make notes towards conclusions throughout the consultation. My technique is to leave a space at the bottom of my blank A4 history-taking sheet, where I jot down very brief notes, usually single words, as they occur to me, in order to provide triggers for discussion at the end of the consultation. A typical example, some of which may be unintelligible even to a fellow phytotherapist, would be:

> *adaptogens; liver; T.rad.; rooibos; upset optional; nerv.troph.; sleep; ↑F&V; meditation?; valeriana; yin e/meal; breathing; Ix liver?; nature; ref. acu?*

These few words relate to a wide range of treatment considerations (T.rad is *Taraxacum officinalis radix*, or dandelion root); dietary advice (↑F&V increase fruit and vegetables); other advice (to spend more time in nature, learn to meditate); treatment focus (liver, nervous system, sleep, breathing); possible referral (for investigation of the liver and for acupuncture in this case); and teaching focus (upset is optional). Each practitioner will evolve their own style of working in this area – the key factor is to find *some* means of keeping focussed on outcomes at the same time as following the patient's lead through the labyrinth of the clinical encounter.

In looking at the issues involved in the final section of the consultation, Silverman et al. (2005) concentrate on 'explanation and planning' as core objectives and summarize these as encompassing:

- Gauging the correct amount and type of information to give to each individual patient
- Providing explanations that the patient can remember and understand
- Providing explanations that relate to the patient's perspective
- Using an interactive approach to ensure a shared understanding of the problem with the patient
- Involving the patient and planning collaboratively to the level that the patient wishes, so as to increase the patient's commitment and adherence to plans made
- Continuing to build a relationship and provide a supportive environment.

Although ostensibly very sound, the phrasing of this agenda has a slightly patronizing edge in suggesting an attempt to build a 'therapeutic alliance' – to bring the patient on side so that they comply with treatment. In its most extreme manifestation, this becomes an adapted form of paternalism dressed up in the language of patient-centred medicine, resulting in little more than asking the patient 'I'm sure you agree, don't you?' and giving them an information leaflet. There is a need to guard against the tendency to see patient participation as a means to making the practitioner feel better about coercing the patient to do what the practitioner wants and instead to be genuinely open to the patient's agenda – and genuinely capable of being flexible to meet it.

Of course some patients do not desire, or are not able, to engage at a high level of participation and expression of preferences, in which case the practitioner must operate in paternal mode as benignly as possible. In another scenario, the patient's agenda may be considered unreasonable, unrealistic, misguided, deluded, dangerous or simply incompatible with the practitioner's approach. In such a situation the practitioner may need to challenge the patient's position and in exceptional cases, recommend that they visit a different practitioner.

Kindelan and Kent (1986) posed a mixed group of general practice patients questions correlating with five territories: diagnosis, prognosis, aetiology and prevention, social effects of the illness and treatment, and asked them to order these in terms of their 'importance for today's visit'. Information on diagnosis and prognosis were deemed most important, followed by treatment and aetiology, with social effects being least important. One reading of this response would be to consider it in terms of knowledge, with an inverse relationship existing between the degree of the patient's knowledge about the area and their need for information about it. 'Social effects and illness' was presented to patients in the form of the question: 'How will it affect your daily life, for example, work, looking after the children?' The patient's knowledge of this, in the case of established illness, is far superior to that of the practitioner – the patient is already an expert in this subject. In the early stages of a condition however, the patient's greatest degree of uncertainty is around the nature of the condition and its degree of seriousness ('prognosis' was posed as: 'The seriousness of your illness, its likely outcome and time before you will be well'), and these are areas where the superior knowledge of the practitioner will usually be recognized. We might surmise, therefore, that although knowledge and information priorities vary between patients, they will tend to lie in the areas where the patient feels greatest uncertainty and anxiety.

Practitioners can use the relation between uncertainty/anxiety and information priorities as a guide but will be best served by asking the patient directly as to the main issues that they would like to discuss. It is important to avoid making assumptions – practitioners may, for example, emphasize information about treatment when that is only of minor immediate concern to the patient; many phytotherapy patients are already in possession of a conventional medical diagnosis but this does not mean that they are disinterested in the topic (some may have a strong desire to gain an alternative rationale); even where the prognosis for a condition is very good patients may still have deep doubts and profound worries about the future and the severity of their state; aetiological uncertainty or controversy (e.g. in fibromyalgia or chronic fatigue syndrome) may be a key focus area; social effects, although well known to the patient, may be the area where there is the greatest need for information providing help, support and enablement; patients in a relatively stable chronic condition may worry that a new treatment could disturb the balance they have found.

We will explore the various issues involved in talking about the herbal prescription later in this chapter but first we will identify and briefly consider a range of other areas of attention (and strategies related to these) in the closing stages of the consultation.

## Awareness of placebo and nocebo effects: facilitating the meaning response

We looked at these phenomena earlier in this volume. The practitioner's manner, language, certainty and so forth will influence the way that advice is received and the effects that it will have. Factors such as being genuine, positive and confident will tend to enhance the potency of advice, whereas a manner suggesting artificiality, negativity or uncertainty may have the opposite effect. Consciousness of how advice is being presented is important at all times but especially so in connection with areas such as prognosis, where triggering a nocebo response is a particular risk. It is not always possible to be positive and it is rarely possible to be completely certain but both capacities should be accentuated to the point that genuineness (a characteristic that *can* be constantly embodied) allows.

### Giving advice

Again, genuineness, positivity and confidence are important qualities to exhibit when giving advice. Clarity can be added to this collection and it is facilitated by avoiding verbosity, being careful to avoid (or explain) technical language or jargon (without being patronizing), and by checking for understanding as you go along: 'Did that make sense?', 'Is there anything you want to ask me about that?', 'Was there anything you didn't get there?' Patients may not voluntarily challenge words or concepts they do not understand, so it is important to provide an opportunity for such challenge to take place by inviting it. Watching the patient's face and attending to other non-verbal cues for signs of lack of comprehension or puzzlement is of great value here. Specific advice tends to be remembered better and to be easier to follow than general advice (e.g. 'try drinking red bush tea in place of regular tea' is better than 'try finding an alternative to tea'). Advice generally needs to be written down in note form or may be easily forgotten – the greater the number of pieces of advice, the more this rule applies. When a wide range of information or advice is being presented, it may help to categorize it into types, e.g. 'I'd like us to talk about your diet, exercise, sleep, and your home life. Can we start with home life?'

#### Talking about diagnosis

The practitioner might begin to summarize by saying: 'So this is what I think is going on …' and end by asking: 'How does that sound to you?' In between, the explanation may loop back into the history and open up new questions and points of clarification. It will frequently be necessary to compare a conventional medical diagnosis with alternative or expanded explanations. In fact, this represents one of the great strengths of herbal practice and the opportunity to provide a pluralist rationale should usually be seized. In doing so, one needs to be careful to avoid overwhelming, and confusing the patient with too many perspectives.

#### Talking about aetiology

Diagnosis and aetiology are closely associated and tend to overlap in practice. In fact they may be conflated in the herbal approach, for example 'stress' may be taken to represent both cause and condition. As for diagnosis, describing alternative or unfamiliar conceptualizations of aetiology (such as the influence of 'damp') needs to be done carefully, with an emphasis on clear explanation. This guidance applies to any technical rationale – whether biomedical or otherwise.

Talking about diagnosis/aetiology naturally leads in to discussing advice and treatment: 'Here's what's going on … and here's what we can do'.

#### Talking about prognosis

Prognosis is a difficult art. As previously mentioned, it is important to be as positive as possible in order to help the patient feel hopeful and optimistic.

If reassurance can be given, then it should be given with emphasis and conviction. Prognostic reassurance does not have to be precise in order to be valuable, e.g. 'I'm sure that over the next few months things are going to get very much better' sounds pretty vague when written on the page but, in chronic conditions, it is typically both as *much* as one can say and *enough* for one to say.

Prognosis is often discussed in connection with the anticipated effects of treatment, and there is commonly a need to speak of this in detail. For example, to a young woman with acne one might be able to say: 'I expect that over the course of the next month your spots will start to look less angry and begin to heal. If you do get any flare up it should be less severe than before and clear up more quickly'. If you have a good degree of certainty that this scenario will take place, it is important to express it clearly and with confidence since placebo effect research suggests this will play a role in activating the healing response.

### Referral: involving others

It may be necessary or desirable to connect the patient with others who are able to offer additional help. This could be for a number of reasons including referral for investigation; for assessment or treatment by another practitioner (see Appendix 3, which considers interprofessional communication); or, using the notion of 'referral' more broadly, to another source of support or information such as an adult education class in tai chi or meditation. It is strongly recommended that practitioners build up a network of contacts (and a portfolio of contact details) for all the sources in the local area that they might need or wish to connect patients with. In doing this, the practitioner puts in place the means to practically enable working with a broad range of advice – and to walk the holistic talk.

Information, activity and support sources that might be considered suitable include:

- Local practitioners and health services
- Specific support service, e.g. bereavement counselling
- Classes and courses, e.g. yoga, tai chi, meditation, anger management, dance, singing, cooking
- Adult education centres
- Healthy food sources, e.g. local farms, organic box schemes
- Fitness centres and sports clubs
- Social groups/clubs, e.g. walking clubs
- Birth and parenting support, e.g. a local breast-feeding counsellor
- Local council services
- Local and national condition specific support groups
- Arts centres
- Citizens advice bureau
- Parks, woods, gardens, etc.
- Aids to explanation.

In communicating explanations in such areas as aetiology and diagnosis, it is useful to have recourse to non-verbal aids such as pictures and anatomical models. Each practitioner can develop these based on the range of conditions they most commonly see. It is also frequently helpful to sketch explanations that are best appreciated visually – my own notes are littered with very rough sketches explaining everything from the heart cycle to nudge theory.

### Aids to providing information

It can be helpful to develop a personal stock of information documents that can be printed off as required. These can cover a vast range of issues, including information regarding: conditions, concepts, dietary advice and recipes, breathing and massage techniques, reading lists, etc.

It is preferable to make such documents personal (do-it-yourself), brief and attractive. I print out postcards with some of the slogans described in Chapter 3 (see the 'Engendering wellbeing' section) such as: ALWAYS CHOOSE BIG MIND! Apparently they end up stuck on a lot of fridge doors.

### Aids to memory

While giving advice or discussing key points, it is helpful, as we have already mentioned, for the practitioner to write notes down for the patient as the need arises. That works well if you can write clearly but since my writing is mostly illegible to others (and occasionally to myself!), I often write notes then post or e-mail them to the patient later (I've even texted them when they have been brief). There seems to be something quite useful about sending brief notes in these ways, following the consultation – certainly it communicates care but also appears to have greater impact.

An alternative strategy is to provide the patient with a sheet of paper (or better still a postcard with your details printed on it, which looks more attractive and is therefore more likely to be kept and used) and a pen to take their own notes. Not all patients like this and it seems to often cause distraction, slowing the momentum and reducing the connection in the encounter. Some patients are glad to be offered the opportunity though and a few have commented that they would have liked to take notes but had not asked in case the request was considered rude.

### Low literacy

The previous item assumes patient literacy however, and Roter et al. (1998) have cautioned against assuming that patients possess this competency. It is not necessarily easy to tell if a patient has difficulties in this regard, since: 'most people with low literacy skills are of average intelligence and function reasonably well by compensating for their lack of reading skills'. However, low literacy might be associated with poor communication skills and this may become noticeable during history-taking. Patients may find it difficult to discuss their predicament and many have never disclosed the degree of their situation, even to their partner. Roter suggests that patient-centred interviewing skills benefits these patients and that their understanding can be helped by the same techniques that work for every patient, namely:

> ... organizing information into logical blocks, simplifying the message, making the message specific rather than general, repeating the message, summarizing, checking understanding by asking patients to give an explanation in their own words, and reinforcing the most important messages.

Good levels of literacy do not guarantee that the patient will understand the practitioner's, or general health messages. Shaw et al. (2008) found that, irrespective of level of literacy skill, many patients still: 'feel unable to access, understand and utilize health information'. The authors called on healthcare professionals to: 'improve their communication skills and ensure that health information is clear and easy to access'.

## TALKING ABOUT HERBAL MEDICINES

We have already mentioned some relevant issues pertaining to the prescription but the list below details the range of factors that may require consideration and discussion:

- The aims of the treatment: what it seeks to achieve
- The content: which herbs are to be used
- The form: which type/s of preparations are to be taken and whether these pose any challenges (e.g. a patient may be able to take a tincture but unwilling to devote time to making decoctions)
- What to expect: what is the patient likely to experience in response to taking the prescription
- How long it will take to gain effects
- Palatability: what it will taste like and whether any action needs to be taken to enable consumption
- Dosage and frequency of taking: e.g. some patients may be able to take medicine once a day but find it difficult to take three doses
- Whether any adverse effects might occur and what to do if they arise
- Compatibility with other medication or treatment (e.g. addressing potential herb-drug interactions)
- Expected length of treatment course
- When the prescription will be received (e.g. immediately on completing the consultation; by post; or by collection at an arranged time)
- What to do if any query arises: how you can be contacted
- Gauging the patient's understanding of the treatment aims and their ability to follow the treatment.

A new patient welcome sheet or short booklet can be developed to deal with frequently asked questions regarding the prescription, addressing the areas we have just listed.

Additional explanations are commonly desirable in the closing stages of the consultation to clarify the nature of herbal medicines and their differences when compared with conventional drugs (Table 7.1); these areas are explored below.

Table 7.1 Differences between herbal and conventional medicines

| Herbal medicines | Conventional medicines |
|---|---|
| Chemically complex: adapts multiple targets | Chemically simple: aims to hit specific targets |
| Generally non-specific: modulates systems performance | Tendency to be specific: can cause precise change |
| Individualized herbal prescriptions tend to change at each consultation, evolving as the condition changes | Fixed courses of treatment with the same medication are the norm |
| Relatively gentle in nature and action | Relatively aggressive |
| Tends to nurture physiological change | Tends to force physiological change |
| Low incidence of adverse effects, which are generally minor when they do occur | Higher incidence of adverse effects, generally of greater severity |
| Slower to accumulate effects but more sustainable as a long-term treatment | Effects more rapid but a less sustainable form of long-term treatment |
| Few issues with tolerance, dependency and withdrawal | Problems associated with tolerance, dependency and withdrawal may be pronounced |
| Ultimate locus of control is the body | Ultimate locus of control is the drug |

## THE NATURE OF HERBAL MEDICINES

Herbal medicines tend to:

- Support, enhance or restore normal physiological function, by facilitating the body's innate self-healing capacities
- Teach, train or 're-programme' the body into better or enhanced patterns of physiological behaviour
- Gently steer the body into more appropriate courses of response and function, with each dose of herbal medicine acting as a small 'nudge' in the 'right direction'
- Render themselves obsolete once they have aided the body in establishing optimal autonomous performance, or
- provide a safe long-term management option when restoration of normal function is not possible
- Work complexly across a number of body systems
- Act quickly in acute conditions but gradually in chronic conditions, accumulating greater effects over time.

## THE PRACTITIONER AS LEADER AND MANAGER

While the patient-centred practitioner will seek to follow the patient's lead and work in response to the patient's agenda, there is still a requirement for the practitioner to convey her own ideas, suggestions and recommendations with regard to such matters as diagnosis, treatment and in the domains of advice. The holistically-minded practitioner needs to reach a point where the broad appreciation of the patient that has been gathered can be translated into particular strategies and actions that can be proposed to improve the patient's situation. In drawing the consultation to a conclusion, a plan of action needs to be negotiated with the patient and its implementation reviewed at subsequent meetings. These various imperatives call for reflection on the notion of the practitioner as 'leader' and as 'manager'.

Herbal practitioners may experience resistance to these terms given that they suggest paternalistic models of control (leaders imply followers; managers imply subordinates) that are usually considered anathema in holistic approaches to medicine such as phytotherapy. Yet, as we shall see, there are alternative readings (of leadership especially) that may enable practitioners to perform these necessary roles in a manner that does not restrict the patient's autonomy. The antipathy that might be felt towards 'leadership and management' by healthcare practitioners can derive from a number of sources including the correlation between leadership and the 'great man' model, or its association with a tendency towards a charismatic or autocratic style; and in connecting management with business and bureaucracy.

Although literature deriving from the business world has traditionally contrasted leadership with management, considering them to represent different though allied roles, there has been a more recent tendency to conflate the two – seeing them as representing different aspects of a continuum. This development appears to be, at least in part, an attempt to redress the balance between management and leadership that has been tilted in favour of the latter, as Gosling and Mintzberg (2003) observe:

*Most of us have become so enamoured of 'leadership' that 'management' has been pushed into the background. Nobody aspires to being a good manager anymore; everybody wants to be a great leader. But the separation of management from leadership is dangerous. Just as management without leadership encourages an uninspired style, leadership without management encourages a disconnected style, which promotes hubris.*

Northouse (2007) draws on early definitions of management as having to do with 'planning, organizing ... and controlling' and insists that, while there are similarities between the two (e.g. both involve the exertion of influence; working with people; and goal accomplishment), management and leadership have distinct differences. In fact, they may be considered to represent antithetical agendas, given that:

*The overriding function of management is to provide order and consistency to organizations, whereas the primary function of leadership is to produce change and movement. Management is about seeking order and stability; leadership is about seeking adaptive and constructive change.*

We may readily see the connections between the definition of leadership given here and our discussion of complexity theory at various points in this book (especially at the end of Ch. 3) and with the assertion made in Chapter 2, that the nature of life (and health) is change. (Wheatley 2006, explores the relationship between complexity and leadership in depth.) We might then be tempted to connect leadership with the holistic phytotherapy approach, in contrast to the management agenda of conventional medicine. This may lead us to reject management in favour of leadership but to do so could risk missing lessons that stand to be learned from the business world:

> ... *if an organization has strong leadership without management, the outcome can be meaningless or misdirected change for change's sake. To be effective, organizations need to nourish both competent management and skilled leadership.*

If we substitute 'practitioner' for 'organization' in this quotation, do the assertions still hold? A final quote from Northouse (in which he draws on Bennis & Nanus 1985) might be helpful in attempting to answer this question:

> *To manage means to accomplish activities and master routines, whereas to lead means to influence others and create visions for change.*

This perspective could be applied such that the patient is cast as self-manager (planning, organizing and controlling their own lives – including implementing and mastering treatment 'activities' and 'routines') with the practitioner acting in a leadership role to catalyse such self-management. Management priorities of 'order', 'consistency' and 'stability' are not incompatible with the leadership imperatives of 'movement', 'adaptation' and 'constructive change' – rather these two groups of qualities define each other because they perpetually engage each other. The patient's urge towards stability drives movement and change just as the atom's desire for electrical neutrality causes it to interact dynamically with other atoms.

The familiar concept of 'case-management' can be justified given that the practitioner must also 'accomplish activities and master routines' (such as those having to do with history-taking, diagnosis, formulating a prescription, etc.) and create 'order' (for instance in regard to setting and keeping appointment times); 'consistency' (such as acting as a source of continuing care); and 'stability' (being there for the patient when needed). In the light of our reflections thus far however, we also need to consider how 'case-leadership' might be enabled and enacted. The rest of this section will therefore focus on leadership rather than management.

The literature on 'leadership' has conventionally viewed the leader as an individual in charge of a team (the leader of an organization), whereas the patient–practitioner relationship is dyadic and the patient-centred version eschews the notion that the practitioner is 'in charge'. A leadership model that fits the values and concepts of patient-centred medicine is therefore required. One approach is to change the 'leader–follower' relationship into one of 'leader–collaborator' (Rost 1995), a concept that emphasizes the active participation of the patient and which can be further democratized by suggesting that the roles of leader and collaborator may be exchanged between practitioner and patient during the course of the consultation. Other models that may inform appreciation of leadership within a patient-centred relationship include those given below.

### FACILITATIVE LEADERSHIP

Facilitative leadership is where the leader facilitates the understanding and development of, or between, others. This fits well with a patient-centred ethos but Schwarz (2005) describes the facilitator–leader as 'a substantively neutral ... party ... who has no substantive decision-making authority'; this is a mode that may be too passive and abstracted for the practice of phytotherapy.

## SERVANT LEADERSHIP

This model has clear resonance with the holistic approach to the consultation. Greenleaf (1982) described servant leadership thus:

> It begins with the natural feeling that one wants to serve, to serve first. Then conscious choice brings one to aspire to lead. The difference manifests itself in the care taken by the servant – first to make sure that other people's highest priority needs are being served. The best test is: do those served grow as persons; do they, while being served, become healthier, wiser, freer, more autonomous, more likely themselves to become servants?

According to Spears (2003) the distinctive qualities, characteristics and behaviours of the servant leader include: listening, empathy, healing, awareness, persuasion, conceptualization, foresight, stewardship, commitment to the growth of people and building community.

## SHARED LEADERSHIP

Although typically applied to leadership within teams, the notion of leadership being shared fits closely with the idea of partnership-centred medicine. Carson et al. (2007) caution that the benefits of shared leadership can only be realized where there is a relationship characterized by 'shared purpose, social support, and voice'. Social support refers to the provision of 'emotional and psychological strength to one another', while voice can be defined as denoting 'participation and input'. One would not normally expect the patient to provide the practitioner with social support – there are limitations to the mutuality of the patient–practitioner relationship.

More general views of the nature of leadership have been expressed. Viall (1996) equates leadership with learning, stating that:

> ... leadership itself is primarily learning. There is nothing static about it, nothing fixed, nothing constant from person to person or from situation to situation. Instead, it is a moment-to-moment process of grasping (learning) the needs and opportunities for influence that are found in situations and realizing (learning) what purposeful things one can do there. [Leaders should cultivate] learning as a way of being.

For Marquardt (2005), the key to learning is to ask questions and he suggests that leaders need 'to resist the impulse to provide solutions' and instead develop the capacity to 'lead with questions'. For phytotherapists, the core of our work lies in asking questions during history-taking – pivotal questions to ask of patients include:

**Table 7.2  A comparison of transactional and transformational leadership**

| Transformational leadership | Transactional leadership |
| --- | --- |
| Builds on a person's need for meaning | Builds on a person's need to get a job done and make a living |
| Is preoccupied with purposes and values, morals and ethics | Is preoccupied with power and position, politics and perks |
| Transcends daily affairs | Is mired in daily affairs |
| Is oriented toward long-term goals without compromising human values and principles | Is short-term and hard data orientated |
| Focuses more on missions and strategies | Focuses on tactical issues |
| Designs and re-designs jobs to make them meaningful and challenging | Follows and fulfils role expectations by striving to work effectively within current systems |
| Aligns internal structures and systems to reinforce overarching values and goals | Supports structures and systems that reinforce the bottom line and maximizes efficiency |

Adapted from Covey (1990).

'What do you think is going on?'

and

'What do you think needs to be done to make things better?'

The patient's views on causes and solutions frequently illuminate and indicate the best way to proceed. The crucial role of the process of questioning returns us to the centrality of the search for meaning in the consultation. Covey (1990) places the need to discover meaning at the core of his distinction between two types of leadership orientation – the transactional and the transformational. These types are contrasted in Table 7.2.

Applied to healthcare practitioners, we can view the transactional mode as representing a reductionist and bureaucratic ethos, whereas the transformational model is holistic and creative. Nonetheless, Cardona (2000) sees transformational leaders as possessing a manipulative potential that needs to be obviated by underpinning with a service ethos along the lines of Greenleaf's servant leadership – this combination leads to what Cardona calls transcendental leadership.

We can suggest, finally, that 'case-leadership' as opposed to 'case-management' might concern itself with learning, meaning and service. Focus on these three key areas in practitioner training and development might result in enhanced outcomes for both patient and practitioner.

## RETURNING TO THE PRACTITIONER AS TEACHER

We touched on the role of the practitioner as teacher in Chapter 3 but our reflections in the last section return us to this theme, since we have now highlighted the need for practitioners to be learners, in fact we may paraphrase Viall (1996) in asserting that practising *is* learning. Learning is a prerequisite for teaching – practising 'learning as a way of being' will incline to generate teaching as an emergent property within the context of the consultation. Although learning and teaching are merged processes we can characterize the fore stages of the consultation as being learning–heavy, while the latter concluding stage is teaching–heavy. Over the course of the clinical encounter, 'leading with questions' builds from information gathering to negotiating solutions and/or honouring and bearing witness to what has been learned. Each follow-up consultation provides an opportunity for continuing learning – on the part of both patient and practitioner. The importance of learning is such that we can propose one functional definition of the therapeutic relationship as follows: relationships are therapeutic to the degree that they enable mutual learning between the parties involved.

The concluding part of the consultation is a space wherein learning can be summarized and made explicit and where teaching can enter a formal mode. In fact teaching may be considered as an attempt to make learning explicit and thereby apparent to others. In this sense, teaching represents a phase, expression or concretization of learning. The contention that 'to teach is to learn twice' is attributed to Joseph Joubert (1754–1824) and attests to the value of teaching for the practitioner particularly. The act of conveying what you have concluded or what you know to another is an opportunity to test and enhance your own understanding; to forge new connections and deepen appreciation – in this way teaching within the consultation serves as a major means of practitioner development.

Theories of learning commonly describe it as a process of change or growth occurring in response to experience, yet defining learning is problematic since it can be applied to a number of ends, as Smith (1982) explains:

> It has been suggested that the term learning *defies precise definition because it is put to multiple uses. Learning is used to refer to (1) the acquisition and mastery of what is already known about something, (2) the extension and clarification of meaning of one's experience, or (3) an organized, intentional ... testing (of) ideas relevant to problems. In other words it is used to describe a product, a process or a function.*

All three of these facets of learning have relevance in the consultation. The first and third relate, for example, to the deployment of a particular herbal protocol in response to the patient's condition (e.g. a treatment for asthma, or for nervous depletion) and the subsequent review and revision of the treatment approach over a series of consultations. In this book, however, we have emphasized the process of 'clarification of meaning of one's experience' as a therapeutic strategy in its own right. In working to achieve this end, the practitioner is likely to find that the teacher's manifestation as facilitator is likely to suit best in aiding the patient's discovery of meaning and in supporting their change and growth. The aim of facilitation is not to instruct, nor to impart knowledge and not even to guide – rather it is concerned with setting the conditions for the patient's self-discovery and self-directed change. Rogers and Freiberg (1994) maintain that the same practitioner characteristics that foster therapeutic growth also define the teacher-as-facilitator, these being genuineness, unconditional positive regard and empathic understanding. Hurst (1987) believes that 'students judge teachers just as patients judge physicians' using the same primary criterion to gauge quality – namely, how much teachers and practitioners 'give of themselves'. The nature of this 'giving', of what is 'given' by the practitioner, relates to Rogers' characteristics and includes: realness, caring, deep listening, and loving concern for the other's growth.

Knowles (1990) considers that the attempt to delineate the specific characteristics that distinguish excellent teachers from mediocre ones represents 'one of the more or less futile quests of educational researchers' but cites Gage (1972) in suggesting that:

> Teachers at the desirable end tend to behave approvingly, acceptantly, and supportively; they tend to speak well of their own students, students in general, and people in general. They tend to like and trust rather than fear other people of all kinds.

That the practitioner–teacher should be a philanthrope, at heart and in word and deed, may appear to be a statement of the obvious yet this happy predisposition is not shared by every healthcare practitioner and it is a posture that can be challenging to maintain. There is a limit to the degree to which practitioners can give of themselves and one of the symptoms of having breached that line is a diminution of the capacity to care for others. Creeping cynicism is one of the features of professional burnout (see Appendix 2). Practitioner self-care combined with the creation of a positive and supportive working environment and a sustainable workload will help to prevent this outcome.

Trait models for teachers, as for leaders, tend to generate detailed lists of desirable characteristics that are unlikely to ever be embodied in a single person. The suggestion of generally useful foundational attributes or orientations (such as those of Rogers) may be more helpful. Knowles (1990) provides 'four variables', derived from research on teaching, that appear to be valuable in developing an effective teaching style:

- Warmth
- Indirectness, i.e. working in such a way that learners are enabled to discover rules for themselves rather than having them made explicit by the teacher
- Cognitive organization, meaning the teacher's 'intellectual grasp ... of what he is trying to teach'
- Enthusiasm.

Enthusiasm links with the issues of confidence and certainty discussed earlier, in conveying the practitioner's conviction about the 'rightness' of advice or treatment in a manner which engenders the patient's trust and belief in the appropriateness and likely efficacy of the course of action proposed. Indirectness is not always an appropriate strategy of course – indeed it may be essential to be *highly* direct and explicit in communicating, for instance, the precise manner in which a particular treatment strategy should be followed. Indirectness will be of greater value in working with patients for whom the phytotherapy consultation represents one method (possibly among several) employed as part of what Tough (1976) denotes as 'learning projects' aimed at creating major personal change. Tough includes CAM therapies as one means by which people seek to achieve personal growth and many CAM consultations might be considered in this light. Bearing this in mind, it is interesting to look at Tough's list of the types of personal changes that people may 'strive for', since it indicates the range of learning imperatives that can become apparent during the clinical encounter. The list (adapted from Tough 1976) includes:

- Improved self-understanding
- Expression of genuine feelings and interests
- Quitting drinking, smoking, etc.
- Coping better with the tasks necessary for survival
- Freeing the body from excessive tenseness and wasted energy; physical fitness
- New priorities: a fresh balance of activities or expenditures
- Reshaping relationships, etc.
- Increased capacity for finding a calm centre of peace and inner strength amidst turmoil
- Achieving adequate self-esteem
- Reducing psychological and emotional problems and blocks that inhibit full human functioning
- Improving awareness and consciousness; becoming more open-minded and inquiring; seeking an accurate picture of reality
- Greater sensitivity to psychic phenomena and alternate realities
- Freedom, liberation, looseness, flexibility
- Competence at psychological processing, at handling own feelings and personal problems
- Increasing zest for life; joy; happiness
- Liberation from female/male stereotyping, or from other role-playing
- Gaining emotional maturity, positive mental health; higher level of psychological functioning
- Achieving spiritual insights; cosmic consciousness
- Finding acceptance of self and others; accepting the world as it is
- Come to terms with own death.

All of the above can be viewed as learning–teaching potentials within the consultation. Many of these agendas may be difficult to deal with unless the practitioner is cognisant of, and comfortable with, the teaching dimension of the consultation. With regard to conventional medicine, Roter and colleagues (2001) maintain that:

> Patient education has evolved from its medically-dominated and narrow origin in patient teaching to a more comprehensive inclusion of the broader empowerment and participation agenda of health promotion and disease prevention.

A disease-centric bias is still betrayed, however, that fails to touch upon many of the territories of development and meaning identified by Tough.

Patient education may be used unethically to manipulate or coerce the individual to follow medical directives that might be inappropriate or faulty. Redman (2008) describes some such instances of 'ethically contested or unethical' practice, including where patient education is used to:

> ... forward a societal goal the individual might not have chosen; assume that patients should learn to accommodate unjust treatment; exclude the views of all except the dominant healthcare provider group; limit the knowledge a patient can receive; make invalid or unreliable judgements about what a patient can learn; or require a patient to change his or her identity to meet a medical need.

The extent to which herbal practitioners are willing and able to engage in the areas of personal development left unacknowledged or unaddressed by biomedicine (and, while doing so, avoiding the dangers identified by Redman) is one determinant of the value of the herbal consultation.

In closing, we can return to the work of Malcolm Knowles, outlining his teaching principles as summarized by Jarvis (1995) who describes them as 'clearly (demonstrating) the facilitative teaching style of a humanistic educator of adults'. This is provided as a model to aid reflection on the components of a teaching approach that is suitable for use by phytotherapists – and indeed by all humanistic healthcare practitioners. In reading this list, try substituting the word 'patients' for 'learners':

The teacher:

- Exposes learners to new possibilities for self-fulfilment
- Helps learners clarify their own aspirations
- Helps learners diagnose
- Helps learners identify life-problems resulting from their learning needs
- Provides physical conditions conducive to adult learning
- Accepts and treats learners as persons
- Seeks to build relationships of trust and cooperation between learners
- Becomes a co-learner in the spirit of mutual enquiry
- Involves learners in a mutual process of formulating learning objectives
- Shares with learners potential methods to achieve these objectives
- Helps learners to organize themselves to undertake their tasks
- Helps learners exploit their own experiences of learning resources
- Gears presentation of his or her own resources to the levels of learners' experiences
- Helps learners integrate new learning to their own experience
- Involves learners in devising criteria and methods to measure progress
- Helps learners develop and apply self-evaluation procedures.

## SHARED DECISION-MAKING AND CO-PLANNING

In order to reach conclusions about how to proceed with regard to treatment and the implementation of advice, and in connection with other issues such as whether to pursue further investigation, decisions have to be made. Gwyn and Elwyn (1999) propose that decisions can be made in one of three ways:

*You can decide for yourself, weighing the options, as an autonomous individual. You can be told, or advised, what's best to do, guided, one hopes, by superior wisdom, experience or expertise. Or, two or more individuals, considering the risks and benefits of the available options, can share decisions.*

Charles et al. (1999) identify the 'three predominant models' of decision-making as: informed (the patient decides based on information); paternalistic (the practitioner decides for the patient); shared (practitioner and patient collaborate).

A partnership-oriented approach to medicine such as is generally applied in herbal practice naturally assumes that decisions will be shared and negotiated between patient and practitioner. Space is available in such a model for the patient's views and preferences to be accorded status alongside the practitioner's opinions, recommendations and guidance. In order for the decision-making process to be shared to a meaningful degree, it will be necessary for both patient and practitioner to explain and justify their positions and for the practitioner to provide the patient with information, although this, as Gwyn and Elwyn (1999) point out, may often be biased and/or incomplete. Even where a profound degree of cooperation in decision-making is achieved, however, the extent of patient and practitioner participation in choices will still be necessarily limited by the ability of each to appreciate the other's position (including limitations of language, experience and technical expertise). For example, the need to use a nervous trophorestorative strategy may be negotiated and agreed but in most cases, the patient will leave the exact choice of herbs to the phytotherapist (although not always, e.g. an experienced patient may report that they do not wish to use *Valeriana officinalis* due to previous adverse reactions to it).

Decision-making presents a territory wherein the true colours of the practitioner's orientation towards the patient are revealed. Paternalism involves making decisions on behalf of the patient, with which the patient is expected to comply, whereas patient-centred approaches value informed patient choice. The issue of where one stands as regards how decisions are to be arrived at is of such weight that some (e.g. Weston 2001) consider that it represents the crux of patient-centred care – shared decision-making (SDM) can only occur in patient-centred approaches. Despite its importance, Makoul and Clayman (2006) showed that there is no generally agreed definition of shared decision-making; rather, they discovered '31 separate concepts used to explicate SDM'. Despite this, we can take the concept of SDM as being generally interpreted as representing some form of combining, or contrasting, two basic elements: (1) the presentation of 'options' by the practitioner, and (2) consideration of the patient's 'values/preferences'.

Charles et al. (1997) provided a model of SDM as including four characteristics:

1. Both the patient and the practitioner are involved
2. Both parties share information
3. Both parties take steps to build a consensus about the preferred treatment
4. An agreement is reached on the treatment to implement.

Although this delineation appears rather straightforward and one might assume that such practice is commonplace, Stevenson et al. (2000) 'found little evidence that doctors and patients both participate in the consultation in this way'. They discovered that there was little participation in sharing information and views about treatment options such that 'there was no basis upon which to build a consensus about the preferred treatment and reach an agreement on which treatment to implement'. This state of affairs might arise for a number of reasons including that the practitioner considers that there is only a single treatment available (i.e. there are no options to be discussed); or that the practitioner has selected what they consider to be the most appropriate treatment option, assuming that the patient would want the practitioner to take this decision for them or that the patient would not possess the appropriate skills or capacities to help make such a decision.

Two studies (Gravel et al. 2006; Legare et al. 2008) have shown that the three most commonly reported barriers to implementing SDM were:

- Time constraints
- Lack of applicability due to patient characteristics
- The clinical situation.

The process of shared decision-making is time consuming (although this may be less of an issue for many herbal practitioners given the tendency to conduct lengthy consultations); not all patients either desire or are able to participate in the process (although practitioners must be wary of making assumptions in this regard); and the clinical situation is not always conducive to the practice of SDM (e.g. some types of acute emergencies). The same studies gave the three most common facilitators of using SDM as:

- Motivation of health professionals
- The perception that shared decision-making will lead to a positive impact on the clinical process
- The perception that shared decision-making will lead to a positive impact on patient outcomes.

In other words, SDM tends to be applied where practitioners are convinced of its value and/or have an ideological commitment to it. Such commitment may occur in the absence of a particularly discernible or rigorously applied method, however. Commonly, the 'method' is fuzzy (and by this I do not necessarily imply criticism), involving a varied amalgamation of practitioner-supplied information and opinion and with the patient's preferences and intuitive 'feel' for what is appropriate for their predicament. Elwyn et al. (2001a) have proposed the statistically-based model of 'decision analysis', originally developed within the discipline of economics, as a suitable means of enabling SDM, claiming that it 'potentially enhances patient autonomy because the patients influence the decision-making process by contributing their own values'. However, it is hard to see how the mathematical neatness of this model can apply in the majority of patient predicaments where huge uncertainty exists around treatment options (particularly when applied to CAM options which commonly have a limited conventional evidence base from which to generate likelihood ratios). It is also difficult to gauge the extent to which the outcome of such a process can be said to constitute a 'shared decision' as opposed to a digitized form of paternalism in that the computed result tells the patient what to do.

SDM initiatives can be construed as a response to patient demand for a more inclusive approach within conventional medicine and, in this context, may represent either genuine attempts to enhance communication and participation or be used cynically to mask old paternalist agendas. Stevenson and Scambler (2005) are among those who have discussed the concept of 'concordance', which is 'based on the idea that patients and practitioners should work together towards an agreement on treatment choice' and 'emphasizes the need for patient involvement and participation'. Concordance may be seen as a development away from notions of compliance and adherence to a more collaborative approach to treatment but Armstrong (2005) shows that it can also be viewed as 'the acceptable face of compliance: the goals remain the same but the technique is more subtle'; at the root however, it may be 'yet another pernicious attempt by medicine to get the patient to behave according to the doctor's wishes'.

In practice the 'method' of SDM often comes down to the practitioner proposing a possible treatment strategy, which the patient is then invited to query. For example the practitioner may say:

'I think this is what's going on ...'

'In the light of this, I think this is what we need to address ...'

'And I think these are the ways in which we could do it ...'

'Alternatively you could ...'

'What do you think about this?'

In proposing possible strategies it can be helpful if the practitioner identifies their own bias. Treatment decisions are not value free and it is down to the patient to decide which option (if options there be) best fits their worldview, health convictions and approach. A typical example from my practice would be the instance where my opinion is being sought regarding a child who is being advised to undergo a tonsillectomy but where the case for the operation seems less than overwhelming. In such a circumstance, my proposals *might* include the following elements:

'I am unconvinced that tonsillectomy is essential ...'

'The tonsils are an important part of the immune system and should be saved if possible ...'

'Your surgeon is unlikely to be aware of the value of herbal medicine in improving the health of the tonsils and there is very little clinical research to prove this, yet it is my experience that herbs can often address this problem effectively ...'

'I think the following risks are associated with losing the tonsils ...'

'And the following benefits might arise from keeping them ...'

'As a herbalist I tend to view the body as sacred and my bias is towards saving the body's organs if at all possible whereas biomedicine views the body more mechanistically and is more comfortable with the idea that certain body parts are relatively inessential ...'

Such a rationale highlights some of the issues attending the concept of SDM. The information provided here is contextualized within an opinion that admits its own bias – this is not a neutral laying out of options but a pitch for a certain take that is motivated by a particular clinician's attempt to act in the best long-term interests of the patient. Such a picture may not be considered to represent an ideal of SDM but it probably reflects the reality of many practice situations. Karnieli-Miller and Eisikovits (2009) question whether practitioners are prone to act as partners or as salesmen and observe that: 'treatment decisions tend to be unilaterally made, and a variety of persuasive approaches are used to ensure agreement with the physician's recommendation'. Persuasive tactics or strategies included:

- Various ways of presenting the illness, treatment and side-effects (e.g. emphasizing the benefits of treatment, frightening patients about the consequences of non-compliance and stressing the ability to control side-effects)
- Providing examples from other success or failure stories
- Sharing decisions only concerning technicalities
- Avoiding reference to alternative approaches
- Using plurals and authority (presenting treatment as an authorized 'we' decision).

In the extreme scenario, the practitioner admits no bias and presents clinical decisions as a 'done deal' based not only on supposed scientific legitimacy but also on an implied moral authority – this is the 'right' way to proceed.

SDM has also been referred to as 'informed collaborative choice' (Elwyn et al. 2001b) but the evidence of those such as Karnieli-Miller and Eisikovits suggests that the potential for achieving genuine decision-making partnerships in clinical encounters is rather limited. Idealized SDM rationales present the clinical situation as a meeting between experts with the practitioner portrayed as an expert in the technical aspects of medicine and the patient as an expert in their personal condition, preferences and values. Yet practitioners also have values and preferences and they hold particular beliefs and convictions about their chosen field of medicine, which will tend to lead to a degree (often a pronounced degree) of directedness. This steering may in fact be welcomed by patients as constituting part of the practitioner's congruence or genuineness. Conversely, attempts made by the practitioner to mask their own opinion may be picked up by the patient and interpreted negatively as a failure of the practitioner to give fully of their self. My own view is that patients prefer practitioners to be 'real' rather than to attempt forced neutrality. What most needs to be 'shared' in the decision-making process then, may be a mutual commitment to 'realness' – a concept that would entail the practitioner acknowledging that they naturally have a bias towards a certain way of conceiving of the patient's predicament and the patient proceeding in full awareness of that bias.

For genuine shared decision-making to occur, it is first necessary for power and authority to be shared. The notion of 'a meeting between experts' implies an equality of authority between practitioner and patient that may be difficult to realize, even when both parties are fully committed to doing so. The nature of each participant's expertise, although deserving of equal respect, is unlikely to be of equal technical capacity. Practitioners can compensate for the patient's lack of expertise in dealing with the minutiae of technical choices by teaching them but this will still reinforce a hierarchy of authority (teacher–student). The locus of authority may also be externalized from the direct patient–practitioner relationship by the practitioner, e.g. the practitioner may use plurals (as described above) to invoke the authority of the whole of the profession ('this is what *we* think') or may refer to the abstracted 'evidence-base'. Such strategies leave the patient with little room for negotiation, since they are unable to bring the whole of the profession into the consulting room or to bring the database into dialogue. Patients, on the other hand, may cite external sources of authority such as internet reference sources. The level at which patients are able to engage with practitioners in discussing decisions will depend on a number of factors including the extent of their medical/illness experience, research and 'health literacy'. Nutbeam (1998) defines health literacy in relation to 'cognitive and social skills' that enable people to 'gain access to, understand and use information in ways which promote and maintain good health'. This amounts to 'more than being able to read pamphlets', rather it denotes: 'a level of knowledge, personal skills and confidence to take action to improve personal and community health by changing personal lifestyles and living conditions'. Edwards et al. (2009) believe that: 'the more health literate the patient is, the more they are likely to become empowered through their engagement with information both inside and outside of the consultation experience'. Patients with substantial ability in terms of health literacy will have greater authority in the consultation and are more likely to be able to participate in SDM. Looking more generally, however, since it is far from easy for authority and power to be shared in the consultation, is it reasonable to expect that decisions be shared? An awareness of the complexities and issues involved will at least make it possible for practitioners to question their own biases and travel as far as they can in the direction of creating real and meaningful partnerships with patients.

Not all patients wish to be highly involved in decision-making. Robinson and Thomson (2001) have referred to research showing that preferences for involvement vary with age, socioeconomic status, illness experience and the gravity of the decision concerned. Stiggelbout and Kiebert (1997) found that older patients, men and 'patients, as compared with non-patients (their companions)' were 'more likely to prefer a passive role regarding treatment decisions'. The authors recommended that practitioners should 'assess every patient to determine what role he or she prefers'. A study by Schattner et al. (2006), however, revealed 'getting more information from the physician and taking part in decisions' as the most desirable patient choices of their study group. The desire for information and participation in decision-making among CAM patients is likely to be high given that people who use CAM tend to be middle-aged, female and of higher than average education (Bishop & Lewith 2008). Such people would also be expected to have high levels of health literacy – though not all.

The person-centred, holistic and extended nature of the phytotherapy consultation naturally inclines towards actively involving patients in shared decision-making and this may represent one of the attractions of the approach for some patients. Although communication around SDM may tend to be naturally fuzzy as opposed to rigorously structured the basic components of the process are straightforward enough. Charles et al. (1999) described the shared decision-making process as involving three phases: information exchange; deliberation; and treatment decision. Maintaining awareness of these three zones of activity within the final stages of the consultation will help to keep a focus on SDM and enable patient participation. In doing so it will also be useful to remember that 'decisions' are not always required to be definitive solutions; patient and practitioner may co-decide to – do nothing; try something; or start with this before trying that. In the relationship of continuing care that characterizes the phytotherapy consultation (see below) SDM is not a one-off event but rather an ongoing process – returned to and refined over a series of visits. This is usually the most appropriate approach to treating chronic disorders, where clarity, focus and results tend to be achieved by a gradual process of testing and checking where shared decision-making is merely one aspect of a mutual journey. In being the best possible companion on that journey, the phytotherapist is advised to disclose and own her own biases and to respect the patient's autonomy.

## REGIMEN: THE TREATMENT PLAN

*[In the eighteenth century] routine dispensing of medication, rather than the formulation of a comprehensive regimen, was frowned upon in best circles, as resembling the short-cut of nostrum-mongers who (according to Cheyne's gibe) 'never dare order a Regimen, and who are continually cramming their patients with nauseous and loathsome Potions, Pills and Bolus's, Electuaries, Powders and Juleps.*

Porter (1995)

In previous chapters, we have described the scope of the therapeutic agenda in phytotherapy, including the strategies for engendering wellbeing covered in Chapter 3; and nurturing the four aspects of being and the six non-naturals in Chapter 5. Such considerations (more commonly reduced to the territories of 'diet and lifestyle') combined with the actual herbal prescription can be conceived in terms of the traditional heading of 'regimen'.

The various elements of the regimen need to be proposed to the patient with accompanying rationale, justification and supporting information; then discussed and deliberated; before being decided upon in conjunction with the patient. In working through this process, the following advice may be helpful:

- Beware of overwhelming the patient with too much advice and too many activities – prioritize the most important strategies (additional or replacement strategies can be added at subsequent consultations)
- Focus on how strategies can be practically implemented in a way that the patient will find achievable
- Remember the advice given in the foregoing sections of this chapter such as to check for the patient's understanding of what is being said; using memory aids; and the various considerations pertaining to discussing the prescription
- Be prepared, as appropriate, to reject, set aside, substitute, modify or further argue the case for strategies which the patient finds unconvincing or inappropriate

- The patient may need time outside of the consultation to reflect on advice before reaching a decision about it; it may be helpful to supply more information (such as printed material, web addresses, etc.) in order to aid the patient in coming to a conclusion
- Check for a sense of completion as you come to the end of deliberating and deciding upon the regimen by asking, e.g.:

    *'Is there anything we've left out?'*

    *'Do you need more information about anything?'*

    *'Are there any other areas we need to address?'*

    *'Is there anything that you can think of that we need to add?'*

    *'Do you want me to go over anything again?'*

The regimen should be conceptualized as a dynamic cluster of treatments and strategies, the elements of which will adapt and change over the course of time. At follow-up appointments, revisions and new interventions will need to be proposed and negotiated according to the patient's response.

## CLOSING THE CONSULTATION

The ideal point at which to move to formally close the consultation is the moment at which both patient and practitioner feel a sense of completion, and of satisfaction that all necessary issues have been properly addressed. Alternatively, the clock may dictate that it is time to end the appointment. One of the finer arts of the consultation involves the ability to steer the encounter to a point of natural completion to coincide with the time allotted. This is not always possible, however, and in such instances, it is important to acknowledge the time limitation and the consequent need to finish the consultation without unduly rushing the patient and leaving them feeling that the consultation ended too abruptly. In order to smooth the transition and assure the patient of your continuing attention and care, perhaps finish with a phrase such as:

*'I'm aware that time is passing and we need to close for today but I'm also aware that we haven't quite covered all that we need to in the depth we would both like – I'm just going to make a couple of notes to remind me about what we need to continue discussing next time.'*

Signposting the movement towards closure earlier can help to avoid such a statement being needed. Keeping a subtle eye on the clock is of inestimable value here.

Silverman et al. (2005) identify four components that can serve as the final movement of the encounter, combining drawing any remaining loose threads together and promoting the sense of completion and satisfaction just described. The four aspects are set within two key final aims:

Forward planning

- Contracting
- Safety-netting.

Ensuring an appropriate point of closure
- End summary
- Final checking.

### Contracting

Contracting seeks to form an agreement about the next steps to be taken by practitioner and patient and to allow 'each party to identify their mutual roles and responsibilities'. The phytotherapist might say, e.g.:

> 'So I will post the herbs to you tomorrow morning and you should receive them by the end of the week. I'll also write up the advice we have discussed and e-mail it to you. Perhaps you can see how you get on with that, focussing on the sleep strategies. Is that okay?'

### Safety-netting

This refers to clarifying contingency plans and how you can be contacted if the patient has any queries. For example:

> 'As I said earlier, I think your skin should start to clear within 3 or 4 days of starting the herbal medicine but if things develop differently contact me. If you have any queries at all you can call me on my mobile – if there's no reply leave a message and I'll get back to you as soon as I can. You can also text or e-mail me – everything comes through to my mobile so I'll be sure to get your message shortly after you send it. Do you have any questions about that?'

### End summary

It is worth formulating a few words to provide a final summary regarding the situation and the plans for its remediation, as you understand it. A succinct statement helps to ensure mutual understanding, promotes a sense of completion for both parties and provides a last opportunity for clarification, if that is required:

> 'So, just to be as clear as possible, and to make sure that I understand things properly, let me try to sum up – and you can tell me if this sounds alright. I think your skin condition is guttate psoriasis and that it should have improved significantly by the time of our next appointment – which is going to be in four weeks time. I am confident that the herbs and advice we have discussed will provide all the treatment you need but if things develop differently you should contact me. I think you are quite depleted; that the various sources of stress that you have experienced over the last year are connected with your skin condition and that it is important that this underlying state is addressed – in the ways we discussed. To that end, I have suggested we work together for perhaps six months, depending on the results we get. Is that a reasonable summary? Have I missed anything?'

### Final checking

It is worth providing an opportunity for the patient to raise any last queries or comments:

> 'Before we finish can I just check whether you have any final queries or comments – about anything at all?'

Interaction with the patient following the formal conclusion of the consultation continues to be important and potentially of therapeutic value. The final exchanges occurring before patient and practitioner part give an opportunity to demonstrate continuing warmth and care. For example, the final scene of the clinical encounter might unfold something like this:

> Practitioner: 'Well, come through to reception and we can book your next appointment'.
>
> Patient: 'Okay'.

The practitioner stands and as the patient is gathering her things says: 'I'm very glad you came; I think it's really important that we spent time looking at things in depth'.

> Patient, now standing: 'It felt that like to me too. I've never discussed my health in such detail with anybody before and it was a very powerful experience – I've got lots to think about now! Thank you'.
>
> Practitioner: 'Thank you too. That's great. But remember to take things gently and be kind to yourself ... Come on through'.

The practitioner holds the door open for the patient and they walk through to reception where the practitioner asks the receptionist to arrange a follow-up appointment for 4 weeks time and says goodbye to the patient before returning to the consulting room.

## CONTINUITY OF CARE

Phytotherapists may practise in a range of settings, most typically within multidisciplinary CAM clinics, but also in: conventional healthcare locations, from home and in specialist centres and clinics such as drug rehabilitation facilities. Although there are some instances of herbal practitioners working at the same location to provide shared care, most work as solo practitioners caring for their own list of patients. The standard mode of herbal practice is therefore continuing care with the same practitioner.

The provision of continuity of care, where the patient sees the same practitioner at every visit ('my doctor'), has long been considered a hallmark of good general practice in conventional medicine (Usherwood 1999). Mainous et al. (2001) contend that the long-term relationship that characterizes continuity of care 'has long been thought to have a beneficial effect on healthcare utilization and outcomes'. The authors go on to provide evidence to support a number of assertions regarding the benefits attending continuity of care:

> *Patients rank continuity of care ... as a high priority. High ... continuity is associated with a decreased likelihood of future hospitalization, as well as decreased emergency department use. In fact ... continuity ... provides health benefits that receiving care at the same site but seeing different providers does not provide. Moreover, discontinuity in the delivery of care has been suggested to play a role in medical errors and patient safety.*

The authors provide evidence that the key explanation for these benefits lies in the tendency of continuing care to lead to 'increased knowledge and trust' between patient and practitioner. Mechanic (2004) views trust as 'the glue that makes cooperation possible without costly and intrusive regulation' and considers that the patient's trust in a practitioner is based on the patient's beliefs that the practitioner is: technically proficient, has interpersonal competence and is their ally (the practitioner is 'on their side'). Interpersonal skills are of particular significance as:

> Central to patients' trust is how doctors communicate and whether they listen and are caring.

The communication of care can be enhanced and potentized when allowed to develop over time. Caring deepens as mutual knowledge, appreciation and understanding grows between the parties involved as a consequence of repeated engagement. Indeed, the propagation of mutual *knowing* through interaction over time distinguishes a relationship from a transaction. As patient and practitioner come to *know* each other, the potential benefits of continuity of care begin to accrue.

Healthcare relationships are not inevitably rendered positive by the fact of their persistence over time. For Haggerty et al. (2003), 'continuity' is not merely a sequence of interactions with the same practitioner, in fact it can only be said to exist as a genuine therapeutic article where the care it provides is 'experienced as connected and coherent' in a manner that is 'consistent with the patient's medical needs and personal context'. Frederiksen et al. (2009) maintain that the key to unlocking the value in continuous relationships lies in 'recognition' – practitioners must both 'respect and remember the patient, in order to create and sustain the trustful relationship'. A continuing relationship with a practitioner who fails to adequately recognize the patient, or who the patient perceives to be uncaring or lacking in some area of competency can have increasingly negative effects over time. Patients need to have choice in order to find a practitioner with whom they feel compatible and confident, as well as the option to remain with the same practitioner once they have found the right one. In herbal practice, where the vast majority of practitioners work privately, this combination of possibilities is generally available.

Although continuity of care may be appreciated by patients across a range of healthcare needs (even by those who are generally well and only need care intermittently, with months or years passing between visits), it appears to be most valued by (and of most benefit to) those with chronic conditions requiring ongoing care and repeated consultations (Love et al. 2000; Cabana & Jee 2004). For such patients, the act of repeatedly telling their story to a range of different practitioners can be tiring, dissatisfying and dispiriting. Brampton (2000) provided a patient's perspective on continuity of care, stating that:

> It is deflating to find a doctor distractedly flicking through your notes to try and gain a sense of your medical history. It is equally frustrating to have to answer the same questions asked just a week earlier, as the doctor tries to come to terms with your condition and character.

It has been quite common in my experience, when recommending a colleague to a patient who is moving to a different part of the country, to hear the patient comment that: 'I don't want to have to tell my story all over again'. From questioning patients about such an observation, I have come to appreciate it as referring to:

- A reluctance to expend (or re-expend) the energy (across all aspects of being) that is required to establish a profound patient–practitioner relationship
- A sense of not personally *needing* to relate or revisit their history
- A sense that 'starting again' with a new practitioner represents a setback; or that it might actually inhibit or delay their progress.

Read from another angle, this interpretation suggests that the provision of continuity of care:

- Saves the patient's energy
- Spares them from engaging in unnecessary activity
- Conveys a stabilizing and progressive force.

Nutting et al. (2003) found that:

*Patients who value continuity tend to be female, at either end of the age spectrum, less educated ... have more health problems, require more medication, and report lower health status.*

This evidence suggests that continuity of care may be especially important for patients who are particularly vulnerable or who have complex health problems. Pereira Gray et al. (2003) consider that 'patients in general have a desire for continuity of care' but some groups value it less, including 'the young, and males' and where 'the disorder is perceived as mechanical'.

Despite the advantages associated with continuity of care and the extent to which it is valued by most patients (and practitioners), conventional medicine, at the management level, has moved some distance towards disavowing it. Guthrie and Wyke (2000) consider that continuity of care: 'is increasingly presented as "old fashioned" and in opposition to the development and modernisation of primary care'. Speaking of change in the UK National Health Service, the authors acknowledge that some developments have benefited both doctors and patients but that most have tended to reduce personal continuity. The types of changes referred to include: larger group practices; the decline of personal lists; sharing out of hours care and the provision of drop-in clinics. Most herbal practitioners operate solo practices (in terms of the modality of herbal practice; meaning, while herbal practitioners may operate within a larger practice they are typically the only herbal practitioner there); operate a personal list; and do not provide out of hours care or drop-in clinics. Although the structure and scope of herbal medicine as a primary care service can be criticized, its current organizational bias, nonetheless, is firmly in the direction of continuity of care. Indeed the emphasis on continuity of care can be considered as representing one of the greatest strengths of phytotherapy and one of its main attractions for many patients. As conventional medicine veers away from providing continuing personal care, herbal practitioners (along with others placed in the CAM bracket) remain oriented to meet the patient's desire to have an ongoing relationship with the same practitioner.

Some of the practical issues involved in providing ongoing care have already been covered in this chapter but the list below provides a re-cap and adds a few more points.

**To be continued ...**

There may not have been time to cover everything in the consultation (e.g. to review the diet in depth or teach a self-care technique such as meditation), so it is important to write down anything that needs to be covered at the next visit and to allow time to do so.

**Keeping promises**

If you have promised to do something between visits then it is essential to do so, or to contact the patient to explain any necessary delays. Again, writing down what needs to be done will help to ensure that it gets done. Trust is partly built on keeping promises – being reliable also increases patient confidence.

**A lot can happen between consultations**

Between visits, patients may experience an exacerbation of their condition; develop a new problem; start other treatments; receive test results; experience a momentous event, and so forth. If you know that something significant is coming up between appointments you may wish to request that the patient updates you as the occasion arises (e.g. 'When you get the test results please send a copy to me'.).

**Recognition**

Earlier we mentioned the importance of 'recognizing' the patient. Part of this is *remembering* them, including their significant events. It is good policy to make a note when the patient tells you that something significant is going to happen in their lives so that you can ask about it once it has taken place: 'So how did the holiday go?'

**Being available**

Patients need to know when you are available to be contacted should they have a query or need to let you know about something. Some practitioners identify a phone-in hour or morning at some point during the week when they are specifically available to be contacted with routine queries. My own policy is to say that I am contactable at any time on my mobile (which receives e-mail as well as calls and texts, so I invite patients to use whichever of those options they prefer).

**Rapid responses**

When patients make contact it is good practice to respond as quickly as is practicable, even if the query is minor and the patient states that there is no rush to get back to them. Dealing with queries efficiently enhances patient trust and confidence. If it is not possible to deal with a detailed request quickly, then a message explaining the situation will usually be highly appreciated: 'I won't be able to sort this out until Friday but I just wanted you to know that I got your message and I am on the case!'

### Additional charges

If you are going to charge patients for time spent dealing with queries between visits (I don't) then it is important that patients know this in advance.

### Modes of communication

Communication between consults may take place via a number of media including: phone, text, e-mail, letter and video-call. Each mode has its pros and cons and if you have a preference for a particular type of communication, this is worth making clear to patients (my own policy is to follow the patient's lead). Mechanic (2001) sees e-mail as being a particularly useful method of maintaining continuity, providing a mechanism for conveying routine information and helping to avoid 'gaps in communication'.

### Re-scheduling visits

Sometimes developments between appointments are so significant that it is necessary to bring an appointment forward rather than attempt to address the situation by means other than a face-to-face visit. Both patient and practitioner may need to change appointments for other reasons, such as an unavoidable circumstance or event of some kind. If I ever need to reschedule an appointment with a patient I always give at least the gist of the reason why – for me this is part of being a genuine practitioner. Other practitioners will prefer to keep a neutral tone: 'I'm afraid I can't make that date, can we rearrange for the following week?'

### Additional prescriptions

It is common for patients to make a request such as: 'I have to rearrange my appointment for the 29th, two weeks later than we had planned, can you send me enough medicine to keep me going until then?' It is important to deal with such requests promptly. Alternatively, a new situation may arise where the patient calls to ask for a revised or different prescription. It will be down to your clinical judgement to decide whether you can make such a change without seeing the patient in person.

### Frequency of visits

The gap left between consultations will depend on the nature of the patient's predicament and the degree of need they have for face-to-face support. Acute episodes may be followed-up within a few days to 1–2 weeks. Long-term treatment of chronic disorders may involve visits spaced anywhere from every 4–6 or 8 weeks apart. Where patients are on continuous treatments over very long time scales (e.g. in osteoarthritis), visits may only take place once or twice a year. Codes of Ethics and Practice tend to advise that patients should be seen 'regularly' or 'periodically' but it is generally left to the practitioner to justify the time period they see as appropriate. My own preference is never to leave more than 6 months between visits at the outside (this length of gap only being appropriate for patients with chronically stable, well-controlled conditions, e.g. patients with inflammatory bowel disease that can be considered as being in long-term remission or 'cured' and where the patient is taking a simple maintenance/preventive tea).

### Changing nature of the patient's predicament

It is important to be alert to recognizing when the nature of the patient–practitioner relationship changes or enters a new stage, e.g. detecting the transition from 'wait and see' to 'time to intervene'; from active treatment to monitoring; or from one form of regimen to another. The point of transition may occur between scheduled visits and it may be necessary to respond to this before the next visit is due. Practitioner qualities of attentiveness, openness, flexibility and responsiveness are therefore as crucial between consultations as they are during them.

### Involving and working with others

Providing continuity of care does not mean providing sole care. The patient may be receiving treatment and/or advice from other practitioners and it is vital to collaborate with these as appropriate. Alternatively you may be in the position of recommending that the patient consult an additional practitioner. Contact with other practitioners regarding the patient's situation may occur between visits and the patient should be apprised of the nature and outcome of such contact.

## REFLECTIVE PRACTICE AND RESEARCH

Between appointments there is an opportunity to reflect on the consultation just passed and to conduct research to gain further insights into the patient's predicament and means of improving it. These activities are, first and foremost, essential in order to provide the patient with the best quality of care but, when discussed with the patient, they also *demonstrate* care – showing recognition and enhancing trust and confidence. For example, you might say: 'I've been thinking about our last meeting and ...'; 'Since I last saw you I've done some research into your condition and ...'. Reflection and research also, crucially, enable practitioner self-development and growth.

The capacity to provide high quality continuing care is one of the greatest assets of the herbal practitioner and is entirely consistent with the approach to the consultation itself, as we have described it. Continuity of care facilitates the evolution of the patient's predicament and their process of discovering meaning and finding and employing strategies for development. It is a cohering practice that demonstrates a profound level of caring and provides patients with a source of security and stability as they go through changes. Returning to our previous discussion of the practitioner as leader, Gosling and Murphy (2004) have pointed out that maintaining a sense of continuity during times of change is the key to successful leadership.

A sense that there is positive change occurring will indicate to both practitioner and patient that the relationship between them is a healthy one and is producing desirable results. Movement, flow, development, growth – these are the characteristics of a dynamically helpful and healing relationship. Conversely, if these factors are absent and the patient's situation is stagnant or in decline, new perspectives and strategies are required which may include the involvement of other practitioners to provide additional insights and fresh impetus. There is a difference between stagnation and stability however, and between inevitable and avoidable decline – chronically or terminally ill patients may reach a point where further physical improvements are unlikely or impossible. In such situations development, growth, and even healing, are still possible in emotional, mental and spiritual terms – in fact this terrain may never have been so fertile. At these times, the practitioner's emphasis will be on bearing witness, providing support, communicating warmth and (let us name what this amounts to) radiating love.

There are obstacles to a practitioner's ability to provide continuity of care – both personal and societal. Providing continuity of care can be overwhelming and unsustainable if the practitioner's caseload is too large. Those who care for others also need care – prioritizing self-care and devoting time and effort to developing and maintaining nurturing relationships with others (outside of the clinic) are essential strategies. The key domain of work in this regard usually relates to time: allotting sufficient time to meet the needs of the working self, the solitary self and the social self. For many of us this represents an ongoing quest, yet one that is not necessarily unobtainable. The pace of societal change drives many of the challenges around 'time'. Societies are in an extraordinary state of flux at the present time. Change is occurring at a greater rate than at any point in history and practitioners cannot stand apart from this. Davies (2004) sees a connection between practitioners changing relationships with their work and changes in relationships at large:

> *The old pattern of lifelong continuous service provided by one person to one population is breaking up ... Just as in the wider society the default relationship is no longer a stable marriage ...*

Both patients and practitioners are subject to the impacts of the nature and accelerating rate of change in society. Patients move home more frequently, travel more, have greater choice of practitioners and treatments but may also suffer more severe fluctuations in income that affect their ability to fund and maintain care. Practitioners are also more mobile; they may wish to work part-time; and to take time out from practice periodically. They may also be less inclined to see medicine (any form of medicine) as a career for life, moving on to other opportunities or experiences in due course. Given these considerations the provision of continuity of care, depending as it does on a longitudinal relationship between one patient and one practitioner, may seem like an 'old fashioned' idea indeed. While the notion continues to be sound its application will inevitably need to change, and, of course, it is already doing so. For one thing the use of technology is enabling *greater* continuity of care between consultations and compensating for some of the societal changes that threaten continuity. I think of a patient (a woman diagnosed with multiple sclerosis) who I saw for around 8 months before she moved to Italy. I have been continuing to care for her for over 4 years now – via e-mail, phone calls, text messaging and video-calls. She also typically visits the UK two or three times a year and I see her in person at those times. She sees no other practitioners for treatment but is in touch with her neurologist in the UK and has access to medical services in Italy should she require them. Our relationship has an informal and creative tonality, which is in keeping with the patient's character and also suits this practitioner. The mutual effort that has been made to maintain continuity in the face of disruption has strengthened the practitioner–patient relationship in this instance.

The therapeutic relationship is not limited to the consultation space, it continues even after the patient and practitioner have vacated each other's presence. The way in which ongoing care is provided between appointments is crucial to the success of the practice of phytotherapy. Continuity of care is central to deepening and sustaining the therapeutic relationship and it is a service that, despite the challenges involved, herbal practitioners are well placed to provide.

## REFERENCES

Armstrong D: The myth of concordance: response to Stevenson and Scambler, *Health: an Interdisciplinary Journal for the Social Study of Health, Illness and Medicine* 9(1):23–27, 2005.

Bennis WG, Nanus B: *Leaders: the strategies for taking charge*, New York, 1985, Harper & Row.

Bishop FL, Lewith GT: Who uses CAM? A narrative review of demographic characteristics and health factors associated with CAM use, *Evidence Based Complementary and Alternative Medicine* 2008; March.

Brampton S: Commentary: a patient's perspective of continuity, *British Medical Journal* 321:735–736, 2000.

Cabana MD, Jee SH: Does continuity of care improve patient outcomes? *Journal of Family Practice* 53(12):974–980, 2004.

Cardona P: Transcendental leadership, *Leadership and Organization Development Journal* 21(4):201–207, 2000.

Carson JB, Tesluk PE, Marrone JA: Shared leadership in teams: an investigation of antecedent conditions and performance, *Academy of Management Journal* 50(5):1217–1234, 2007.

Charles C, Gafni A, Whelan T: Shared decision-making in the medical encounter: what does it mean? (or it takes at least two to tango), *Social Science & Medicine* 44(5):681–692, 1997.

Charles C, Gafni A, Whelan T: Decision-making in the physician-patient encounter: revisiting the shared treatment decision-making model, *Social Science & Medicine* 49(5):651–661, 1999.

Covey SR: *Principle-centered leadership*, Toronto, 1990, Summit Books.

Davies P: The non-principal phenomenon: a threat to continuity of care and patient enablement? *British Journal of General Practice* October:730–731, 2004.

Edwards M, Davies M, Edwards A: What are the external influences on information exchange and shared decision-making in healthcare consultations: a meta-synthesis of the literature, *Patient Education and Counseling* 75:37–52, 2009.

Elwyn G, Edwards A, Eccles M, et al: Decision analysis in patient care, *The Lancet* 358:571–574, 2001a.

Elwyn G, Edwards A, Mowle S, et al: Measuring the involvement of patients in shared decision-making: a systematic review of instruments, *Patient Education and Counseling* 43:5–22, 2001b.

Frederiksen HB, Kragstrup J, Dehlholm-Lambertsen G: It's all about recognition!

Qualitative study of the value of interpersonal continuity in general practice, *BMC Family Practice* 10:47, 2009.

Gage NL: *Teacher Effectiveness and Teacher Education,* Palo Alto, 1972, Pacific Books.

Gosling J, Mintzberg H: The five minds of a manager, *Harvard Business Review* 2003; November.

Gosling J, Murphy A: *Leading continuity,* Working paper, Centre for Leadership Studies, 2004, University of Exeter.

Gravel K, Legare F, Graham ID: Barriers and facilitators to implementing shared decision-making in clinical practice: a systematic review of health professionals' perceptions, *Implementation Science* 1:16, 2006.

Greenleaf RK: *The servant as leader,* New York, 1982, Greenleaf Center.

Guthrie B, Wyke S: Does continuity in general practice really matter? *British Medical Journal* 321:734–735, 2000.

Gwyn R, Elwyn G: When is a shared decision not (quite) a shared decision? Negotiating preferences in a general practice encounter, *Social Science and Medicine* 49:437–447, 1999.

Haggerty JL, Reid RJ, Freeman GK, et al: Continuity of care: a multidisciplinary review, *British Medical Journal* 327: 1219–1221, 2003.

Hurst JW: Foreword. In Schwenk TL, Whitman N, editors: *The physician as teacher,* London, 1987, Williams and Wilkins.

Jarvis P: *Adult and continuing education: theory and practice,* ed 2, London, 1995, Routledge.

Karnieli-Miller O, Eisikovits Z: Physician as partner or salesman? Shared decision-making in real-time encounters, *Social Science and Medicine* 69(1):1–8, 2009.

Kindelan K, Kent G: Patient's preferences for information, *Journal of the Royal College of General Practitioners* 36:461–463, 1986.

Knowles M: *The Adult Learner: a neglected species,* ed 4, New York, 1990, Gulf Publishing.

Legare F, Ratte S, Gravel K, et al: Barriers and facilitators to implementing shared decision-making in clinical practice: update of a systematic review of health professionals' perceptions, *Patient Education and Counselling* 73(3):526–535, 2008.

Love M, Mainous A, Talbert J, et al: Continuity of care and the physician-patient relationship, *Journal of Family Practice* 49(11), 2000.

Mainous AG, Baker R, Love MM, et al: Continuity of care and trust in one's physician: evidence from primary care in the United States and the United Kingdom, *Family Medicine* 33(1):22–27, 2001.

Makoul G, Clayman ML: An integrative model of shared decision making in medical encounters, *Patient Education and Counselling* 60(3):301–312, 2006.

Marquardt MJ: *Leading with questions,* New York, 2005, Wiley.

Mechanic D: How should hamsters run? Some observations about sufficient patient time in primary care, *British Medical Journal* 323:266–268, 2001.

Mechanic D: In my chosen doctor I trust: and that trust transfers from doctors to organisations, *British Medical Journal* 329:1418–1419, 2004.

Northouse PG: *Leadership: theory and practice,* ed 4, London, 2007, Sage.

Nutbeam D: Health promotion glossary, *Health Promotion International* 13(4): 349–364, 1998.

Nutting PA, Goodwin MA, Flocke SA, et al: Continuity of primary care: to whom does it matter and when? *Annals of Family Medicine* 1(3):149–155, 2003.

Pereira Gray D, Evans P, Sweeney K, et al: Towards a theory of continuity of care, *Journal of the Royal Society of Medicine* 96:160–166, 2003.

Porter R: The eighteenth century. In Conrad LI, Neve M, Nutton V, et al., editors: *The Western Medical Tradition: 800BC to 1800AD,* 1995, Cambridge University Press.

Redman BK: When is patient education unethical? *Nursing Ethics* 15(6):813–820, 2008.

Robinson A, Thomson R: Variability in patient preferences for participating in medical decision making: implication for the use of decision tools, *Quality in Healthcare* 2001; 10(Suppl I): 34–38.

Rogers C, Freiberg HJ: *Freedom to learn,* New York, 1994, Merrill.

Rost JC: Leadership: a discussion about ethics, *Business Ethics Quarterly* 5(1): 129–142, 1995.

Roter DL, Rudd RE, Comongs J: Patient literacy: a barrier to quality of care,

Journal of General Internal Medicine 13:850–851, 1998.

Roter DL, Stashefsky-Margalit R, Rudd R: Current perspectives on patient education in the US, *Patient Education and Counselling* 44:79–86, 2001.

Schattner A, Bronstein A, Jellin N: Information and shared decision-making are top patients' priorities, *BMC Health Services Research* 6:21, 2006.

Schwarz R: *The skilled facilitator fieldbook*, San Francisco, 2005, Jossey-Bass.

Shaw A, Ibrahim S, Reid F, et al: Patients' perspectives of the doctor–patient relationship and information giving across a range of literacy levels, *Patient Education and Counseling* 75(1):114–120, 2008.

Silverman J, Kurtz S, Draper J: *Skills for communicating with patients*, ed 2, Oxford, 2005, Radcliffe Publishing.

Smith RM: *Learning how to learn: applied theory for adults*, Chicago, 1982, Follett.

Spears LC: Introduction: Understanding the growing impact of servant-leadership, In Beazley H, Beggs J, Spears LC, Greenleaf RK, editors: *The servant-leader within: a transformative path*, Mahwah, 2003, Paulist Press.

Stevenson FA, Barry CA, Britten N, et al: Doctor-patient communication about drugs: the evidence for shared decision making, *Social Science and Medicine* 50(6):829–840, 2000.

Stevenson F, Scambler G: The relationship between medicine and the public: the challenge of concordance, *Health: an Interdisciplinary Journal for the Social Study of Health, Illness and Medicine* 9(1):5–21, 2005.

Stiggelbout AM, Kiebert GM: A role for the sick role: patient preferences regarding information and participation in clinical decision-making, *Canadian Medical Association Journal* 157(4):383–389, 1997.

Tough A: Self-planned learning and major personal change. In Smith RM, editor: *Adult Learning: issues and innovations*, 1976, Northern Illinois University.

Usherwood T: *Understanding the consultation: evidence, theory and practice*, Buckingham, 1999, Open University Press.

Viall PB: *Learning as a way of being*, San Francisco, 1996, Jossey-Bass.

Weston WW: Informed and shared decision-making: the crux of patient-centred medicine, *Canadian Medical Association Journal* 165:438–440, 2001.

Wheatley M: *Leadership and the new science: discovering order in a chaotic world*, San Francisco, 2006, Berrett-Koehler.

# Appendix I
# Considerations attending the psychotherapeutic stance

This book has argued that the practice of phytotherapy tends to incline towards psychotherapeutic dimensions. This arises from factors including the extended nature of the consultation and the attempt made within it to discern meaning. It should be noted that there are implications associated with working in this way that call for an awareness of the limitations of one's competence to work psychotherapeutically; and a familiarity with the appreciations and safeguards that psychotherapists have developed to support their work. Such territories include:

- Understanding interpersonal dynamics (e.g. from the perspective offered by transactional analysis)
- The concepts of transference and counter-transference
- The supportive and developmental roles of supervision and debriefing.

It is beyond the scope of this book to explore these issues in any detail. They are however, mentioned here within an appendix in order to emphasize their importance. It is vital that the education of herbalists (under- and postgraduate) engages with the experience and strategies of psychotherapists in informing the therapeutic relationship.

## RECOMMENDED READING

Balint M: *The doctor, his patient and the illness* ed 1, 1957, Edinburgh, 2000, Churchill Livingstone.

Budd S: Transference revisited. In Budd S, Sharma U, editors. *The healing bond: the patient–practitioner relationship and therapeutic responsibility*, London, 1994, Routledge.

Casement P: *On learning from the patient*, London, 1985, Tavistock.

Crown S: Contraindications and dangers of psychotherapy, *British Journal of Psychiatry* 143:436–441, 1983.

Kahn M: *Between therapist and client*, New York, 2001, Holt.

Stewart I, Joines V: *TA today: a new introduction to transactional analysis*, Chapel Hill, 1987, Lifespace.

# Appendix 2
Self-care

Developing therapeutic relationships involves utilization of the self. The approach to the consultation described in this book calls for an intensity of concentration in listening to, and appreciating, the patient's narrative and predicament that can be very demanding. *Living and being* the attitudes and practices described in this book (such as learning as a way of being; genuineness, empathy and unconditional positive regard; ongoing reflective practice; working holistically and phenomenologically; and providing continuity of care) can be tiring and potentially draining. Caring for ourselves is essential if we are to make our work not only sustainable but also enjoyable, exciting and developmental – a source of energy generation rather than depletion.

## BURNOUT

The term 'burnout' is used to refer to practitioners who have become exhausted by their work. Although different authorities define burnout in different ways, the same keywords tend to recur: fatigue, frustration, disengagement, stress, depletion, helplessness, hopelessness, emotional drain, emotional exhaustion and cynicism. Skovholt (2001) observes that: 'These words point to a profound weariness and haemorrhaging of the self as key components of burnout'.

In a key work on burnout, Maslach and Leiter (1997) defined it as: 'the index of the dislocation between what people are and what they have to do. It represents an erosion in values, dignity, spirit and will – an erosion of the human soul'. They contrasted three key areas in which one could feel either burnt out or its opposite pole – fully engaged (Table A2.1).

Practitioners can readily get a sense of their position on the spectrum between burnout and full engagement by questioning where they stand with regard to these pairings. However, Dyrbye et al. (2009) caution against relying on neat diagnostic models in determining burnout, given their view that:

> ... burnout is a complex, continuous, and heterogeneous construct that manifests itself differently in different individuals. Emotional exhaustion, depersonalization, and inefficacy are symptoms of the syndrome. These symptoms can manifest in differing degrees resulting in burnout being best considered a continuum rather than a dichotomous variable.

Maslach and Leiter (1997) diagnose six specific causes of burnout focussing on workplace related issues; these can be contrasted to suggest six sources of burnout prevention (Table A2.2).

**Table A2.1** Three key areas when burnt out or fully engaged

| Burnt out | Fully engaged |
|---|---|
| Exhaustion | Energy |
| Cynicism | Involvement |
| Ineffectiveness | Efficacy |

**Table A2.2** Six sources of burnout creation and prevention

| Burnout creation | Burnout prevention |
|---|---|
| Work overload | Sustainable workload |
| Lack of control | Feelings of choice and control |
| Insufficient reward | Recognition and reward |
| Unfairness | Fairness, respect, justice |
| Breakdown of community | A sense of community |
| Value conflict | Meaningful, valued work |

Irving (2009) provides evidence to support the assertion that: 'burnout is endemic in health care professionals'. Herbal practitioners are not immune to burnout, although the factors above may be modulated by the typical independent, as opposed to institutionally employed, status of phytotherapists. Nonetheless, it is still very much possible for herbal practitioners to experience all the factors that create burnout, e.g. to be overloaded with work; to feel insufficiently rewarded (including financially); and to become isolated (lack of community).

Skovholt (2001) distinguishes between two types of burnout:

1. Meaning burnout: this occurs when the meaning of the work has been lost and the existential purpose for the work is gone: 'Why am I doing this?'
2. Caring burnout: where 'dehumanized responses' are a core feature. The practitioner ceases to care (sometimes called 'compassion fatigue').

## SUSTAINING THE SELF AND PREVENTING BURNOUT

Skovholt recommends a number of strategies for practitioner sustenance and burnout prevention. It is essential, he contends, to support and sustain both the personal and professional selves, for example by using the strategies listed below.

### SUSTAINING THE PERSONAL SELF

- Constantly invest in a personal renewal process:
    - Search for and find positive life experiences. Seek: zest, euphoria, peace, excitement, happiness, pleasure. Keep the energy flowing.

- Be aware of the danger of one-way caring relationships in one's personal life:
  - Cultivate relationships where care is mutual in order to counterbalance this.
- It is important to attend to, and to nurture, each aspect of one's self:
  - The emotional self
  - The financial self
  - The humorous self
  - The loving self
  - The nutritious self
  - The physical self
  - The playful self
  - The priority-setting self
  - The recreational self
  - The relaxation-stress reduction self
  - The solitary self
  - The spiritual or religious self.

Reflection on these aspects of the self and whether they are being cared for will quickly reveal which dimensions of our being require attention or adaptation (and may reveal some that are being over-emphasized). Practitioners tend to accept that they need to sacrifice care for themselves in certain areas in the short-term while undergoing initial practitioner education and training (Ratanawongsa et al. 2007a) but commonly, self-sacrifice continues once in practice, becoming perceived as an ongoing necessity as opposed to a short-term strategy. The notion of 'self-sacrifice' may be underpinned and maintained by profound influences such as religious orientation or conviction; or by negative conceptions of self-worth and low self-esteem. Such influences may be large enough to constitute shadow motivations for being in practice that stand in need of assessment. Ratanawongsa et al. (2007b) maintain that: 'career resilience requires that physicians reflect on and define the sources of their own intrinsic motivation'. Practitioners should seize 'opportunities to maximize self-awareness' since these may serve to 'maximize meaning and fulfilment over the long term'. We have previously discussed the fit between the practitioner's search for self-meaning and their attempt to help the patient achieve the same goal. When the practitioner is alive and responsive to this dual quest, then practice may become a process of growth, learning and healing for all parties.

With regard to sustaining the professional self, Skovholt advises practitioners to:

- Avoid the grandiosity impulse, and relish small 'I made a difference' victories
- Think long term: see the long-term map while meeting short-term goals
- Find healthy ways of maintaining a strong sense of self, since this is a prerequisite for effective functioning as a professional helper
- Cultivate professional social support (participate in activities with colleagues)
- At work, learn how to be playful, have fun, tell jokes and laugh
- Be a 'good enough practitioner'

- Increase intellectual excitement and decrease boredom by reinventing oneself
- Learn to set boundaries, create limits, and say no to unreasonable helping requests.

Skovholt urges practitioners to become aware of the difference between genuine development and pseudodevelopment ('stagnation'). The latter state is present when the practitioner believes they are developing due to the fact that they have been in practice for some time, whereas they are actually doing little more than repeating stuck patterns over and over again. In order to facilitate real development:

> *Reductionistic and simplistic conceptions of reality, attractive to practitioners because they offer clarity, must be resisted. Rather, an attitude of adventure into the complexity must take hold. One must have an openness to all of the information and feedback that comes to the practitioner. To develop rather than to stagnate, the practitioner must tolerate not knowing and ambiguity. Sound easy? It is not. The achievement and mastery culture of the professional world treasures knowing and clarity. Not knowing and ambiguity are considered undesirable. Consequently, it is hard for practitioners to seek the undesirable. Yet, such seeking, on the road less travelled, leads to practitioner growth.*

## TAKING OUR OWN ADVICE

Caring for the self and caring for others should be complementary rather than opposed or mutually exclusive activities. By living the advice we give our patients, with the same blips in consistency that they experience, we increase our capacities both to be well and to be helpful. The need for practitioners to address, for example, the six non-naturals and the four aspects of being (physical, emotional, mental, spiritual), is of course as fundamental as it is for patients.

Phytotherapists are well placed to support their own wellbeing with herbal medicines – drawing on appropriate strategies (commonly adaptogens, nervines and immunomodulators) to support or optimize function. In treating ourselves, we learn how to treat others.

In 'practising what we preach' and taking seriously the injunction: 'physician, heal thyself', it is important to operate with an appreciation of the counterbalancing concept of the wounded healer. The aim is not to attempt to embody a vision of super-health but rather to be true to one's own path – acting with integrity in attempting to sustain and realize the self, and demonstrating a commitment to creativity and learning as we journey along.

Irving et al. (2009) propose meditation as one of the most useful techniques that practitioners can utilize in order to enhance self-care. They urge meditation as a means of achieving 'mindfulness', citing Kabat-Zinn's (2003) definition of mindfulness as: 'the awareness that emerges through paying attention, on purpose, in the present moment, and non-judgmentally to the unfolding of experience moment by moment'. Adopted as a default *way of being*, mindfulness enables us to make continual positive adjustments to our thoughts and actions, carefully attending to the self and our impact on others.

It needs to be emphasized that self-care does not mean doing things alone – full care of the self necessarily involves others, including other practitioners, both within and without our own disciplines. It should also be grasped that self-care can be a delight rather than a chore. Ackerman (1999) emphasizes that ongoing self-care is best when composed of small joyful episodes of self-nurturing and enablement and attests that: 'Rituals of self-care, planned and savored, can rise up like a shimmering oasis at the end of a long dry day'.

# REFERENCES

Ackerman D: *Deep play*, New York, 1999, Vintage.

Dyrbye LN, West CP, Shanafelt TD: Defining burnout as a dichotomous variable, *Journal of General Internal Medicine* 24(3):440, 2009.

Irving JA, Dobkin PL, Park J: Cultivating mindfulness in health care professionals: a review of empirical studies of mindfulness-based stress reduction (MBSR), *Complementary Therapies in Clinical Practice* 15:61–66, 2009.

Kabat-Zinn J: Mindfulness-based interventions in context: past, present and future, *Clinical Psychology: Science and Practice* 10:144–156, 2003.

Maslach C, Leiter P: *The truth about burnout: how organizations cause personal stress and what to do about it*, San Francisco, 1997, Jossey-Bass/Wiley.

Ratanawongsa N, Wright SM, Carrese JA: Well-being in residency: a time for temporary imbalance? *Medical Education* 41(3):273–280, 2007a.

Ratanawongsa N, Howell EE, Wright SM: What motivates physicians throughout their careers in medicine? *Comprehensive Therapy* 32(4):210–217, 2007b.

Skovholt TM: The resilient practitioner, Boston, 2001, Allyn & Bacon.

# Appendix 3
# Interprofessional communication

There are numerous instances where it may be either appropriate or necessary for herbal practitioners to communicate with other healthcare practitioners or related services – whether of conventional medicine or otherwise. Relevant scenarios include:

- Recommendation to another practitioner for assessment or treatment
- Referring a patient to their GP to carry out investigations, etc.
- Querying a prescription or other treatment
- Alerting the practitioner to an issue
- Seeking the practitioner's opinion
- Suspicion that the patient is being abused
- Concern that the patient may be at risk, e.g. of harming themselves.

The degree of severity and urgency of the patient's predicament will influence the means of communication used, e.g. telephone in acute situations or letter in routine or formal communications.

At the time of writing, herbal practitioners in the UK are not yet statutorily regulated and therefore usually operate outside of formal channels of medical communication. This situation can pose risks for patients and challenges for practitioners but it does not serve as an excuse for inadequate communication.

Phytotherapists need to proceed with particular care and communicate as appropriate in the following types of situations:

- Where patients are taking conventional medication, especially where the patient's health crucially depends on this or where there is a known risk of a herb–drug interaction occurring
- In vulnerable or high-risk patients such as the elderly, the very young, in pregnancy and in the critically ill
- Where a notifiable disease is suspected.

Phytotherapists, as non-statutorily regulated practitioners, have the same duty as members of the public to report if they suspect that the law is being broken, e.g. in suspected child abuse. Herbal practitioners are advised to make contact with their local child protection services to know who to contact should a case of suspected abuse arise.

When communicating with other practitioners, phytotherapists should strive to ensure that communication is:

- Clear (e.g. written in language that the target practitioner will understand; and that it is legible)
- Concise (i.e. brief but comprehensive)
- Identifies the patient accurately and clearly (e.g. providing the patient's name, address and date of birth)
- Respectful of patient confidentiality
- Courteous and respectful to the person being addressed
- Easy to respond to (i.e. contains details of how to reply to the phytotherapist: name, address, telephone number, e-mail, time of availability, etc.)

Interprofessional collaboration leading to shared responsibility for patient care between CAM practitioners such as phytotherapists and conventional medical practitioners lies beyond the scope of this book, but Peters (1994) provides a good introduction to this topic. For wider issues pertaining to ethics and professional behaviour in CAM see Stone (2002).

To access the UK National Professional Standards for Herbal Medicine, visit: www.ehpa.eu – the address of the European Herbal and Traditional Medicine Practitioners Association.

## REFERENCES

Peters D: Sharing responsibility for patient care: doctors and complementary practitioners. In Budd S, Sharma U, editors: *The healing bond: the patient–practitioner relationship and therapeutic responsibility*, London, 1994, Routledge.

Stone J: *An ethical framework for complementary and alternative therapists*, London, 2002, Routledge.

# INDEX

abstraction 143–144
*Achillea millefolium* (yarrow) 12–13
acid taste 3
activity–passivity model 44–45, 51
activity–rest balance 112
acupuncture 27
acute conditions
  assessment and diagnosis 192–193
  focus of biomedicine on 150, 200
  frequency of visits 381–382
  herbal treatment 199–200
  as medical emergency 200
adaptogens 4, 82–83, 124, 188–189, 194
address, patient's 275–276
adenosine triphosphate 10–11, 82–83
adherence 371
adverse effects 11–12
advice
  giving 120, 356–357
  mode of presenting 355–356
  taking our own 392–393
aetiology
  notions of 92–93
  talking about 356
agape 58
age, patient's 276
ageing 248–249
agenda forms 141
agendas
  patient 134–142
  practitioner 137–138
AIDS *see* HIV/AIDS
alcohol dependence and abuse 292–294
alcohol use 291–294
alkaloids 10
allergies 286
allopathic approach 3, 302
allostasis 107
American Indians *see* Native Americans
amygdala 10
analytic philosophy 159–160
ancient times, physicians of 19
animal products, in traditional medicines 19

animals, co-evolution with plants 8
annual health examination 328–330, 329f
answers
  limitations to 228–229
  listening to 227–240, 263–264
antioxidants 124
Antonovsky, Aaron 97
appointments
  contacts between 380–381
  re-scheduling 381
  *see also* consultation(s)
arts, engagement with 63–64
Asheninka people 211–212
assessment 149–158
  four aspects of being 253–256
  Hippocratic tradition 210–211
  questioning prior 271
  traditional Chinese medicine 209–210
  *vs* diagnosis 155–156
*Astragalus membranaceus* (huang qi) 4
astringency 3, 8
atheism 31
audiovisual technology 163
auditory sensory input, reducing 110
authentic self 164–165
authority, shared 372–373
automythology 179–180
autonomy
  patients 45, 47–48, 49t, 50–51
  practitioners 45, 47–48
availability to patients 380
*Avena sativa* (oat straw) 4
Ayurvedic medicine
  correspondences 14–15, 16t
  origins 1–2
  physical examination 336, 339
  taste 7–8

bedside medicine 345, 346t, 348
behaviour
  during the consultation 165–166
  observing own 101
being, four aspects of 253–256, 257t

beliefs, shaping physiology 112
Belize 17
beneficence 47
Bernard, Claude 21–22
big-mindedness 106
bilious taste 3
biographical disruption, chronic illness 197–198
biographical work 197
biomedicalization of herbal medicine 29–30, 145–146
biomedicine/conventional medicine 7–8, 89
  continuity of care 379
  distinction of phytotherapy from 147–148
  focus on acute conditions 150, 200
  Illich's critique 45–46, 86
  limitations and failures 87–89, 94–95
  management of chronic conditions 198–200
  physical examination 327–328, 336
  referral to 272–273
  reliance on 46, 86–87
  utopian vision 94
biopsychosocial model 114–115, 157–158
biopsychosocial perspective 51
bitterness 3, 8–10
blandness 3–5
blank sheet approach 225, 270–271
bodily felt sense 58, 69–71
body
  impact of beliefs on 112
  phytotherapist's view of 122
body clock, Chinese 299–300, 300f
body language (non-verbal activities) 226–227, 232–233, 262
body-typing schemas 170
Bone, Kerry 24
boundaries, placing 101
breast cancer 181
*British Pharmacopoeia* (1948) 18
burnout, professional 48, 389–390, 390t
  caring 390
  meaning 390
  prevention 390–393
'by the way …' situations 268

CAM *see* complementary and alternative medicine
Campbell, Joseph 180–181
cannabis use 290, 294
Cannon, Walter 21–22, 56–57, 129
cardiovascular system 314
carminatives 124
case history-taking 142, 205–321
  aims 209
  allergies, intolerances or sensitivities 286

asking questions and listening to replies 227–240
assessing four aspects of being 253–256
children 246–248
comprehensive 317
definitions 212–213
diet 306–310
drug and treatment history 288–289
energetic assessment 301–304, 303t
family history 287–288
follow-up consultations 264–269
formats 261–264
general considerations 207–261
hearing, speaking, moving and recording 224–227
history of 209–212
history of presenting complaint 283–284
initial consultations 269–273
medical textbooks 149, 213–214
older patients 248–250
patient's expectations 284–318
personal details leading into 282
personal style 306
practitioner's tasks during 221–222
presenting complaint 283
previous medical and life history 284–286
relative weight 142–144
six non-naturals and prioritizing the individual 256–261
social history 289–298
systems enquiry 311–317
temperament, personality, mood and outlook 304–306
terminology 212–214
transiting to physical examination 317–318
vitality 298–301, 299t
case notes *see* notes, case
case-leadership 362, 364
case-management 362
Catholicism 184–185
cause of illness *see* aetiology
certainty 59–60, 62–63
certainty-agreement model, Stacey's 127–128, 191–192, 191f
challenges, reactions to life's 106
chamomile 18
change
  follow-up consultations 268–269
  in nature of life 14–16, 97
  openness to 107
  types of personal 366–367
chaos
  edge of 127
  Golbin & Umantsev's theory of adaptive 190–193

chaos narratives 175–176, 179, 187
  challenges of working with 177–179
  complexity of consultation 128
chaos theories 82, 124–125, 127
chaotic systems 125
chaotic zone 127–128, 191–192, 191f
checking, final 376–377
*Chelidonium majus* 341
chemicals, plant
  defence 9–10
  utilization by animals 10
  variability 13
child abuse 248, 395
child-centred 242
child-friendly 242
children 242–248
  adults accompanying 244–246
  asking questions 246
  case history-taking 246–248
  consultation times 116–117
  developmental stages 244
  enquiring about patient's 279–280
  physical examination 342
child-safe 242
Chinese body clock 299–300, 300f
Chinese medicine, traditional 99, 341
  acute conditions 192
  assessment methods 209–210
  bland flavours 4–5
  categories of taste 3
  classification and diagnostic approach 167–168
  complexity and 127
  correspondences 14–15, 15t
  energetic assessment 301
  *I Ching* 16
  nature of health 97–98
  non-vegetable herbal medicines 19
  physical examination 327, 336–341
  use of colour in diagnosis 334
  vs ancient Greek medicine 334–335
*Chionanthus virginica* 341
choices 160–161
choleric temperament 169–170, 169f
Christian perspective, cause of illness 92–93
chronic conditions 193–195, 197–200
  continuity of care 378
  as disruptive experience 197–198
  frequency of visits 381–382
  practitioner's role in public aspects 195–200
  reviewing case notes 266
  role of diagnosis 149–150
  types of work involved 197
  *see also* follow-up consultations
chronic fatigue syndrome (CFS) 150–151, 181, 189, 190f, 195–197

chronic unhappiness 175–176
Cilliers, P. 124–126
circulatory stimulating herbs 82–83, 124
classification
  changing approaches 170
  suggested 186–187
  traditional approaches 167–170
  types 187
client-centred therapy, Rogers' 57–58
clinic setting 113–114
clinical examination 149
  *see also* physical examination
clinical expertise 28, 66, 219
clinical hermeneutics 217–218
clinical iatrogenesis 83–85
closing the consultation 375–377
  aims and strategies 353–359
  moving towards 352–353
co-evolution, plants and animals 9–11
coherence
  Antonovsky's sense of 97
  at conclusion of consultation 353–359
cold picture 168–169
  case history-taking 301–303, 303t
  physical examination 341–342, 341t
College of Phytotherapy 24–25
colour 334
communication
  asking questions and listening to replies 227–240
  of care 378
  interprofessional 382 395–396
  methods, between consultations 381
  non-verbal *see* non-verbal cues
community support 87–89
competence, awareness of one's own limitations 272–273
complementary and alternative medicine (CAM) 7, 24–27
  attacks on 31
  Hyland's extended network theory 187–189
  practitioner–patient relationships 46–48
  therapeutic relationship 74
  university courses 144–145
complex systems
  definitions 124–125
  *vs* chaotic systems 125
  *vs* complicated systems 125–126
complex zone 127–128, 191–192, 191f
complexity 81–82
  consultation and 124–130, 273
  definitions 124–125
  herbal medicines 11–14
  ill effects of too little 129
  limitations of evidence-based medicine 65–67
compliance 371

complicated leads 240
complicated systems 125–126
computers 225–226
concluding stage of the consultation, 351–386
concordance 371
conditions, medical, nature of 187–200
confidence 59–60, 62–63, 174–175, 356
congruence, therapeutic 57
consciousness 24
constitutional approaches, categorizing patients 170
consultation(s), 79–132
  aims 80–91
  to be continued ... 271, 380–382
  children 242–248
  closing *see* closing the consultation
  complexity and 124–130, 273
  complexity of herbal medicines and 13–14
  concluding stage, 351–386
  environment (setting) 113–116, 240–242
  follow-up *see* follow-up consultations
  frequency 381–382
  fully present status of patients 136–138, 140–141
  guiding principles/practices 123–124
  initial *see* initial consultation
  as labyrinth 119–124
  moving towards a conclusion 352–353
  partially present status of patients 135–136
  storytelling basis 42
  structure 116–119
  therapeutic nature 119
  time allowed 116–119
  updating between 380
  weighing the three classic strategies 142–144
  welcoming 273–317
  *see also* appointments; case history-taking
consulting room 241
  basic requirements 242
  symbols 241
  as theatrical space 115
contacts
  with other practitioners 382
  by patients between appointments 380–381
context-sensitive medicine (CSM) 66–67
continuity of care 382–384
contracting 376–377
control system theory 189–191
conversation, case history-taking as 214
conversational leads 239
conversion, in psychoanalysis 158
cooking 309
Copernicus, Nicolaus 184–185

co-planning 368–374
counter-irritation 188
Counter-Reformation, English 184–185
counter-transference 387
Cronbach, L.J. 182–183
cues, non-verbal 224, 226–227
cultural iatrogenesis 84–85
cure perspective 89
cycles, natural 14, 97
cytokines 34–35

damp state 340
date of birth, patient's 276
Davies, M.L. 181–182
Dawkins, Richard 7, 31
death
  concepts of ideal 249
  perspective on 85–86, 111
debriefing 387
decision analysis, statistically-based 370–371
decision-making
  different methods 368–369
  role of intuition in rapid 252
  shared *see* shared decision-making
deficiency picture 301–302
deliberative model, doctor–patient relationship 49–50
diagnosis, 133–203
  key omissions 153
  non-conventional 155
  patient's views/perspective 153–154, 271–272
  questioning prior 154, 271
  relationship to treatment 151
  relative importance 149–158
  significance to patients 150–151
  talking about 356
  as tool of political control 151–153
  traditional approaches 167–170
  triple 157–158
  uncertainty in 156–157
  *vs* assessment 155–156
  weighing the three classic strategies 142–144
diamorphine 5
diaphoretics 188
diatetica 19, 33–34
diet 306–310
  financial limitations 310
  general questions 308–310
  in herbal practice 19
  intake 307–308
  origin of herbal medicine and 1–2
  sense of taste and 110
  six non-naturals and 258–260
  *see also* eating; food
dietetics 19

'difficult' patients 176–178
difficulties 106
digestive system 311–312
directional questions 240
discomfort 101
discourse analysis 221–222
disease 92
  concept 91
  factors affecting expression 93–94
  as part of the family 92
  *see also* illness
'dis-ease' 91, 101
doctor-as-person 51
doctor–patient relationships *see*
  practitioner–patient relationships
doctor–phytotherapists 21, 29
domestic medicine 18
dopamine 56
doshas 7–8
drug history 288–289
drug use, illicit 294–295
drugs, conventional
  adverse effects 11–12
  as chemical compounds 13
  derived from plants 18
  herb interactions 194
  herbs as 5–7
  non-complex nature 82
  *vs* herbal medicines 147–148, 148t, 360t
dryness 302–303
dustbin diagnoses 150

earth foods 4–5
eating
  pattern of 307–308
  setting and manner 309–310
  *see also* diet; food
Ebers Papyrus 9
ECG recordings 108f, 327
*Echinacea* 35, 82–83, 199–200
echoing 230
education
  patient 367–368
  practitioner 144–145
Egnew, T.R. 89
Egypt, ancient 9, 51, 336
elder abuse 250
elements 301–302
*Eleutherococcus senticosus* (Siberian ginseng) 10–11
e-mail 380–381
emergent phenomenon, patient's predicament as 285–286
emotional aspect of being 253–256, 257t
emotional stability (neuroticism) 183, 185
emotions, listening to 106–107
empathy 57–58
end summary 376

endobiogenic phytotherapy 347–348
energetic assessment
  case history-taking 301–304, 303t
  physical examination 333, 338–342
energy
  deficiency and excess 298–299, 299t
  follows thought 112–113, 266
environment, consultation 113–116, 240–242
epistemology 348
ethnobotany 17–18
Europe, mainland 21–23
European Herbal Practitioners Association (EHPA) 27
everyday life-work 197
evidence, best research 28, 219
evidence-based medicine (EBM) 27–30, 166
  definition 28
  doctor–patient relationships and 50
  doctors' concerns about 28–29, 65–66
  intuition and 251
  as mode of meaning 61–62
  therapeutic relationship and 67–68
  *vs* narrative-based medicine 219
evidence-based physical examination 330–332
examination, physical *see* physical examination
excess picture 301–302
excuses, distinction from reasons 103
exercise 295–297
expectations, patient 52–53, 59
  enquiring about 284–318
  having realistic 102
  making assumptions 134–142
  *vs* patient requests 134
experienced practitioners
  instrumental, authentic and transpersonal modes of being 165
  intuition 127, 253
explanations, providing 354
explanatory models
  patient's 72–73
  practitioner's 73, 99
extended network generalized entanglement theory 187
extended network theory 187–189, 190f
extracts, herbal 12
Eysenck, Hans 169–170, 169f
Ezzy, D. 181–182, 184

facilitative leadership 362–363
faith, healing influence 86
family 92
family history 287–288
fatty taste 3

fear(s)
  correspondences 110t
  discouraging 107–109
  voicing 102
felt presence of the (body in the) moment 67–73, 90
felt sense, bodily 58, 69–71
fibromyalgia 129, 150, 189
final checking 376–377
first consultation *see* initial consultation
flavonoids 10
flexibility 273
focusing-oriented psychotherapy 58
follow-up consultations 143, 264–269
  'by the way …' situations 268
  change and recollection 268–269
  enactment 266–268
  four territories of information 268
  opening questions 263, 266–267
  outline format 116–119
  physical examination 333
  preparation for 265–266
  time allowed 116–117
food 1–2, 7–9
  history 310
  intolerances 286
  preferences, attitudes and beliefs 310
  preparation 309
  *see also* diet; eating
food-stuffs 9
Foucault, M. 92, 127, 133–134, 216, 261, 334
four aspects of being 253–256, 257t
four humours model, Eysenck's 169–170, 169f
frame of reference, practitioner's 98–99
France 21–22
Frank, A. 128, 172–175, 177–181

Gadamer, H.G. 214–215
Galen 8, 255–256
gardening 105–106
gaze, direction of practitioner's 224–226
gender, patient's 277
Gendlin, Eugene 58, 69–71
general practitioners (GPs)
  details, patient's 281
  evidence-based medicine and 65–66
  as phytotherapists 29
  referral to 142, 272–273
generalized quantum entanglement theory 187
generalizing about individuals 166–172
genuineness 355–356
Germany 21–22
Gibson, George 32
ginger *(Zingiber officinale)* 82–83, 168
*Ginkgo biloba* 2

ginseng
  Chinese or Korean *(Panax ginseng)* 10–11, 35, 82–83
  Siberian *(Eleutherococcus senticosus)* 10–11
'go-along' interview 115–116
goals, achieving 103
Golbin, A. 190–193
Goldacre, Ben 46
governments 28–29
GPs *see* general practitioners
Greaves, D.
  on acute conditions 150
  on diagnostic investigations 344–345
  on Illich 86–87
  on physical examination 325–326, 328–330
Greece, medicine of ancient *see* Hippocratic–Galenic medicine
greeting patients 274
guidance–cooperation model 44–45, 51

hair 303, 312–313
hands, shaking 274
happiness
  cultivating 104–105
  as network phenomenon 91–92
  *see also* unhappiness
Hatfield, Gabrielle 18
headache, tension 326
healing 89
healing plant, phytotherapist's view 122–123
healing relationship 72–73
health 87, 91–98
  Antonovsky's model 97
  changing expectations 94–95
  factors affecting expression 93–94
  Illich's concept 97–98
  in traditional medical systems 97–98
  World Health Organization definition 96
health examination, annual 328–330, 329f
health literacy 372–373
Health Professions Council (HPC) 27
healthcare practitioners, sociocultural influences 45–46
healthism 94–96
hearing 323–324
heart rate recordings 107, 108f
'heartsink' patients 176–178, 266
*heilpraktikers* 21
Heraclitus 14
herb–drug interactions (HDIs) 194
herbal medicine
  biomedicalization 29–30, 145–146
  development as practice 14–20
  distinctive features 146–148
  integration and regulation 24–27

normalization 30
organization in the UK 20
origins 1–14
university courses 144–145
herbal medicines
  arriving at a prescription 124
  availability in Europe 21
  meaning 74–75
  nature of 360
  phytotherapist's view 122–123
  range of effects 82–83
  specific effects 74
  talking about 359–360
  vs conventional drugs 147–148, 148t, 360t
  wholeness and complexity 11–14
herbal practitioners 18–21
  in UK 23–24
herbalists 18–20
  Thomsonian 20
  traditional 20
Herbalist's Charter 184–185
hermeneutics, clinical 217–218
Hippocratic–Galenic medicine
  classification and diagnostic approach 168–169
  correspondences 14–15, 15t
  energetic assessment 301
  four humours 234
  patient assessment 210–211
  physical examination 336–338
  qualities of taste 3
  six non-naturals 256–261
  spirituality 255
  vs Chinese medicine 334–335
history 214
  defined 212–213
  nature of 214–216
  of the presenting complaint 283–284
  taking see case history-taking
HIV/AIDS 181–182
Hoffman, David 23–24
holism/holistic approach 24, 45, 133–134
  defined 137
  diagnosis and assessment 156–157
  illness narratives and 179
  polyphonic nature 184–185
home
  circumstances, patient's 280, 297–298
  visits 113–115, 241–242
homoeodynamism 107–109, 125–126
homoeopathy 3, 188
homoeostasis 21–22, 107–109, 125–126, 129
Hooke, Robert 344
hormone replacement therapy (HRT) 151
hospital medicine 150, 345, 346t, 348

hot picture 168–169
  case history-taking 302–303, 303t
  physical examination 341–342, 341t
House of Lords Select Committee Report (2000) 27
'how did you hear about me?' 281
humans, co-evolution with plants 9–11
humoral approach, ancient 15t, 21–22, 169–170, 234
humour 234–235
Husserl, Edmund 68–69, 71
*Hydrastis canadensis* (golden seal) 4
Hyland, M.A. 43, 57–58, 74
Hyland, M.E. 187–189, 190f
*Hypericum perforatum* (St John's wort) 6–7
hypertension 154
hypochondriasis 151

*I Ching* 16
iatrogenesis 83–85
iatroplacebogenic effect 54
iatrotherapeutic effect 54
ibuprofen 8
idiosyncratic conditions 151
Illich, Ivan
  concept of health 97–98
  concepts of iatrogenesis 83–85
  criticisms of 86
  critique of conventional medicine 45–46, 86
  on diagnosis as a political tool 151–152
  on generalization of research results 166
  placebo effect and 56–57
  on practitioner–patient relationships 46–47
  on religion and suffering 86
illicit drug use 294–295
illness 91–98
  cause of see aetiology
  factors affecting expression 93–94
  as teacher 101
  teleological interpretation 92
  vs disease 91
  see also disease
illness narratives, Frank's 172–181
  complexity of consultation 128
  higher order construct 186–187
  vs Davies' forms of temporal orientation 181–182
illness work 197
immoderate way of life 5
immune system 314–315
immunomodulators 188–189, 195
implication leads 240
Indian medicine see Ayurvedic medicine

indigenous peoples 17–18
  relationships with nature 92–93, 105
  sacred worldview 254–255
  shamans 211–212
individuals
  generalizing about 166–172
  getting to know 171–172
  prioritizing 256–261
indulgent lifestyle 5
inflammation 34–35
information
  aids to providing 358
  asking for more 229–230
  four territories, follow-up visits 268
  patient's needs 354–355
  providing 354–355
information technology 161–162
informative model, doctor–patient relationship 49–50
initial conditions, sensitivity to 285–286
initial consultation 118, 143, 269–273
  to be continued … 271
  blank sheet approach 270–271
  complexity, non-linearity and flexibility 273
  opening questions 263
  outline format 116
  questioning prior conceptions 271–272
  recognizing limitations 272–273
  time allowed 116–117
instrumental self 164–165
integrity, body and its components 298
integumentary system 312–313
interests 297
interpersonal relationships
  enquiring about 278–280, 287–288
  practitioner's agenda 138
  tending 104–105
interpretive model, doctor–patient relationship 49–50
interpretive philosophy 157–160
interprofessional communication 382, 395–396
  *see also* referral
interrogation 213
interruptions 232–233
interview 149, 213–214
intolerances, food 286
intuition 126–127, 251–253
investigations 142, 224–227
  relative weight 142–144
  *vs* physical examination 326–330, 327t
*Iris versicolor* 341
irritable bowel syndrome 150, 189, 190f

jangle fallacy 184
Japan 152–153
jargon, avoiding 356

Johns, Timothy 2
Jonas, W.B. 53–55, 74
Judge, T.A. 182–186
Jullien, Francois 4–5
Jung, Carl 166–167, 178–179

*kapha* 7–8, 16t
*karoshi* 152–153
Kiecolt-Glaser, Janice 43–44
Klein, R. 27–28
knowing, tacit 252–253
knowledge, tacit 252–253
Kuriyama, Shigehisa 209–210, 228, 255, 327, 334–337

labelling 150
laboratory medicine 345, 346t, 348
labyrinth
  the consultation as 119–124
  life as a 112, 180–181
landscape
  of the consultation 115–116
  therapeutic 105–106
language, avoiding technical 356
leader, practitioner as 360–364
leadership 360–364
  facilitative 362–363
  relationship to management 361–362
  servant 363
  shared 363–364
  transactional 364, 364t
  transformational 364, 364t
leading questions 239–240
learning
  defining 365
  leadership and 363–364
  lifelong 109–110
  and teaching 364–365
*Leptandra virginica* 341
life history, previous 284–286
lifelong learning 109–110
lifestyle
  bland/moderate 4–5
  in herbal practice 19
  history-taking 289–298
  overstimulated/indulgent 5
  six non-naturals and 258–260
liking, in practitioner–patient relationship 58
limitations, recognizing one's own 272–273
linear narratives 182, 184, 186
listening
  active 227–228
  to answers 227–240, 263–264
  to one's own stories 103
  polyphonic/monophonic modes 184–185

sympathetic 229
  to your heart 106–107
literacy
  health 372–373
  patient 358–359
literature 63–64
locus of control 183, 185–186
love
  choosing 107–109
  correspondences 110t
  therapy of 58
low dimensional dynamical chaos 189–191
lumpers, Cronbach's 182–183

al-Majusi, Ali ibn Abbas 8–9
manager, practitioner as 360–364
marital status 278–279
Maslow, A.H. 159
*materia medica* 18
*Matricaria recutita* (chamomile) 18
maze 112
McKenna, Terrence 90, 105, 163, 180–181, 210–211, 223
meaning
  herbal medicines 74–75
  medical encounters 54–55
  working with 60–63, 61b–62b
meaning response 54–56
  facilitating 355–356
  *see also* placebo effect
media, mass 31–32, 162
medical conditions, nature of 187–200
medical cosmologies 345, 346t
medical culture, dominant 5–7
  *see also* biomedicine/conventional medicine
medical history, previous 284–286
medically unexplained symptoms (MUS) 156–158
medicine, conventional *see* biomedicine/conventional medicine
medicines, conventional *see* drugs, conventional
Medicines Act 1968 23–24
meditation 392
melancholic temperament 169f
melatonin 301
memory aids 358
menopause 151
mental aspect of being 253–256, 257t
*Mentha piperita* (peppermint) 18
mettle, Illich's concept 98
microscope 344
mild flavours 4
*milieu interieur* 21–22
milk thistle *(Silybum marianum)* 35
Mills, Simon 23–26, 33, 188–189
moderate way of life 4–5

Moerman, Daniel 17, 53–55, 74
monophony 184–185
mood 301, 304–306
movement in the body, direction of 302, 304
multidimensional health locus of control (MHLC) 185–186
musculoskeletal system 313
mutual participation model 44–47
  origins 51

nails 303, 312–313
name, patient's 275
narrative-based medicine (NBM) 42, 66–67, 218–223
  *see also* storytelling
narratives
  factors influencing 219–220
  illness *see* illness narratives, Frank's
  initiating 220–221
  interpretation 221–222
  linear 182, 184, 186
  non-linear 175, 222–223
  older patients 249
  polyphonic 182, 184, 187
  *see also* chaos narratives; quest narratives; restitution narratives
National Association of Medical Herbalists (later the National Institute of Medical Herbalists) 20, 23–24
National Health Service 23–24
Native Americans 14, 17, 343
nature
  cultivating a relationship with 105–106
  tendency to change 14–16, 97
naturephilic standpoint 92–93
naturephobic standpoint 5–6, 92–93
naturopaths 21
naturopathy 19
Needham, Joseph 84–85
negative encounters 41
nervines 6, 124, 194
nervous system 315
nervous trophorestoratives 188–189
Nettleton, S. 45, 128, 195, 197
neuroendocrine phytotherapy 347–348
neuroticism (emotional stability) 183, 185
New Age 24, 180
nocebo effect 56–57, 68
  awareness of 355–356
non-linear approach, consultation 119–124, 273
non-naturals, six 256–261
non-self 163–164
non-verbal cues 224, 226–227
  *see also* body language
non-verbal questions 240

notes, case
　blank sheet approach 225, 270–271
　closing stage of consultation 353–354
　at end of consultation 380–382
　review at follow-up 265–266
　taking 224–225, 263–264
novel experiences, seeking 109
nudge theory 188–189

objectification of the person 143–144
objective assessment 142–144, 207–208
observation
　own behaviour 101
　patients 324
occupation, patient's 277–278
Okasha, S. 32
older patients 248–250
oleo canthal 8
open-handedness 112
open-heartedness 112
open-mindedness 112
opioids, endogenous 56
*Organic Materia Medica* (Southall) 18
orientation
　of patient to phytotherapy 282–283
　practitioner's 98–99
outlook 304–306
overwork, death from 152–153

pain, unrealistic expectations 102
*Panax ginseng* (Chinese or Korean ginseng) 10–11, 35, 82–83
*Papaver somniferum* 5
Paracelsus 12
paradigm shift 24–25
parents
　accompanying child patients 244–246, 342
　enquiring about 287
Parker, Malcolm 24–25, 27
partnership-centred medicine 50, 369
　quest narratives and 179, 186
　shared leadership and 363
　transpersonal mode and 165
　*see also* shared decision-making
partnerships with patients 46–48
Pascal, Blaise 69
Pasteur, Louis 22
pastimes 297
paternalism 48–52, 369
　evidence-based medicine and 66–68
　in herbal practice 354
　illness narratives and 172–173, 179
　medical rationalism as 95–96
　origins 51
　shift away from 47

patient(s)
　aspirations 59
　conventional medically-orientated 96
　engendering well-being 98–113
　expectations *see* expectations, patient
　getting to know 171–172
　healthist 94–96
　'how did you hear about me?' 281
　information needs 354–355
　low literacy skills 358–359
　moving with 200
　nature of 172–187
　personal details 275–281
　phytotherapy orientation 282–283
　possessing credible medical diagnoses 150–151
　relationships with practitioners *see* practitioner–patient relationships; therapeutic relationship
　rights and obligations 150–151
　values 28, 49t, 219
　welcoming 273–317
　without credible medical diagnoses 151
patient-as-person 51
patient-centred approach 47, 51–52, 157–158, 165
　conceptual dimensions 51
　herbal medicine 354
　patient expectations and 53
　shared decision-making 369
patient-centred communication 156–157
patient's predicament
　appreciating, 133–203
　changing nature 382
　comprehension 317
　as emergent phenomenon 285–286
　history-taking 283–284
Payer, L. 22–23
peppermint *(Mentha piperita)* 18
personal details, patient's 275–282
personal growth, types of 366–367
personal relationships *see* interpersonal relationships
personal style 306
personality
　assessment 304–306
　traits 183–185
person-centred therapy, Rogers' 57–58
perspectives, shifting 102–103
pharmaceutical companies 6–7, 28–29, 151
pharmacological perspective 7–9
pharmacopoeias 18
phenomenology 67–73, 90
phlegmatic temperament 169f
physical aspect of being 253–256, 257t
physical examination 120, 142, 323–350
　aims and potentials 333–334
　directed 324

energetic assessment 333, 338–342
evidence-based 330–332
general 325
implementation in practice 335
levels of competence 330–331
in medical textbooks 149
nature 323–326
periodic/annual 328–330, 329f
practical techniques 342
relative weight 142–144
therapeutic potential 325–326
touching and knowing 335–338
transiting to 317–318
varieties of clinical gaze 334–335
*vs* investigation 326–330, 327t
physician-healer 89–90
physiology, shaping by beliefs 112
physiomedicalists 34
phytotherapist 20
phytotherapy 21–36
beyond scientism 30–33
distinctive features 146–148
evidence-based medicine and 27–30
integration and regulation 24–27
personal view 33–36
in UK 23–24
varieties 21–23
Pietroni, Patrick 60–62, 61b–62b, 64
*pitta* 7–8, 16t
placebo 53–54
placebo effect 30, 53–57
awareness of 355–356
defined 53–54
failure to learn from 67
as meaning response 54–56
mechanisms 54–55
negative *see* nocebo effect
physiological mediators 56
practitioner qualities enhancing 59–60
plan, treatment 374–375
play 234–235, 247
pluralist approach 32–33, 84–85, 338
pneuma 255
poisons 9
political control, diagnosis as tool of 151–153
polyphonic narratives 182, 184, 187
polyphony 184–185
positive encounters 41–42
positive manner, behaving in a 355–356
positivist science 30–31
approach to herbs 6–7
disease and illness 91
engagement of herbal practitioners with 26–27
evidence-based medicine and 68
generalizing about individuals 166–167
powders, herbal 12

Power, Henry 344
power, shared 372–373
practitioner-centred care 165
practitioner–patient relationships
continuity of care and 378
contribution to placebo effect 54
evolution over time 51
instrumental, authentic and transpersonal modes 165
internal and external contexts 240–241
models of 44–45, 48–50, 49t
physical examination and 326
*see also* therapeutic relationship
prayer, healing influence 86
predicament, patient's *see* patient's predicament
prescription
additional 381
arriving at 124
talking about 359–360
*see also* herbal medicines
presenting complaint 283
history of 283–284
primary care
diagnosis in 150
practitioners, phytotherapists as 272
*see also* general practitioners
problems 106
profane world 254
profiling, patient, 133–203
prognosis 210–211, 356–357
promises, keeping 380
psychoactive plant chemicals 10
psychologists, splitters and lumpers 182–183
psychoneuroimmunology (PNI) 22, 34–35, 35t, 43–44
Hyland's extended network theory and 187–189
placebo effect 55–56
psychotherapeutic stance 387
psychotherapies
patients requiring 178–179
therapeutic relationship 43, 74
public expression (of patient's condition) 195–200
public influence (on patient's condition) 195–200
public reception (of patient's condition) 195–196
pull therapies 188–189
pulse
Ayurvedic medicine 339
conventional medicine 327–328, 339–340
theory, Greek 337
traditional Chinese medicine 209–210, 327–328

pungency 3
push therapies 188

qualitative research methods 40
quest narratives 179–181, 187
    complexity of consultation 128
    inviting 220–221
questions
    asking for more information 229–230
    child consultations 246–248
    clarifying 52–53, 230
    closed 236–239
    eliciting patient agendas/expectations 136–137, 139–140
    erratic sequence 237f, 239
    follow-up visits 266–268
    funnel sequence 237–238, 237f
    getting to know the patient 171–172
    inverted funnel sequence 237f, 238
    leading 239–240
    limitations of answers 228–229
    non-verbal 240
    open 236–239
    opening 261–263
    open-to-closed sequence 237–238, 237f
    posing, and listening to replies 227–240
    separation 236
    sharing thoughts 230
    simplicity and clarity 236
    six non-naturals approach 259–261
    tunnel sequence 237f, 238–239

randomized controlled trials (RCTs) 7, 40
Rangel's Systemic Theory of Living Systems 35
Rasa 7–8
rationalism, medical 95–96
reasons, distinction from excuses 103
receive, ability to 102
recognition (of patients) 378, 380
records, patient *see* notes, case
red flag scenarios 272–273
referral 154–155, 192, 272–273, 357–358, 395
reflection
    enabling patient autonomy 141
    making space for 103
reflective practice 64–65, 253
    between appointments 382–384
    reviewing case notes 266
Reformation, English 184–185
regimen 258–260, 374–375
registration 25
regulation of herbal medicine 24–27
*Rehmannia glutinosa* (Sheng di Huang) 168
relationship status, patient's 278–279
relationships *see* interpersonal relationships; practitioner–patient relationships
relaxation 295–297

religion
    Illich on 86
    monotheistic 184–185
    recent attacks 31
    sacred and profane worlds 254–255
remedial food-stuffs 9
remedies 9
remembering patients 378, 380
repetition 230
reproductive system 315–317
requests
    ability to decline 101
    patient, *vs* expectations 134
research
    between appointments 384
    evidence, best 28, 219
    generalizability of results 166–172
    scientific methodology 25–26
resilience, Antonovsky's model 97
resins, plant 10
respiratory system 314
rest–activity balance 112
restitution narratives 173–175, 179, 186
    complexity of consultation 128
    inviting 220–221
retirement 248, 277–278
rheumatoid arthritis 197
risks, of exploring patient agendas 136–137
rituals 241
Robinson, George Canby 114–115
robust therapy 188–189, 190f, 192
Rogers, Carl 40–41, 43, 57–58, 250, 365–366

Sackett, David 28
sacred world 254–255
safety-netting 376
saltiness 3
salutogenesis 97
sanguine temperament 169f
scientific research methodology 25–26
Scientific Revolution 184–185
scientism 30–33
    challenges to 31–32
    concept 30–31
    new 27–28
secondary metabolites, plant 8, 10
self
    concepts of 158–166
    increased revelation 161–162
    plasticity 160
    practitioner's use of 164–165
    sustaining the professional 390–392
self-care
    facilitating patient 98–113, 362
    professional 389–393
self-esteem 183, 185
self-healing 40, 55–56
    extended network theory 188–189
self-limiting conditions 151

self-organizational change, extended network theory 187–189, 190f
self-sacrifice 391
Selye, Hans 106
senses, exercising one's 110–111
sensitivities 286
sensitivity to initial conditions 285–286
servant leadership 363
setting, for the consultation 113–116, 240–242
sex, patient's 277
sexual orientation 279
shamans 210–212
shape-shifting 5–7
shared decision-making (SDM) 50, 368–374
  barriers to implementing 370
  definition/concept 369
  patient preferences 373
  *see also* partnership-centred medicine
shared leadership 363–364
sharing power and responsibility 51
Sharma, U. 47–48
Sheldon, William 170
Sheng di Huang *(Rehmannia glutinosa)* 168
sick-role 150, 172–173, 195–196
silence 103, 233–234
*Silybum marianum* (milk thistle) 35
simple leads 239–240
simple zone 127–128, 191–192, 191f
six non-naturals 256–261
skin 303, 312–313
sleep 299–301
small-mindedness 106
smell
  patient's 324
  sense of 110–111
Smohalla 92–93
smoking 290
snoring 300–301
social history 289–298
social iatrogenesis 83–85
sociocultural influences 45–46
somatization 157–158
somatotyping 170
sourness 3, 8
South Africa 17
specialism, move towards 32–33
speech
  disrupted and disconnected 224
  performance, when summarizing 231–232
spiritual aspect of being 253–256, 257t
spirituality 24
splitters, Cronbach's 182–183
Stacey's certainty-agreement model 127–128, 191–192, 191f
standardization, herbal preparations 13–14
steady state 129
stethoscope 344

stinging nettle *(Urtica dioica)* 188
storytelling 42
  initiating 220–221
  listening to own 103
  open approach to 120–121
  *see also* narratives
stress
  induced conditions 151
  personality traits and 183, 185
strong flavours 4
subjective assessment 142–144, 207–208
substance abuse 293
substance dependence 292–293
subtle leads 240
subtle therapy 188–189, 190f
suffering 85–89, 94
summarizing 230–232
summary, end 376
supervision 387
surrender, ability to 111
Svenaeus, F. 68–69
Sweeney, Kieran 88
sweetness 3, 8
symbols
  consulting room 241
  patient's 241–242
symptoms 100–113
Systemic Theory of Living Systems, Rangel's 35
systems enquiry 311–317

Tao Te Ching, of Lao Tsu 97–98
Taoism 223
tasks, working at 103
taste 2–5, 7–8
  associated properties 3, 7–8
  categories or qualities 3, 7–8
  developing sense of 110
  in pharmacological detection 8
  strength of 4
  unpleasant 9–10
teacher
  illness as 101
  practitioner as 113, 364–368
technology 328, 343–345, 348
teleological interpretation of illness 92
telephone
  contacts, between appointments 380–381
  number, patient's 276
temperament
  assessment 304–306
  Eynsenck's concept 169–170, 169f
temporal orientation, Davies's three forms 181–182
tension headache 326
terrain 21–23
tests *see* investigations
theory of generalized quantum entanglement 187

therapeutic alliance 43–44, 51, 354
therapeutic attitude 43, 57–58, 64–65
therapeutic intent 43, 57–58
therapeutic relationship 35, 39–77
  challenge of 39–41
  conceptualization 41–44
  definition 56–57
  evidence-based medicine and 65–67
  new perspectives on placebo effect 53–57
  patient expectations 52–53
  phenomenology 67–73
  practitioner factors influencing 57–64, 61b–62b
  reflective practice 64–65
  relevance in phytotherapy 74–75
  variety of models 44–52
therapeutic window 147
Thomson, Samuel 20
Thomsonian herbalism 20
thoughts, sharing 230
time
  consultation 116–119
  patient's experience of 71
tinctures, herbal 12
tongue
  diagnosis, Chinese 337–338, 340–341, 340f
  indications, herbal medicines 341
Toombs, S.K. 71–73
torture 213
touch 111, 324, 335–338, 348
Tower of Babel problem 184
traditional healers 17
traditional systems of medicine
  classification and diagnostic approach 167–170
  energetic approaches 338–339
  physical examination 336, 339–341
  use of animal products 19
transactional analysis 387
transference 177, 387
transition towns movement 35–36
transpersonal self 164–165
transsexual (transgender) people 277
treatment
  decision-making 368–374
  history 288–289
  monitoring response to 333
  patient's views 271–272
  plan 374–375
  professionally prescribed or applied 40
  relationship to diagnosis 151
  talking about 359–360
  *see also* herbal medicines
trickster methods 232
triterpenoid saponins 10–11
trophorestoratives 4, 188–189, 195
trust
  continuity of care and 377–378
  engendering 59–60

Umantsev, A. 190–193
uncertainty 50, 127, 343
unconditional positive regard 58, 261
understanding, at conclusion of consultation 353–359
unhappiness
  chronic 175–176
  incoherent narratives 223
  *see also* happiness
United Kingdom (UK)
  phytotherapy 21, 23–27
  professional self-organization 20
  traditional and Thomsonian herbalists 20
United States of America (USA) 22, 26
universities, CAM courses 144–145
unpleasant taste 9–10
urinary system 312
*Urtica dioica* (stinging nettle) 188
utopian visions 94

vaccinations 289
*vata* 7–8, 16t
Vesalius, Andreas 184–185
vipaka 7–8
virya 7–8
visual knowledge 334
visual sensory input, reducing 110
vitality 298–301, 299t
voice, tone of 231–232
voodoo death 56–57
vulnerability 107–109
vulneraries 107–109

waiting room, meeting patient in 273–274
Warhol, Andy 163
water 274–275
welcoming patients 273–317
wellbeing, engendering 98–113
wellness adviser 26
wetness 301–303
Wheen, Francis 31
whole plant herbal medicines 11–14
working life, patient's 297–298
workplace, consultations at patient's 114–115
World Health Organization (WHO), definition of health 96
worried well 91

yarrow *(Achillea millefolium)* 12–13
yin deficiency 337–338

Zen philosophy 97
*Zingiber officinale* (ginger) 82–83, 168
zoopharmacognosy 9
Zulu herbal medicines 17

www.ingramcontent.com/pod-product-compliance
Ingram Content Group UK Ltd.
Pitfield, Milton Keynes, MK11 3LW, UK
UKHW020148230226
468272UK00005B/26